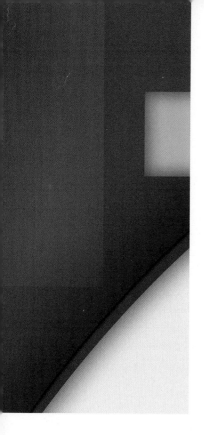

Understanding Nursing Research

Using Research in Evidence-Based Practice

Second Edition

Carol L. Macnee, RN, PhD
Professor
University of Wyoming Fay W. Whitney School of Nursing
Laramie, Wyoming

Susan McCabe, RN, CS, EdD
Associate Professor
University of Wyoming Fay W. Whitney School of Nursing
Laramie, Wyoming

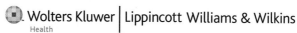

Wolters Kluwer | Lippincott Williams & Wilkins
Health

Philadelphia · Baltimore · New York · London
Buenos Aires · Hong Kong · Sydney · Tokyo

Senior Acquisitions Editor: Peter Darcy
Managing Editor: Michelle Clarke
Production Project Manager: Cynthia Rudy
Director of Nursing Production: Helen Ewan
Senior Managing Editor/Production: Erika Kors
Art Director: Joan Wendt
Manufacturing Coordinator: Karin Duffield
Production Services/Compositor: TechBooks
Printer: R.R. Donnelley–Crawfordsville

2nd edition

9 8 7 6 5 4 3 2

Library of Congress Cataloging-in-Publication Data

Macnee, Carol L. (Carol Leslie)
   Understanding nursing research: using research in evidence-based practice/Carol L. Macnee, Susan McCabe. –2nd ed.
      p. ; cm.
   Includes bibliographical references and index.
   ISBN-13: 978-0-7817-7558-8
   ISBN-10: 0-7817-7558-2
   1. Nursing—Research.   I. McCabe, Susan, RN.   II. Title.
   [DNLM: 1. Nursing Research.   2. Evidence-Based Medicine— methods.   WY 20. 5 M169u 2007]
   RT81.5.M235 2007
   610.73072—dc22

                                          2006028269

Care has been taken to confirm the accuracy of the information presented and to describe generally accepted practices. However, the authors, editors, and publisher are not responsible for errors or omissions or for any consequences from application of the information in this book and make no warranty, express or implied, with respect to the content of the publication.

The authors, editors, and publisher have exerted every effort to ensure that drug selection and dosage set forth in this text are in accordance with the current recommendations and practice at the time of publication. However, in view of ongoing research, changes in government regulations, and the constant flow of information relating to drug therapy and drug reactions, the reader is urged to check the package insert for each drug for any change in indications and dosage and for added warnings and precautions. This is particularly important when the recommended agent is a new or infrequently employed drug.

Some drugs and medical devices presented in this publication have Food and Drug Administration (FDA) clearance for limited use in restricted research settings. It is the responsibility of the health care provider to ascertain the FDA status of each drug or device planned for use in his or her clinical practice.

LWW.com

REVIEWERS

Nezam Al-Nsair, RN, PhD
Assistant Professor
College of Mount St. Joseph, Nursing Program
Cincinnati, Ohio

Linda Bugle, RN, PhD
Associate Professor
Southeast Missouri State University
Cape Girardeau, Missouri

Maureen Dever-Bumba, RN, DrPH(c), MSN, CFNP, PNP-C
Assistant Professor and Coordinator, NP Programs
Medical College of Georgia
Augusta, Georgia

Betsy Frank, RN, PhD
Professor
Indiana State University, College of Nursing
Terre Haute, Indiana

Lynette M. Gibson, RN, PhD
Assistant Professor
Clemson University, School of Nursing
College of Health, Education, and Development
Clemson, South Carolina

Vincent P. Hall, RN, PhD
Department Head of Nursing
Western Carolina University
Cullowhee, North Carolina

Hendrika Maltby, RN, PhD, FRCNA
Associate Professor
University of Vermont
Burlington, Vermont

Joan C. Masters, RN, MA, MBA
Assistant Professor of Nursing
Bellarmine University, Lansing School of
    Nursing and Health Sciences
Louisville, Kentucky

Karin Morin, RN, DSN
Professor of Nursing
Western Michigan University,
    Bronson School of Nursing
Kalamazoo, Michigan

Beth Perry, RN, PhD
Professor
Athabasca University
Athabasca, Alberta, Canada

Sharon J. Thompson, RN, PhD, MPH
Assistant Professor of Nursing
Gannon University, Villa Maria School
    of Nursing
Erie, Pennsylvania

We believe that learning should be fun and that learning happens best when students can relate new knowledge to something relevant to them. We also believe that when students are not expected to be researchers, they can enjoy learning how to read and use research as one important form of evidence on which to base practice. We both love research, and we are both fundamentally practitioners who find excitement and challenge in tackling new information to fill in the gaps in our knowledge about practice. We hope that some of our enthusiasm is communicated in these pages.

Understanding Nursing Research: Reading and Using Research in Practice differs from existing undergraduate research textbooks in a number of important ways. The first premise of this book is that nursing students need to understand the language of research and the underlying concepts of the research process, but do not necessarily need to be prepared to conduct a research study. The second premise is that nursing students and practicing baccalaureate-prepared nurses are motivated to read and use research evidence only as it relates to their practice. Given these two premises, it is logical that many nursing students and nurses read only the abstract and the conclusion sections of research reports. Those two sections usually contain less of the technical language of research and address most directly the clinical meaning of a research study, so they are viewed as both understandable and useful for practice. Following that reasoning, we organized this book around the sections of a research report rather than the steps of the research process. It starts with what most practicing RNs are interested in—the conclusions—and then moves forward to the beginning of a research report. We believe that this will help the student recognize the relevance of each section of a typical research report in understanding and using research in evidence-based practice. In addition, five questions that a nurse might ask when reading research are used to further organize the text, and throughout the chapters the emphasis is on reading, understanding, and using research in practice. In keeping with this, each chapter of the book begins with a clinical case that identifies what information the nurse is seeking from research literature to answer a clinical question. One or two published research articles that directly relate to the clinical case are discussed throughout the chapter to provide specific examples of the concepts addressed; they are reprinted in full in Appendices A-1 through A-9.

It is a challenge to represent the breadth and depth of nursing practice and nursing research in a single textbook. A real effort has been made to include clinical cases that reflect nursing practice in a variety of settings, ranging from acute care to public health, and across a range of specialties. This text also differs from other undergraduate research texts in that we use the research articles as exemplars to discuss both qualitative and quantitative research methods. As nursing science evolves, we recognize the need to use a variety of methods from both the positivist and naturalist viewpoints to develop knowledge that reflects nursing's holistic perspective. Both qualitative and quantitative methods are used to build knowledge in nursing, and rather than artificially separate the discussion of these two approaches, we contrast the approaches while identifying the broader conceptual base that is common to both. However, because combining quantitative and qualitative methods in each chapter may be confusing at times, icons are used to identify the method being described within a paragraph.

Learners learn best by doing, so each chapter of this book ends with a specific learning activity that prepares students for the concepts addressed in the following chapter. The learning activity is directly related to the examples and the clinical case in the chapter. To provide an opportunity for students to be active learners, an in-class questionnaire that can be used as a mini-research study is included in Appendix C, and Appendix B is a fictional article that could have been based on the results from the in-class questionnaire. It intentionally contains flaws that are slightly more glaring than any likely to be found in a published, peer-reviewed research report. The fictional article is used throughout the text as an example, along with the authentic research reports.

The goal of this text is that students finish it being able to read and comprehend published research, so that they can make professional decisions regarding the use of research reports in evidence-based practice. Associated with this goal is the hope that students will develop their interest and confidence in reading research, rather than avoiding it. Our text is designed to be user-friendly, taking a more casual tone than some research texts do, to minimize the intimidating nature of the language and concepts of research. For easy reference, each term in the glossary includes its chapter and page number in the text.

The sign of a successful textbook is that students decide to keep it to use in the future, rather than sell it after they complete their course. We hope ours will be one they keep. We believe that learning to understand and use published research can be fun, interesting, and useful for students if they can see its direct relevance to their practice. The organization of this book is unconventional and the tone conversational, addressing the subject from the perspective of a reader and user of research, rather than from a creator of it. Students tell us this is a helpful perspective and one that they enjoy. As nurse researchers, our greatest goal is to foster appreciation and enthusiasm for the process that we find so challenging and so clinically meaningful. We hope this text contributes to accomplishing that goal. And we hope you have some fun!

Carol L. Macnee
Susan McCabe

ACKNOWLEDGMENTS

I would first like to acknowledge and thank the many students I have taught in Kentucky, Tennessee, and Wyoming, who have patiently but stubbornly insisted that they were in nursing to practice, not to be researchers, and in so doing have pushed me to make my case for the relevancy of nursing research to their practice. I also want to acknowledge my colleagues who, like me, recognize that if we fail to instill a valuing of research in the baccalaureate student, we do a great disservice to our profession and its growth as a science. I want to thank the three most important mentors in my career: Jean Goeppinger, Lauren Aaronson, and Carol Loveland-Cherry. Each has shared with me her excitement and love of knowledge development, along with many practical opportunities to learn the research process. I hope this book passes some of that enthusiasm and knowledge on. Finally, I want to thank the many people at Lippincott for taking a risk with a new author and a new idea. Without them, this book would not have happened.

Carol L. Macnee

With gratitude to my parents, who were the first to introduce me to the wonders of intentional inquiry; to my students, who never let me forget why structured inquiry matters; and to my partner, who supports and inspires me to excellence in the pursuit of research.

Susan McCabe

CONTENTS

CHAPTER 9

Research Designs: Planning the Study 193

CHAPTER 10

Background and the Research Problem 226

CHAPTER 11

The Research Process 250

1

EVIDENCE-BASED NURSING: USING RESEARCH IN PRACTICE

LEARNING OBJECTIVE:

The student will describe evidence that can serve as the basis for nursing practice.

KEY TERMS

Abstract
Electronic databases
Evidence-based nursing
   (EBN)
Internet
Key words
Knowledge
Printed indexes

CLINICAL CASE

A.K. is a 20-year-old woman who is incarcerated in a minimum security prison to serve a 10-month sentence for shoplifting. She is 5-months pregnant with her first child and has tested positive for the human immunodeficiency virus (HIV). When A.K. entered the prison system, her prenatal care was up-to-date, but she was very anxious about the baby's health. The RN in the prison clinic recognizes that A.K. needs both education and support in preparation for her maternal role. The RN completes a literature search and finds two research articles that appear to relate to A.K. and her pregnancy. The first is titled "Motherhood in the context of maternal HIV infection" (Sandelowski & Barroso, 2003), and the second is titled "Complex physical and mental health needs of rural incarcerated women" (Kane & DiBartolo, 2002). You can find these articles in Appendices A-1 and A-2 of this text.

INTRODUCTION

Understanding Nursing Research discusses how you can use nursing research in your nursing practice. Its goal is to teach you, a practicing nurse, to find answers to clinical questions you may have by using nursing research. Another way to phrase this goal is that this book is about practice based on research evidence, or evidence-based practice. To base your practice on research evidence, however, you must be able to understand the research language as well as the research process.

Because answering clinical questions is important for a practicing nurse, this book begins at the end of the research process, with the conclusions, and moves forward through the process. While this may seem unusual, research study conclusions often lead to further questions. You may wonder, for example, why the author(s) reached these conclusions. That question may lead to the results section of the study, where specific numbers and measurements are described. You also may wonder to what types of patients these research results apply. That question may lead you to the description of the study sample. If you wonder why a certain patient was studied, or how the author(s) measured some aspect studied (eg, pain), you must read and understand the methods section of the research study. Finally, the methods section may direct you to review what has been done before and what nursing theory and other theories may suggest about this clinical question. That information is in the beginning or background section of the research report.

Therefore, this book begins at the end of and moves forward through a research report to understand both the research language and the process underlying it. The five general questions that are described in the paragraph below are used to organize the end-to-beginning approach. Each chapter discusses a different component of the research report and how that component can help to answer the five questions. These questions also can be used to organize your own reading and understanding of research. They are:

- What is the answer to my practice question—what did the study conclude?
- Why did the author(s) reach these conclusions—what did they actually find?
- To what types of patients do these research conclusions apply—who was in the study?

- How were those people studied—why was the study performed that way?
- Why ask that question—what do we already know?

This book focuses on assisting you to read and understand research reports and to use them intelligently as evidence to guide your clinical practice. Therefore, each chapter begins with a clinical case that raises a clinical question that can be addressed by nursing research. A published research report that is related to the clinical case is part of the required reading for the chapter, and each chapter focuses on what can be decided about practice based on an understanding of the article. To help bring the language and process of research to a practical level, you and your classmates also may participate in a small practice "study" that will be used in the text as a concrete example of different aspects of the research process.

When you finish reading this book, you will be prepared to read nursing research critically and use it intelligently. Critically reading research means reading it with a questioning mind: knowing what information should be presented in a report, understanding what is reported, and asking yourself whether the research is good enough for you to accept and use in your practice. You will not be prepared to be a researcher yourself, but you will understand some of the processes of nursing research and how that research can help you in your practice.

QUESTIONS FOR PATIENT CARE

In the clinical case at the beginning of this chapter, the nurse has a clinical question and needs answers. She is questioning how she can best meet the complex needs of a woman who is pregnant, is about to become a mother for the first time, is in jail, and is HIV positive. The nurse knows that she will need to implement educational and supportive interventions and help prepare A.K. for motherhood, while addressing her positive HIV status. The nurse wonders if A.K.'s stress of knowing she is HIV positive, or the stress of jail, will in any way alter her bonding with the baby. The nurse also knows that she will need to consider other complex issues, including psychosocial issues, physiological issues, health promotion issues, and referral procedures for specialized care if needed for this incarcerated woman. The nurse wonders which factor to focus on first and whether there might be a way to plan nursing care that would promote A.K.'s sense of being a mother, and also focus on several different issues at the same time, given the nurse's busy workload.

This nurse's question is just one example of the kinds of practice-related questions nurses face each day. Any nursing student knows that not all nurses do everything the same way. Therefore, the questions arise, and you may already have had many questions yourself, such as which is the best way to flush a percutaneous endogastric (PEG) tube, maintain an indwelling urinary catheter, or prepare a patient for surgery? And then there are questions about the differences in patients. Why do male patients have a quicker postoperative recovery from coronary artery bypass grafts than do female patients? Why do some patients quit smoking when they are pregnant and others do not? Why do some patients with AIDS keep recovering from infections, when others seem to weaken and die as soon as the first severe complications occur? Which is more helpful to patients with major depression—to urge them to get up and moving each day or to urge them to listen to themselves and follow their own natural schedules? Although nursing knowledge has grown steadily and we know a great deal about providing optimal health care, there are still more questions than there are answers about how to promote health.

Finding Answers to Patient Care Questions: Evidence-Based Nursing

How do you, as a nurse, find answers to clinical questions such as those listed in the previous section? Traditionally, four approaches have been taken, including:

1. Consulting an authority or trusted individual.
2. Using intuition and subjective judgment.
3. Turning to experience.
4. Reading textbooks and other authoritative material.

As you might guess, using these four traditional approaches to answering clinical questions can produce a wide range of answers, some useful and some not so useful. Relying too much on experience or on intuition may prevent new knowledge or understanding from being applied to clinical problems. Consulting with just one trusted person may not bring a range of thoughts and may result in a biased sense of perspective. Because of these concerns, a newer approach is being developed to standardize a nurse's clinical decision-making process and to provide a framework for planning care that answers the kinds of clinical questions nurses may have. This approach is called evidence-based nursing.

Evidence-based nursing (EBN) practice is the term used to describe the process that nurses use to make clinical decisions and to answer clinical questions. Like traditional approaches, EBN also has four approaches to answer questions. But unlike the traditional approach in which you could choose to use an expert opinion or you could use a textbook, EBN uses ALL of the approaches all of the time for every clinical question. The approaches include:

1. Reviewing the best available evidence, most often the results of research.
2. Using the nurse's clinical expertise.
3. Determining the values and cultural needs of the individual.
4. Determining the preferences of the individual, family, and community.

To answer clinical questions using EBN strategies, the nurse must know how to access the latest research, be able to correctly interpret the research findings, be able to apply the findings to the clinical problem using his or her nursing judgment and experience, and take into account the cultural and personal values and preferences of the patient (STTI, 2002). As more nursing research is conducted, there is more and more evidence that practicing nurses can turn to in order to answer clinical questions. Using EBN allows a nurse to determine the meaningfulness of the available evidence for the patient he or she is caring for and assists the nurse to make decisions about nursing interventions, based on research evidence, that are justified as part of clinical practice.

EBN implies that one of the roles of a professional RN will be to frequently seek out the available evidence in order to plan and implement the best nursing care possible. While the bulk of this book will focus on assisting you to know where to find research evidence, and how to interpret it in order to have the research evidence influence your care, it is worth taking a minute to discuss when you should seek evidence. It is ideal to say that you will seek evidence for every patient care situation, but that may be unrealistic. Routine care is often based on protocols or procedures that apply evidence. But there will be moments in your clinical practice when you should actively and independently seek out evidence to inform your care.

Situations in which you should actively seek out research evidence on which to base your care include such times as when something in your clinical practice is out of the ordinary. It may be out of the ordinary because you are caring for a patient with a disease or health need you have not encountered before. An example of this would be if you were caring for a pregnant patient who is newly diagnosed with HIV, and although you had cared for maternity patients, you had never cared for a patient with HIV before. Or it may be a situation in which a patient has a characteristic that you have never encountered before, such as a cultural or religious characteristic. An example of this would be if you were working on a step-down unit for postrenal transplant patients and were assigned to care for a Hasidic Jewish patient who has just emigrated from Russia. If you were unfamiliar with the patient care situation, this would be an ideal time to seek research-based evidence in order to improve care.

Another time that you should seek evidence is when the outcomes of the care you are delivering seem to differ in one or more patients without clear reasons. An example of this is given in the clinical case in Chapter 3. It describes a postsurgical patient whose rate of recovery is different from the typical patient the nurse deals with in her care setting. In this case, a search for research-based evidence may well provide increased knowledge, allowing the nurse to provide the best care possible. Another time when an RN should seek out evidence is when she is attempting to develop policy or plan standards for care. An example of this may be a nurse who is a unit manager in an ambulatory care unit. Her hospital has decided to initiate universal assessment for domestic violence for every patient, male and female, who presents for care. In deciding how to best initiate this change in routine care, the nurse will find that a search of the available literature is very helpful.

While there are four approaches used in EBN, it starts with the ability to locate and then interpret evidence, most often the results of research. This book focuses on how to review the best available evidence. The other pieces of EBN—using the nurse's clinical expertise; determining the values and cultural needs of the individual; and determining the preferences of the individual, family, and community—also are very important and should always be considered (STTI, 2002).

DEVELOPING AN EFFECTIVE CLINICAL QUESTION

We have been talking about EBN and the professional responsibility of RNs to identify and understand research-based evidence. We have used a clinical case as an example of the common nature of clinical questions that can be answered by examining research. But not every question can be answered by examining research evidence. Sometimes no researcher has studied anything similar to your question, or sometimes even though the health problem has been researched, the aspect of the clinical problem you are most interested in has not been studied. So it is important to be able to state your clinical question effectively and know when you can expect research-based evidence to be of help to you. An effective clinical question for EBN is one that has been asked before by someone else and, at least in part, has been explored by a researcher. In addition, a good clinical question has to focus on a health care issue that can be measured or described in some consistent manner. Finally, a good clinical question that may be answered by examining research-based evidence has to provide information about what nurses want or need to do.

An example of an effective clinical question would be "What is the best patient teaching method for newly diagnosed adolescent diabetic patients treated in ambulatory care clinics?" This question is effective because it clearly focuses on what nurses need to do. Diabetes in adolescents is an area that has been researched, and it can be described or measured. We can use blood sugar levels to measure someone's diabetes. We can interview patients to describe how they learned to cope with their diabetes. A clinical question that is less effective would be "How can I help my young diabetic patient feel better?" While this question is nursing-related, it is less effective because it asks how a nurse can make someone "feel better." Feeling better may mean different things to different people, and it is not easily measured. Another example would be the question "Which insulin pump delivers the most consistent and accurate level of drug to adolescent diabetic patients?" While this is a much more specific and measurable question, it is less effective because it is not directly nursing-related. This type of question is most likely physician-related or pharmacist-related; it does not directly relate to nursing actions.

CORE CONCEPT 1-1

An effective clinical question for evidence-based nursing includes a concern that someone else has studied, focuses on a concern that can be measured or described, and is a concern that is relevant to nursing. The question also addresses Who, Where, What, and When in terms of the clinical concern.

In addition to being related to an area of nursing that has been researched and can be either described or measured, an effective clinical question includes a few other things. It identifies *Who* you are interested in. In our example, the *Who* are adolescent diabetic patients. An effective clinical question also identifies the *Where*. In our example, the nurse identifies his or her interest in adolescent diabetic patients treated in ambulatory care clinics. In addition to *Who* and *Where,* the effective question will identify the *What* and the *When.* The *What* is the health problem of interest or the desired outcome of nursing care. In our example, the *What* is patient teaching. The *When* is often the least identified element of a clinical question, but an important one. The *When* identifies where in the course of the clinical problem the question arises. In our example, we asked, "What is the best patient teaching method for newly diagnosed adolescent diabetic patients treated in ambulatory care clinics?" Our *When* is "newly diagnosed." We are focusing our clinical question on patients who have just been diagnosed. As you can imagine, the patient teaching needs of individuals who have had diabetes for many years are different from those of patients who have just been diagnosed. We could have asked in our example, "What is the best patient teaching method for diabetic patients experiencing neuropathic pain treated in an ambulatory setting?" In this case, our *When* focus is on a time in the course of diabetes that a person has begun to experience the complications of the chronic illness; therefore, the health needs of this person are different from what they were at the start of the illness. Using the *Who, What, When,* and *Where* approach to forming your clinical question will do a great deal to help you search for the best available evidence to answer your question. For each clinical question in this text, we will identify the *Who, What, When,* and *Where* in a table following each clinical vignette.

Determining the Best Available Evidence

Practicing EBN implies that nurses use evidence to answer clinical questions. But what is evidence, and is all evidence equally useful for guiding a nurse's decision making? Evidence should be thought of as information that provides a point of view or contributes to finding the solution to a clinical question. But all information is not always equally useful. Some information is from informal sources and is collected under less than rigorous conditions. Other information is obtained from very rigorous procedures, through formal methods. While both kinds of information may be useful, the more formally and rigorously the information is collected, the stronger it is considered as evidence on which to make EBN clinical decisions.

In considering what the best available evidence is, a nurse needs to look at how the information that makes up the evidence was collected, how rigorous the method used to develop the evidence was, and what source was used to share the evidence. In this sense, evidence can be placed into two categories: research-based and nonresearch-based. Figure 1-1 shows examples of both. We will discuss nonresearch evidence first.

Let us say that you have a clinical question regarding the transmission of the common flu virus. In order to plan how best to prevent the transmission of the flu, you could directly ask people who have had the flu recently how they think they got it. As you ask several people, you may notice some common answers that provide you with information (evidence). But it may not be the strongest evidence on which to base clinical interventions. You could consult a textbook. As a nursing student, you will often use authorities, a type of nonresearch evidence, to answer your patient care questions. As a student nurse, you will regularly seek answers to questions from authoritative sources such as reference books, practice journals, other members of

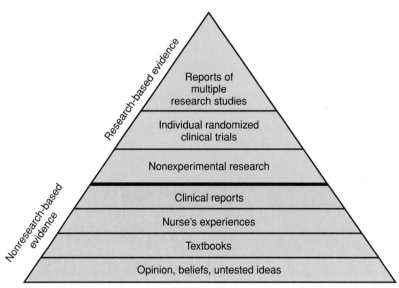

FIGURE 1-1 • Sources of evidence.

the health care team (such as the pharmacist), and patients. Notice that all these sources of evidence reflect the traditional approaches discussed earlier.

Another approach to answering clinical questions is to use your intuition or subjective judgment. This type of evidence is based on your own experience. Nursing is both a science and an art, and intuition or subjective judgment can be an important way of knowing what to do in clinical situations. Intuition can be a source of indirect evidence that is not explicit and articulated fully. Intuition can be thought of as a form of nonresearch evidence. It differs from common sense or arbitrary choice because it is knowledge—but knowledge that we cannot explicate in detail. Intuition may tell you that a particular day is not the day to push a depressed patient to get out of bed. Intuition may tell you that one patient with AIDS has given up and will not survive a hospitalization, whereas another who is equally ill is determined to live. Such intuition will guide your care for each of these patients, perhaps leading to a focus on social support and spiritual care for the first patient and a focus on independence for the second patient. In this sense, intuition is evidence to consider in clinical decision making.

Other approaches to answering questions about nursing care depend on your own experience as evidence. Experience may indicate that patients who had their indwelling urinary catheters changed every 72 hours had fewer urinary tract infections (UTIs) than did those who had theirs changed every 48 hours. Experience may also indicate that depressed patients who were strongly encouraged to get out of bed and follow a daily morning routine were discharged sooner than those who were not encouraged. Personal experience with a health problem may also provide answers to clinical questions. You may know what worked for you or your family, so that is what you will offer or do for your patient.

Clinical reports are another source of nonresearch-based evidence for clinical decision making. This type of evidence is less personal, representing instead the formal experience of someone else. You may find a published article in a practice journal that discusses another nurse's experience with a clinical issue. Or you may find an article that discusses the outcome of a particular approach to patient care. These case reports can provide a rich source of evidence, but the evidence is limited because it may pertain only to that one case and not reflect the unique needs of your patient or the factors that are present in your clinical question.

Each of these sources of nonresearch evidence can assist in answering clinical questions and can be helpful and appropriate. However, sometimes you cannot get the answer from an authority, and you have no intuitive or experiential basis on which to answer the question. Or there may not be a case report on the clinical problem you face. Sometimes the answers from these diverse sources of evidence may differ and lead to a more confusing picture. Take the question about how the RN at the correctional facility can best assist A.K. to be ready for her maternal role, given that she has tested positive for HIV. The nurse in the clinical case could talk to a peer who works in a larger jail and see if they have any protocols for this type of care. The nurse could also check the standardized care plan for patients diagnosed with HIV to see if maternal needs are addressed and if they seem helpful to such patients. The nurse's experience with her 15-year-old niece who is newly diagnosed with HIV after a blood transfusion might tell her that patients with HIV do not respond well to interventions such as "lecturing," but sharing concerns and ideas may work. However, all of these sources of evidence are biased, reflecting subjectively held beliefs or opinions. Despite using these forms of evidence, the question of how to best implement maternal planning care for A.K. remains.

Finding Answers Through Research

Research-based evidence, in the form of nursing research, may provide the nurse with an answer to her question that avoids the subjective concerns or the informal nature of nonresearch evidence. Often it is exactly the types of questions that are not answered in textbooks, and that everyone has a different idea about or experience with, that are the questions studied in nursing research. However, while very useful, reading and analyzing research is not necessarily the easiest way of gathering evidence for answering clinical questions.

Just as there are several sources of nonresearch-based evidence, there are several kinds of research-based evidence. Research-based evidence is considered to be stronger evidence on which to base decisions about nursing care. It is the result of carefully designed and implemented research that has been thoughtfully and precisely conducted to answer a specific question. The research process, as you will learn in this book, involves a set of systematic processes that formalize the development of evidence, which is why this type of evidence is stronger than nonresearch evidence.

The sources of research-based evidence are discussed in depth in later chapters. They include nonexperimental research and randomized clinical trials. The strongest forms of research-based evidence are reports that combine multiple research studies such as metasynthesis, meta-analysis, and systematic reviews. We will discuss these further in this chapter, as well as in later chapters.

In our clinical example, the nurse asks the clinical question of how to best implement care to prepare A.K., a patient with HIV, for her impending maternal role. She can look to research to find answers. To look for answers in research, the nurse must:

1. Identify research in the area of interest.
2. Access the research report(s).
3. Read and understand the research report(s).
4. Decide whether the research is relevant and useful in answering the question.
5. Decide whether to accept and use what is found in the research.

Rather than completing all of these steps, it is easier to ask someone who is an expert or an authority, hoping that he or she has read the research. However, it is not uncommon for the answer to the question to be "I do not know," or for the answer to differ among sources. As a professional nurse, you will be an authority from whom others will be seeking answers. This book gives you the skills needed to use research intelligently in your practice, whether for answering direct clinical care questions based on systematic reviews or individual research reports, or for developing and evaluating quality of care standards. However, to read and understand research, you first must know more clearly what research is.

Identifying Applicable Research Reports

Finding research reports is the first step in using research in clinical practice. Identifying research has become easier with the widespread use of the Internet and the increasing numbers of journals that are published electronically. In the clinical case for this chapter, the nurse used the jail's computer to search for research about preparing a patient with HIV for motherhood. Not every article about a health condition is a research article. In fact, most information one can access through journals, texts, and the World Wide Web is not research. So, what is nursing research?

CORE CONCEPT 1-2

Nursing research is the systematic gathering of information to gain, expand, or validate knowledge about health and responses to health problems. Evidence-based nursing uses research-based evidence to plan and implement quality care.

The definition of nursing research includes two key components. First, for a written report or a Web site to be considered research, it must describe the systematic gathering of information to answer some question. Systematic means that a set of actions was planned and organized. The information-gathering actions may include interviews, observations, questionnaires, or laboratory tests, but they must have been guided by a plan and administered methodically or systematically.

Second, the information must have been gathered to answer a question that addresses a gap in our knowledge about nursing. **Knowledge** is what is understood and recognized about a subject. Information can be gathered for many other purposes, including evaluation, reporting, or accounting for resources. Research seeks to gather information so that we can understand or learn something about which we do not yet have knowledge. Research begins with a question—an unknown—and develops new knowledge. In contrast, evaluation, reporting, and accounting usually describe or validate something that is already known or occurring.

An article found by our nurse working with A.K. describes, for example, the complex physical and mental health needs of rural incarcerated women. The article mentions that the number of incarcerated women in U.S. jails has "nearly doubled since 1990" (Kane & DiBartolo, 2002, p. 210). While this number is of interest, it is from other sources and would not be considered a research report. Even if the article provided statistics or numbers about characteristics of incarcerated women, it still would not be a report of research. A research report about the risks of complications in HIV-positive mothers would formulate a question about those complications and then describe the process and results of a systematic effort to answer that question. Therefore, facts and numbers alone do not make a source of information a report of research. A research report provides a description of the systematic gathering of information to gain, expand, or validate knowledge.

Not only is it important to differentiate research reports from those that are not research, but also it is important to identify and find primary sources of research. A primary source is a report of the research written by the original author(s). Professional newsletters and journals often include summaries of research that have been presented at a conference or published elsewhere. Although these summaries are a quick source of information, they do not allow you to fully understand and evaluate the actual research because they are another individual's summary of that research. These summaries are helpful, however, for identifying research studies that may be potentially interesting and important in your practice. To use research intelligently, you must find and read the original research.

As you read more research, the difference between reports of research and other scholarly and informative work becomes clearer. In fact, many of the computer sources used to find research reports have an option that allows you to select only reports that are research, eliminating the need to even decide if an article is a research report. But it is important to understand that what you find when you read a research report is not just a description of facts, ideas, theories, or procedures, but also is a question and a systematic effort to gain information to address that question.

Accessing Research Reports

Once you know what you are looking for, the next step in finding research reports is knowing where to look. As a nursing student, you are probably already aware of numerous nursing research reports. One of the obvious sources is a journal that includes the words "nursing research" in its title (ie, *Research in Nursing and Health* or *Nursing Research*). Most professional nursing journals, even those whose primary purpose is not publishing research, often do include research articles, usually specifically labeled as research in the table of contents. However, simply picking up and scanning journals at the library or at a hospital is a somewhat hit-or-miss approach if you are interested in a specific clinical question. Three primary sources that allow you to search for research on a specific question or topic are (1) printed indexes, (2) the Internet, and (3) electronic databases. Table 1-1 lists examples of these three primary sources.

Printed Indexes. **Printed indexes** are written lists of professional articles that are organized and categorized by topic and author, and they cover articles written from 1956 to today. They usually can only be found in formal academic libraries and are being used more infrequently since the development of computerized electronic databases. Printed indexes are, however, the only source that lists and categorizes research that was done before 1982. Because indexes are tedious to use, are not as available as other sources for finding research, and provide a catalog of studies that are older and thus not current, they should be considered a last resort for research. However, indexes can be helpful in providing ideas for key words to use in a computer search on a topic as well as indicating the kinds of research that have generally been done in your area of interest.

The Internet. The **Internet** is the worldwide network that connects computers throughout the world. Programs called *search engines* can be used to search the Internet; they often come already loaded on the hard drive of a new personal computer. Because the Internet is a source of information from computers throughout the world, a tremendous and potentially overwhelming amount of information can be found on it. However, because almost anyone can put information on the Internet, the accuracy, completeness, and even honesty of information found there must be considered carefully.

When you use the Internet to look for research, it may help to use the word "research" in the search in addition to words that describe your question. Initially, you will probably get thousands of results, or "hits." These vary from connections to large databases, specific journals or newsletters, and organizations, to connections to individuals' Web pages. You then narrow the search to specific links that will give you research reports. Examples of sites that may provide links that could be helpful in answering clinical questions are the CDC (http://www.cdc.gov) and the National Institute for Nursing Research (NINR) (http://www.nih.gov/ninr). Links to large and well-established health-related organizations such as these can assure you high-quality information, and many of these sites provide selected research reports. Links to little-known organizations or sites, however, should be used cautiously because the information may be incorrect or incomplete.

When the RN in our clinical case used the Internet to search for ideas about helping A.K. prepare for motherhood, her search led to a link with a site that discussed the benefits of HIV testing for pregnant women (http://www.doh.wa.gov/cfh/mch/HIV.htm). Another site provided her with a practical overview of the incidence and prevalence of HIV in incarcerated women and some of the problems they encounter (http://hivinsite.ucsf.edu/InSite.jsp?page=kb-07&doc=kb-07-04-13). Another site provided information about a number of programs that are being developed related

TABLE 1-1

Sources to Search for Nursing Research About a Specific Clinical Topic

Type of Source	Specific Examples
Print	
Indexes: provide lists of articles that are organized by topic and author from a range of journals; include all types of articles, including research articles published as early as 1956	Printed *CINAHL* (*Cumulative Index to Nursing and Allied Health Literature*), also known as Red books *Index Medicus* *International Nursing Index*
Card catalogs: list all materials held by the library, including books, audiovisuals, theses, and dissertations organized by topic and author	
Abstract reviews: summaries of research studies and prepared bibliographies	*Dissertation Abstracts International* *Psychological Abstracts* *Sociological Abstracts*
Electronic	
World Wide Web (WWW): an information service that provides access to the Internet using numerous programs called *search engines*	Popular search engines include: http://www.yahoo.com http://www.go.com http://www.altavista.com http://www.dogpile.com http://www.google.com Relevant nursing-related Web sites include: http://www.ana.org/—American Association of Nursing http://www.nih.gov/ninr/—National Institute of Nursing Research http://www.cdc.gov/—Centers for Disease Control and Prevention http://www.dhhs.gov/—Department of Health and Human Services http://www.nursingsociety.org/—Sigma Theta Tau International Nursing Honor Society http://www.cna-nurses.ca/—Canadian Nurses Association
Electronic databases: categorized lists of articles from a range of journals, organized by topic, author, and source	CINAHL—includes articles from 1982 to the present MEDLINE (medical literature analysis and retrieval system) PsycInfo (psychology information) PubMed (database provided by the National Library of Medicine)

to perinatal care of HIV positive women (http://www.cdc.gov/hiv/projects/perinatal/) and gave her some ideas about what she might consider when planning care for A.K.

Electronic Databases. Besides using search engines on the Internet, you also can use the Internet to make a connection with academic libraries through most university Web sites. Once you make that connection, you can usually access the large electronic databases available at these libraries. **Electronic databases**, the most commonly used source to find research reports, provide categorized lists and complete bibliographic citations of sources of information in a broad field of knowledge. Examples of computer databases include the Cumulative Index to Nursing and Allied Health Literature (CINAHL), which categorizes information that relates to the practice of nursing and allied health professions, and PubMed, which is a database provided by the National Library of Medicine that provides access to more than 11 million health-related and medicine-related citations. Electronic databases can be found in CD-ROM format as well as online. Most are organized similarly so that you can initiate a search for information using **key words**, terms that describe the information you are interested in getting. In the case of the clinical example, the nurse might have used key words like "pregnancy," "HIV," "incarcerated," "maternal role," and "health promotion." Sometimes the most difficult part of using an electronic database is determining which key words to use to narrow your search. As mentioned, a quick look at printed indexes may help identify appropriate key words.

Electronic databases also allow you to search for information written by a specific author, or for a specific article using its title. Searches can be limited by date of publication or type of information sought, such as research only. The results of an electronic search include a list of references with bibliographic citations and, usually, an abstract or summary of the article. Again, remember that not all articles found in a search will be research articles unless you have specified that you only want research articles. Although occasionally the title of an article alone may clearly tell you that it is relevant to the question you are asking, you may also need to read the abstract to decide whether it is relevant. Abstracts are discussed in detail later in this chapter.

After finding a citation for a possibly relevant research report, the next challenge may be to acquire a copy of it. Copies of research reports may be acquired in several ways. One way is to subscribe to those journals that usually print the types of research articles that are of interest to you. This allows the article you are interested in reading to be available in your home. A second way is to join one or more professional organizations that provide subscriptions to their journals as a membership benefit. For example, membership in Sigma Theta Tau International includes a subscription to *The Journal of Nursing Scholarship,* which includes many research reports. Another option for acquiring research reports is by obtaining them from your place of practice, as most health care organizations subscribe to several professional journals.

Because numerous journals are now published online as well as in print format, a third way to acquire a research report is to get it online. Although most online journals provide full-text articles only to subscribers, many academic libraries have subscriptions to both print journals and online journals. As a nursing student, you may be able to get articles online. You also may be able to request an interlibrary loan of an article from a journal to which your library does not subscribe. If you do so, be sure to find out whether there is a charge for the article. Finally, you can acquire articles by visiting the closest academic library that subscribes to the journal that you need.

Reading and Understanding Research Abstracts

The nurse in our clinical case will read the published online abstract to decide whether to take the time and trouble to acquire the entire text of the research article. However, reading and understanding the abstract to decide whether the report is potentially useful may be a challenge. Because the abstract for a research report is frequently available when a nurse uses one of the different sources to find research, let us examine what usually is included in an abstract of a research report.

An **abstract** is a summary or condensed version of a research report. Although one meaning of *abstract* is "to summarize," another is "to take away." Because an abstract is a condensed summary, it does "take away" from the total picture or information about a research study and gives only limited information about the study itself. Therefore, the abstract should not be depended on for understanding a research study or making decisions about clinical care. However, if you are trying to decide whether to acquire the full report of a research study, the abstract can certainly be useful. Abstracts vary from journal to journal in format and length. They also vary depending on the type of research performed. Abstracts may be organized by headings, such as Background, Problem, or Results, or they may be written as a single paragraph. However they are organized, almost every abstract identifies the general problem or research question and the general approach taken to implement that research. Most abstracts also briefly describe the people included in the study (called the *subjects* or *participants*) and one or two of the most important findings. Abstracts vary in length from 100 to 500 or more words; those that are more limited in the number of words obviously provide less information. Even longer abstracts, however, provide only a "skeleton" of the key ideas from the research report.

Despite the abstracts' limitations, they still can be useful in determining whether the research study reported is one that you want to acquire and read. The abstract usually provides a clear idea about two important factors: (1) whether the research addressed the clinical question of interest and (2) whether it studied patients or situations that are similar to your clinical case, so that the research is relevant.

Often you can determine from reading an abstract whether the study addressed is the topic you are interested in exploring. For example, a search of the CINAHL database using the key words "pregnancy" and "HIV" might return a citation for an article titled "Prediction of acceptance of maternal role in HIV patients using MMPI testing," a fictional title simply used as an example. This title suggests that the research might be relevant to caring for pregnant HIV patients. The abstract for this article, however, might indicate that the purpose of the study was "to describe the relationship between the acceptance of HIV positive status and maternal personality type." Because the nurse in our clinical case is sure that her jail clinic will not be using a personality test on patients, a review of the abstract would allow her to conclude that this article is not worth acquiring at this time. It is also possible that although the purpose of this study does not fit with the clinical question, the RN may choose to acquire this research report anyway because of its general clinical interest. Besides giving you information about the purpose of a study, most abstracts include information about who was included in the study. Regarding the question about HIV-related care, if an abstract tells you that the people (subjects) in the study were all adults who were vegetarians, you may decide that this study will probably not be helpful for your specific purpose. But if it said the people (subjects) in the study were all women who were in jail settings, it might be very helpful. Be careful, because searching for research on a topic of interest can be a bit like eating peanuts—each one leads to yet another. It is easy to become distracted from the clinical question of interest by related studies. Because you may have limited time and resources, it is important to have as clear an idea as possible regarding the clinical question of interest before you begin searching and reading abstracts of research reports.

PUBLISHED ABSTRACT: WHAT WOULD YOU CONCLUDE?

To better understand the usefulness of reading and understanding research report abstracts, read the abstract of the article found by the nurse in our clinical case, "Complex physical and mental health needs of rural incarcerated women" (Kane & DiBartolo, 2002). You can find this article in Appendix A-2. Remember that the nurse in the clinical case is trying to plan care to assist her pregnant patient who is HIV positive to best adjust to her impending role as a mother. Consider the following questions as you read the abstract:

1. What do you understand or not understand in the abstract?
2. Do you believe that reading the entire report will be helpful in deciding what nursing care would be necessary to assist A.K. in her adjustment to motherhood? Why or why not?
3. Based on the abstract alone and what you know about the clinical question, can you make a decision about what would go into a care plan for A.K.? Why or why not?

It is likely that you will not understand all the language in the abstract; do not be discouraged. The goal of this book is to help you learn to understand that language, and the next chapter directly addresses that topic. However, it is likely that you will understand some of the abstract, and reading even limited information about the research will add to your knowledge about pregnancy and the complex needs of individuals with HIV. Some abstracts are organized by major headings, such as Methods or Subjects, that can be helpful to your understanding, but our example is not. The abstract indicates that little is known about the unique physical and mental health needs of incarcerated women. It states that the researchers worked with 30 incarcerated women in a rural detention center and provided the research participants with a detailed physical and mental health assessment. It tells you that the study found that 63% of participants reported a drug problem, and 84% reported a history of physical or sexual abuse. The results indicate that there is a need to "develop a brief objective mental health screening for this population"

(Kane & DiBartolo, 2002, p. 209). So even if you did not understand the entire abstract, you can see that this research report is relevant to planning for the patient in our clinical case.

CORE CONCEPT 1-3

Abstracts from research reports are an important source of evidence and can be helpful in narrowing down or focusing on the appropriate research to acquire and read. They cannot, and should not, be depended on to provide a level of understanding of the research that would support clinical decision making.

Good, solid, practice-related decisions cannot, however, be based on information gleaned only from the abstract of a research report. Specifically, the research abstract does not give enough information for you to:

1. Understand all the results of the study.
2. Identify who was in the study.
3. Recognize how the results fit or do not fit with existing knowledge.
4. Decide intelligently whether the study was performed in a way that makes the results realistic for clinical practice.

For example, the abstract from the Kane & DiBartolo article (2002) does not tell you that most of the research participants were in a county detention center designed for incarceration not to exceed 18 months or that some of them were released from the center within hours of their participation in the research. The abstract also does not tell you what was meant by "detailed physical and mental health assessment." Because the RN in the clinical case is interested in how to implement care to assist her patient in the complex work of adjusting to the role of motherhood, it is important to determine what is meant by "detailed physical and mental health assessment." The RN must read the entire research report to find the answer to these questions and to decide if the study's findings can be helpful to her in planning care for A.K.

SYSTEMATIC REVIEWS IN EVIDENCE-BASED NURSING

This book treats evidence-based nursing in the broadest sense by including all types of research, as well as other sources of knowledge, as evidence. Currently, however, there is a particular emphasis in nursing on a process of evidence-based practice that addresses clinical questions by searching the literature, evaluating evidence, and choosing an intervention. The product of this process is a systematic review of the research regarding a particular clinical question, and is considered by many as one of the strongest forms of evidence for EBN. Thus, there is a *process* that is often referred to as implementing a systematic review as a basis for evidence-based practice, and there is a *product* that also is often referred to as a systematic review. Although it might be easier to refer to the process of implementing a systematic review as the process of evidence-based practice, doing so significantly limits the breadth of evidence that may be used in nursing. Therefore, throughout this text whenever the term *systematic review* is used, the specific usage of the word will be made explicit to avoid confusion. An example of a systematic review titled "Non-somatic effects of patient aggression on nurses: A systematic review" (Needham, Abderhalden, Halfens, Fisher, & Dassen, 2005) will be used in Chapter 10 and can be found in Appendix A-9.

Like individual research reports, a systematic review includes an abstract and a statement of the problem. However, rather than developing a systematic plan to directly gather information from patients about that question, a systematic review gathers reports of research studies that have already been completed that address the problem. The review summarizes these studies, considering aspects of the research process (such as designs and samples), and then draws conclusions about what is known about the clinical question based on the entire group of studies. Here, as with abstracts of individual studies, a nurse can review the abstract to decide whether the review is directly related to the question of interest. Again, even reviewing the abstract requires a basic understanding of the research language.

SUMMARY

This chapter starts you on the way to critically reading, understanding, and intelligently using research in practice by: (1) defining research, (2) describing sources of research reports, and (3) discussing how to use abstracts to select which research to read. You should now have a working sense of what is meant by EBN and how you might format a clinical question that could be answered through EBN strategies. The next chapter discusses the language of nursing research as well as the components of published research reports and how they can guide your understanding and decisions about using the research in clinical practice.

OUT-OF-CLASS EXERCISE

Get Ready for the Next Chapter

To prepare for the next chapter and to give you a concrete example of the components of a research report, read the fictional research report titled "Demographic characteristics as predictors of nursing students' choice of type of clinical practice" in Appendix B. This report describes a fictional study similar to one in which you may participate during your first class period. As you read this report, make two lists—one containing important words or ideas that you understand in the report, and one listing important words or ideas that you do not understand. Once you have read the report, you are ready to read the next chapter. Also, make sure you read the Discussion and Conclusion sections of the two articles that our nurse found in the clinical case (Kane & DiBartolo, 2002; Sandelowski & Barroso, 2003).

References

Kane, M., & DiBartolo, M. (2002). Complex physical and mental health needs of rural incarcerated women. *Issues in Mental Health Nursing, 23,* 209–229.

Needham, I., Abderhalden, C., Halfens, R. J. G., Fischer, J. E., & Dassen, T. (2005). Non-somatic effects of patient aggression on nurses: A systematic review. *Journal of Advanced Nursing, 49*(3), 283–296.

Sandelowski, M., & Barroso, J. (2003). Motherhood in the context of maternal HIV infection. *Research in Nursing and Health, 26,* 470–482.

Resources

Agan, R. D. (1987). Intuitive knowing as a dimension of nursing. *Advanced Nursing Science, 10*(1), 63–70.

American Nursing Association (ANA). (1989). *Education for participation in nursing research.* Kansas City, MO: Author.

Burns, N., & Groves, S. K. (2002). *Understanding nursing research* (3rd ed.). Philadelphia: W. B. Saunders.

Carper, B. A. (1978). Fundamental patterns of knowing in nursing. *Advances in Nursing Science, 1*(1), 13–23.

Cronin-Stubbs, D. (1992). Publishing research for staff nurses' use. *Applied Nursing Research, 5*(4), 157.

Heath, H. (1998). Reflection and patterns of knowing in nursing. *Journal of Advanced Nursing, 27,* 1054–1059.

Huycke, L. I. (2001). Evidence-based nursing practice. *Southern Connections, 15*(2), 2.

LoBiondo-Wood, G., Haber, J., & Krainovich-Miller, B. (2002). Overview of the research process. In G. LoBiondo-Wood & J. Haber (Eds.), *Nursing research: Methods, critical appraisal, and utilization* (5th ed.). St. Louis: Mosby.

Polit, D. F., & Beck, C.T. (2002). *Nursing research: Principles and methods* (7th ed.). Philadelphia: Lippincott Williams & Wilkins.

Nahas, V. L., Chang, A., & Molassiotis, A. (2001). Evidence-based practice: Guidelines for managing peripheral intravascular access devices. *Journal of Nursing Administration, 31*(4), 164–165.

Sigma Theta Tau (2002). Sigma Theta Tau International's position statement on evidence-based nursing. Retrieved 08/16/2005 from http://nursing society.org/research/main.html.

Stevens, K. R., & Long, J. D. (1998). Incorporating systematic reviews into nursing education. *The Online Journal of Knowledge Synthesis for Nursing* [On-line serial], *5*(7). Retrieved 08/16/2005 from http://www.nursingsociety.org/library.

Thompson, C., McCaughan, D., Cullum, N., Sheldon, T. A., Mulhall, A., & Thompson, D. R. (2001). Research information in nurses' clinical decision-making: What is useful? *Journal of Advanced Nursing, 36*(3), 376–388.

THE RESEARCH PROCESS: COMPONENTS AND LANGUAGE OF RESEARCH REPORTS

LEARNING OBJECTIVE:

The student will differentiate the terminology in and the components of research reports.

KEY TERMS

Conclusions	Meta-analysis	Quality improvement study
Data	Metasynthesis	Quantitative methods
Data analysis	Methods	Results
Descriptive results	Multivariate	Sample
Hypothesis	Problem	Significance
Limitations	Procedures	Systematic review
Literature review	p value	Themes
Measures	Qualitative methods	Theory

CLINICAL CASE

The RN described in the case in Chapter 1 begins to read two research reports she found regarding maternal HIV and incarcerated women. It has been a long time since she has read research reports, and she finds herself struggling with some of the language. But she is reminded of the overall similarity in the organization of research reports. The two articles the RN found are available in Appendices A-1 and A-2. If you have not done so, read through them quickly to make the best use of the examples that are provided in this chapter. Do not worry about fully understanding the articles right now, but do keep a list of words or ideas that you do not understand.

INTRODUCTION

This chapter provides an overview of the major components or sections in most research reports as well as some of the unique research language that identifies these different sections. As you probably discovered when reading the articles in Appendices A-1 and A-2, not understanding certain terms in a research report is frustrating and creates barriers to your ability to use evidence-based nursing intelligently in practice. This chapter discusses the meanings of some of the language of research and gives an overview of the research process. The remaining chapters will walk you through the individual sections of a research report and will elaborate on definitions of terms used in those sections. Viewing the entire report first will allow you to see the whole "picture" and will help you to understand where each section fits when we begin to review each specific part. Recognizing and understanding nursing research language will make it easier for you to start reading and comprehending the research and to use it in your practice.

The language and style of research reports are unique and, therefore, can be difficult to read. They are generally written in a scientific writing style, the goals of which are to be clear, precise, and succinct. Like health care language, research language is formal, technical, and terse, with many ideas compounded into each sentence. This makes research reports reliable methods of communication for anyone immersed in the language of science, but it also makes them inscrutable to the novice who is just beginning to learn the language of research.

Learning to read research reports is similar to learning to read a patient's chart. The first time that you read a sentence such as "The patient is a 64 yo m w m, presenting c̄ RUQ abd pain, post a MVA yesterday a.m.; denies LOC or pain at time of accident," it probably made little, if any, sense to you. Now, however, you know that this sentence refers to a patient being a 64-year-old married white male who has come to seek health care because he has pain in the upper half and right side of his belly. He was in a motor vehicle accident yesterday morning but says that he did not lose consciousness or have pain at the time of the accident. Notice that it took two sentences and many more words to say the same thing in everyday prose. The language of research is much like the language of health care—it, too, is packed with meaning in every sentence and uses unique terms that communicate clearly to anyone familiar with it. Just as you have mastered or are mastering the language of health care, you can master the basics of the language of research.

THE LANGUAGE OF RESEARCH

This chapter presents several terms that are unique to research. Each will be defined in this chapter, but do not be discouraged if you are not completely clear about all of them. They are also included and defined in the glossary, and we will revisit these terms as we discuss the different sections of a research report in more detail in the following chapters. The learning outcome for this chapter is that you differentiate the different sections or components of a research report and the language associated with each of those sections, not that you understand each of the terms in depth. Table 2-1 provides a summary of the sections of a research report and their associated language.

You were asked at the end of Chapter 1 to read the fictional article from Appendix B and compile a list of terms that you did and did not understand. Hopefully, this chapter will touch on some of the terms that were not clear to you and, perhaps, add to your understanding of those that you believed you already understood. Again, you can think of reading research as being similar to reading a patient's chart. The first time you read a patient's hospital chart, a great deal of the information in it may not have made sense to you, and you may not have even known which section to look in for different types of information. With time, however, you learned the unique language of the health care field and found your way around a chart with ease. The same thing will happen with research reports. Just as you learned where to look for physicians' orders as well as the unique language used

TABLE 2-1	
The Sections of a Research Report and Associated Terms	
Research Report Section	**Associated Terms**
Problem or Introduction: describes the gap in knowledge that will be addressed in the research study	■ Literature review ■ Theory ■ Research question ■ Hypothesis
Methods: describes the process of implementing the research study	■ Qualitative ■ Quantitative ■ Measures ■ Sample ■ Procedures
Results: summarizes the specific information gathered in the research study	■ Data ■ Data analysis ■ Themes ■ Descriptive ■ Significant ■ Multivariate
Conclusions: describes the decisions or determinations that can be made about the research problem	■ Limitations ■ Implications for practice

in those orders, you will learn where to look for specific information about a research study and to understand its unique research language. For example, you will learn where to look for information about procedures in a research study and some of the unique language used to describe those procedures so that you will have a good start at reading and better understanding research reports. As you read the different research reports used in this book, keep adding to your list of words or ideas that you do not understand, then periodically review it and cross out those words you believe you understand. You can use the list to guide your own reading and can share it with your fellow students and your faculty to assure clarification of the words to facilitate your own and fellow students' learning.

COMPONENTS OF PUBLISHED RESEARCH REPORTS

In addition to an abstract, almost every research report has at least four major sections:

- Introduction or Problem
- Methods
- Results
- Conclusions or Discussion

Table 2-1 describes each of these sections and lists some of their associated research terms. Because this book discusses research by beginning at the end or the conclusions of a research report and moving to the beginning of the report or introduction, we will look at each of the sections of a report, starting with the end.

Conclusions

The word **conclusions** is used in research reports much as it is generally used outside of the research setting. Conclusions identify what was found and complete a report by identifying an outcome. They specifically describe or discuss the researcher's final decisions or determinations regarding the research problem.

In nursing research reports, conclusions usually include a description of implications for nursing practice. That is why practicing nurses often start with the conclusions of a report. That section provides the "so what" by providing the meaning of the research for practice. What distinguishes conclusions in a research report from those in other reports is the expectation that they contain either new knowledge or confirmation of previous knowledge. This is a core concept. The goal of the research process is to generate knowledge that can be used in practice. In the conclusions section of a research report, the findings or results of a study are directly translated into that new knowledge. So you should expect that the conclusions go beyond simply saying what was found in a study; they present the implications or meaning of those findings for future practice. As such, the conclusions of research reports are powerful because they are the evidence for EBN. They are used as the basis for decisions about direct patient care, whether in program planning, or in one-to-one direct patient care, such as that being planned by the RN.

CORE CONCEPT 2-1

What distinguishes conclusions in a research report from those in other reports is the expectation that they contain either new knowledge or confirmation of previous knowledge.

Because of the power and importance attached to them, the statement or decisions described in the conclusions of a research report are carefully worded and should list any relevant cautions or limitations. This cautious presentation may, however, make the conclusions weak or not helpful to the nurse who is looking for clear and direct answers to clinical questions.

For example, the RN in our clinical case is looking for specific advice about how to promote healthy adaptation in A.K. in her maternal role and finds the conclusions of the two reports described in sections labeled "Discussion" and "Conclusions." From reading these sections, she learns that mothers who are HIV positive experience contradictions in the process of pregnancy, including both a buffering and an intensification of the negative effects of HIV infection (Sandelowski & Barroso, 2003). She also learns that 84% of the women in the incarcerated women study reported being either physically or sexually abused and that 70% of the women were in the "clinical range" for mental health problems (Kane & DiBartolo, 2002). This is useful information for the RN, but it does not provide her with specifics about how to assist A.K. as she goes through her pregnancy or how to facilitate the positive maternal attachment and safe care for the baby once it is born. The discussion in the maternal HIV article goes on to state: "This motherhood (study) was also performed mostly before the advent and use of new drug therapies that have transformed HIV infection in the United States." (Sandelowski & Barroso, 2003, p. 478). The incarcerated women article states that the study has "obvious limitations both in terms of sample size and the . . . convenience sample" (Kane & DiBartolo, 2002, p. 224). The authors of both articles clearly express their conclusions cautiously and may do so for several reasons. Chapter 3 examines in more detail why conclusions often are constrained or hesitant.

The conclusion section of a research report usually has fewer unique research terms than does the rest of the report. This is probably another reason why the conclusion section is sometimes the first part read by nurses. One term that regularly appears in the conclusions section is *limitations*. **Limitations** are the aspects of how the study was conducted that create uncertainty concerning the conclusion that can be derived from the study as well as the decisions that can be based on it. These limitations often address the information presented in the beginning sections of the report, such as the study's methods and sample.

Just as the cautious language used in the conclusions section can be frustrating when you are looking for practical answers to clinical questions, the limitations described may make you wonder whether you can use conclusions as evidence on which to practice. That is why the limitations are included in the conclusions: to remind the reader that there are constraints or limits to the knowledge being

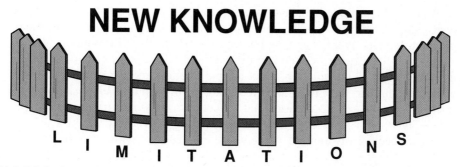

FIGURE 2-1 • Limitations of the research process constrain knowledge acquired.

reported. Limitations do not mean that the results of a study are flawed or meaningless. They do, however, indicate the boundaries of or constraints to the knowledge generated by the research. One might view the limitations as the fence that surrounds and "limits" the new knowledge in the report. To decide whether to use the knowledge described in a research report and how it will be used, you must understand not only the knowledge but also the "fence" that surrounds it (Fig. 2-1). This requires understanding of other aspects of the research process, such as sampling or methods that may fence or boundary the new knowledge.

Finally, the conclusions section of a research report usually contains recommendations for future research regarding the problem of interest. These recommendations often directly address the limitations that have been described and suggest additional studies that are needed to further build on the new knowledge generated and stretch the boundary of that knowledge.

Results

The **results** section of a research report summarizes the specific findings from the study. Almost no research report can give all of the information that was gathered during a research study, so the results section contains a summary or condensed version of what the authors believe are the most important findings. *Data* is a word that is often used and has specific meaning in research. **Data** are the information collected in a study. Organizing and compiling data is called *data analysis*. **Data analysis** pulls elements or information together to present a clear picture of the information collected, but it does not interpret or describe the implications for practice of that picture of the information.

CORE CONCEPT 2-2

The difference between results and conclusions is that results are a summary of the actual findings or information collected in the research study, whereas conclusions summarize the potential meaning, decisions, or determinations that can be made based on the information collected.

Some of the unique language found in this section is a result of how the data were analyzed and what analysis methods were used to summarize the information collected. Results or findings may be reported in the form of numbers, words, or both. Which form is used depends on the type of information or data collected. If the study collected information about people's beliefs and experiences, the results section summarizes the words collected using terms such as *themes, categories,* and *concepts*. **Themes** are abstractions that reflect phrases, words, or ideas that appear repeatedly when a researcher analyzes what people have said about a particular experience, feeling, or situation. A theme summarizes and synthesizes discrete ideas or phrases to create a picture from the words collected in the research study. For example, the maternal HIV article identifies seven major findings that are reported in Table 1 of their research report found in Appendix A-1. Similarly, in the fictional research report about nursing students' choices of type of clinical practice, the results section mentions "three distinct themes that represent the meaning of life experiences related to choice of field of nursing." The authors of these two articles do not list the answers given by 30 different nursing students or within each of the 56 reports used in the synthesis; rather, they have looked for recurring ideas or words in those answers and have categorized them into themes or findings.

In contrast, the research study on incarcerated women primarily collected information in the form of numbers, such as scores on the Brief Symptom Inventory (BSI) and the Multidimensional Scale of Perceived Social Support (MSPSS). Again, the authors do not list all the responses from 30 different women who completed the scales; rather, they summarize the numbers in several different forms, such as means and percentages. The language that describes data analysis of information in numbers is called *statistics,* and the language of statistics is often some of the most intimidating language to readers of research. We do not have to be statistical experts to develop a greater understanding of that language, and we will focus on the language of statistics in Chapters 4 and 5. However, a few key terms are worth highlighting here to help us get started.

Almost all research reports, even those that are mostly reporting results of interviews in the form of words, include descriptive results. **Descriptive results** summarize information without comparing it with other information. For example, descriptive results may state how many people were in a study, the average age of those studied, or the percentage who responded in a specific manner. In the incarcerated women article, almost all of the results presented are descriptive. In Box 2-1, the paragraph describing

---

Box 2-1 **Descriptive Results of the Incarcerated Women Study**

"Seventeen of the participants were in jail for drug offenses or drug-related offenses (stealing, violation of probation by using drugs, taking a possession charge for a friend, etc.). While only 13 openly admitted to a drug problem at the time of the arrest, 16 noted that they had a current alcohol problem. As one might expect, a larger percentage reported a history of drug (63.3%) and alcohol problems (80%). Only 30% of the participants had ever been in an addictions treatment program." (Kane & DiBartolo, 2002, p. 219)

alcohol and drug use from the article is repeated. Here, the authors describe the number of women who had been in jail for drug offenses, the number who acknowledged a type of drug problem, and the percentage with histories of drug problems.

Thus far, we have talked about descriptive results, but the authors of the incarcerated women study also provide some correlation statistics in the paragraph headed "Social Support" (Kane & DiBartolo, 2002). Here, the authors are doing more than just describing the findings because they are looking for connections between the variables in their study. Specifically, the authors are looking for a connection between the women's BSI scores and their MSPSS scores. The computation of a correlation statistic to look for connections between variables requires consideration of two important statistical concepts: significance and p values.

Let us look at what *significance* means first. The second sentence in the Social Support section of the incarcerated women report indicates that, "The total scores (mean = 4.71) on the MSPSS were *significantly* negatively correlated with the Global Severity Index on the BSI ($r = -.377, p = .04$)" (Kane & DiBartolo, 2002, p. 220). **Significance** is a statistical term indicating a low likelihood that any differences or relationships found in a study happened by chance. In research, we often try to make decisions about clinical care for a large group of patients based on what we have found in a small group of patients. Statistical significance is important because we need to be sure that what was found in the small group of patients studied is not something that happened by chance rather than because of some factor we are studying. The correlation described as $r = -.377$, which the authors of the incarcerated women study tell us is significant, indicates that the connection between the women's level of psychological distress and their level of social support probably did not occur by chance alone. Thus, we could expect that in another group of incarcerated women, we would find some relationship between psychological distress and social support. This significant relationship has a p value equal to .04, which leads us to the second important statistical concept.

So if significance is indicated by p values, what is a p value? **P values** indicate what percentage of the time the results reported would have happened by chance alone. For example, a p value of .05 means that in only 5 out of 100 times would one expect to get the results by chance alone. If it is unlikely that the results happened by chance, then we can summarize the findings by saying that the results are statistically significant. In order to consider if the results of a study help to answer your clinical question, and in order to practice EBN, you will need to look for these p values, For example, the p value given for the correlation between the MSPSS and the BSI is "$p = .04$" (Kane & DiBartolo, 2002). This tells us that the connection found between these two scores would happen by chance alone in only 4% of samples. What that connection means and how it affects our clinical planning are not discussed until the conclusions section of the report. However, summarizing and reporting the finding of a connection that is not likely to happen by chance alone is important so that the reader knows why the researchers reached their conclusion.

Another term that is often found in the results section of a research report is *multivariate*. If you think about this term, it is easy to figure out that **multivariate** indicates that the study reports findings for three (multi) or more factors (variate) and includes the relationships among those different factors. The fictional article in Appendix B reports multivariate results because it looks at relationships and differences between more than two factors. The article does not use the word *multivariate,* but it does describe results of a statistical procedure called a *logistic regression,* which included the three factors of age, rating of health, and choice of field of nursing. Now that you know what the word means, you can count the number of factors analyzed and identify that this study is, indeed, multivariate. Logistic regression is a statistical procedure that allows us to look at relationships between more than two factors and test whether those relationships are likely to occur by chance. Statistical language such as this is discussed further in Chapters 4 and 5.

The information summarized in the results section of a report depends on who was studied, how the study was conducted, what the research question asked, and how the researcher(s) analyzed the information. To understand more completely what was implemented in a study and who was studied, we must look at the methods section of the research report.

Methods

The **methods** section of a research report describes the overall process of how the researchers went about implementing the research study, including who was included in the study, how information was collected, and what interventions, if any, were tested. Remember from Chapter 1 that one of the things that distinguishes research from other ways of answering questions is its systematic collection of information. The methods section of a research report should describe those procedures used to collect information. Chapter 8 examines, in detail, the variety of research methods, along with the many names used for them. For now, remember that research methods can be broadly categorized under two major headings: qualitative and quantitative methods. Because qualitative and quantitative methods are used both separately and together in nursing research, both methods are discussed throughout this text. To assist you in understanding the differences between them and how the differences may affect your use of the research in practice, the following eight chapters will be organized so that general information relating to both approaches is described first, followed by specific information related to qualitative and then to quantitative methods. These sections will be identified by use of an icon, just as the two following paragraphs are identified. Be sure to read carefully and note the icons, as it is easy to get the two approaches confused. At this point, we will briefly differentiate qualitative and quantitative methods.

Qualitative

Qualitative methods focus on understanding the complexity of humans within the context of their lives. Research that uses qualitative methods attempts to build a complete picture of a phenomenon of interest. Therefore, qualitative methods involve the collection of information as it is expressed by people within the normal context of their lives. Qualitative methods focus on subjective information and never attempt to predict or control the phenomena of interest. As an example, the maternal HIV article used in Chapters 1 and 2 is an example of a metasynthesis of a number of studies using qualitative methods.

Quantitative methods focus on understanding and breaking down the phenomenon into parts to see how they do or do not connect. Therefore, quantitative methods involve collecting information that is specific and limited to the particular parts of events or phenomena being studied. Quantitative methods focus on objective information and can yield predictions and control. The incarcerated women study used in Chapters 1 and 2 is a study using quantitative methods.

Quantitative

Figure 2-2 illustrates the differences between knowledge building using qualitative versus quantitative methods: qualitative research assembles the pieces of a

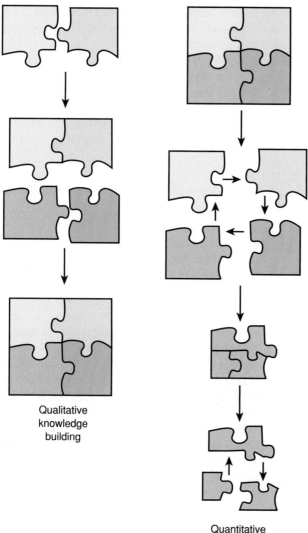

Qualitative
knowledge
building

Quantitative
knowledge
building

FIGURE 2-2 • The differences between qualitative and quantitative methods.

puzzle into a whole picture, whereas quantitative research selects pieces of a completed puzzle and breaks them down into their component parts.

Methods sections of research reports, whether they use qualitative or quantitative methods, usually include information about three aspects of the research method: (1) the sample, (2) the data collection procedures, and (3) the data analysis methods.

Sample

A **sample** is a smaller group, or subset of a group, of interest that is studied in a research. Using the incarcerated women study as an example, you will see that the researchers were interested in gaining knowledge that could help a provider do a better job of caring for incarcerated women, but they only had the time and resources to study a group of 30 such women from one jail.

Therefore, in planning care for A.K., the RN must consider whether the 30 women from rural Maryland described in the research report are similar to women in her clinic. The effort to assure that the subgroup or sample and what happens to them is similar to the other patients or people being studied is emphasized in quantitative research methods. However, describing the sample, that is, who was studied, is important for understanding the results of a qualitative study as well as those of a quantitative study.

CORE CONCEPT 2-3

Most research attempts to gather information systematically about a subset, or smaller group of patients or people, to gain knowledge about other similar patients or people. Many of the methods in research are aimed at assuring that what happens in the subgroup or sample studied is as similar as possible to what would happen in other larger groups of patients or people.

The sampling subsection in the methods section of a research report describes how people, or studies in the case of the metasynthesis, were chosen, what was done to find them, and what, if any, limits or restrictions were placed on who or which research could be done in the study. It also usually describes how many patients or people declined to be in the study, withdrew from it, or were not included in it for specific reasons. For example, the fictional article states that the sample was one of convenience, meaning that no special efforts were made to get a particular type of student to participate. The students chose whether or not to participate in the study and did not provide identifying information on the questionnaire. Therefore, no restrictions were placed on who would participate; all the researcher did was approach a class of students and ask them to volunteer. This is an example of a simple sampling procedure.

In contrast, the maternal HIV article states that, "Of the 114 reports in the bibliographic sample, 56 contained motherhood findings, and these comprised the primary data for this report" (Sandelowski & Barroso, 2003, p. 471). These authors go on to say that some of the reports had been published and others not, and they describe a complex process of assuring that there were no important differences in these two types of reports. This is a more complicated sampling method, involving the analysis of information about each report in order to identify the sample of reports that best met the criteria of the study. Understanding samples and sampling is an important part of making intelligent decisions about the use of research in practice and is discussed in more detail in Chapters 6 and 7.

Procedures

In addition to information about samples, the methods section usually includes information about procedures used in the study. Nurses are familiar with procedures within the context of health care. Research **procedures** are similar because they are the specific actions taken by researchers to gather information about the problem or phenomena being studied. Research procedures in qualitative and quantitative studies differ because the purposes of the two approaches to research differ.

Because the systematic collection of information in a qualitative study involves looking as much as possible at the whole phenomena being studied, procedures for qualitative studies are systematically planned activities—such as observations or open and unstructured interviews of people in their natural life situations—to see and hear as much as possible of the complexity of those situations. A qualitative researcher may videotape or audiotape interviews with individuals so that every word, expression, and pause can be carefully considered and studied. In addition, qualitative researchers keep detailed notes of their observations of the environment where the information is collected as well as the expressions and actions of those being studied. This is not a haphazard process but an organized, systematic, and intensive process to collect and then analyze the complexity of experiences.

Qualitative

In contrast, because the methods used in a quantitative study involve identifying specific aspects of a problem, the procedures involve actions to isolate and examine those particular aspects or pieces. The focus of a quantitative study is on clearly defining and examining that which is believed to be relevant to the problem being studied. Therefore, procedures may involve carefully defined repeated observations at set time intervals, such as taking a blood pressure reading immediately before and after a patient is suctioned. Another example may be a specific protocol for teaching each patient, in exactly the same manner, to use visualization to relax before surgery.

Quantitative

In summary, quantitative and qualitative methods lead to different approaches and procedures. Control and objectivity are hallmarks of quantitative methods, whereas naturally occurring conditions and subjectivity characterize qualitative methods.

Often, the procedures in a quantitative study involve taking measurements, sometimes directly, such as taking a blood pressure reading, but often indirectly, such as in a written questionnaire. **Measures** are the specific method(s) used to assign a number or numbers to an aspect or factor being studied. For example, in the article about incarcerated women, the authors used a 53-item questionnaire to collect information about the women's psychological symptoms. They did not do extensive mental health testing on the women; rather, they depended on the women's self-report of how much distress they experienced in relation to a number of situations. The final numbers used in this study are the average or mean scores on this self-report of level of distress. Thus, the abstract concept of psychological distress is converted into a number that can be analyzed.

Another example of the use of measures is found in the fictional article in Appendix B. The study examines factors that cannot be directly observed. The article has a section labeled "Measures," which describes a three-part written questionnaire. This questionnaire was used to assign numbers to aspects that were studied, such as perceived well-being or choice of field of study. So again, abstract concepts are converted into a number that can be analyzed using statistical procedures. Based on the previous discussion of qualitative and quantitative studies, it should make sense that the incarcerated women study used a quantitative method because its goal was to break down and describe aspects of the health of incarcerated women. It carefully defined the factors to be studied and established a clear, easily reproduced approach to get information. Similarly, the fictional article describes measures used to translate the factors that were studied into numbers, indicating a quantitative approach, but also includes what the author calls a "qualitative question." By using the word *qualitative,* the author indicates that this part of the research attempted to look broadly or holistically at the students' experiences, without selecting specific pieces and asking focused questions. Therefore, the fictional article describes the use of both qualitative and quantitative procedures in its methods section.

An important point to understand is that although this book describes and defines many of the terms used in the research process and found in research reports, the terms can have various meanings and can, at different times, be used broadly or more specifically. This can be frustrating or discouraging because the words or ideas are new, and you are just beginning to understand them. However, the more experience you gain from reading and learning about research, the easier understanding it will be. You will find the same situation with many of the words used in the health care field. For example, "normal" body temperature is defined as 98.8°F. Fever is clearly present when a patient has a temperature of 100.8°F or higher, but a temperature between 99.8°F and 100.8°F is not considered either febrile or "normal," and a patient can feel "feverish" with a "normal" temperature. With practice, nurses learn to recognize these variations in the meaning of the words *fever* and *feverish.* Similarly, with practice, you will learn to recognize and be comfortable with the variations in meanings or use of research terms. Although we have said that quantitative and qualitative methods usually look different, which suggests that an individual research study will use only one of the two broad approaches, at times, researchers use a combination of the two methods to address the same research problem. The fictional article is an example of such a study.

CORE CONCEPT 2-4

Many of the terms used in research have a range of meanings rather than a single, discrete, locked-in meaning.

Data Analysis Plan

In addition to describing the sample and procedures used in a study, the methods section often includes a description of the data analysis. Remember that data are the information collected in a study, and data analysis is a description of what was done with that data to obtain a clearer picture of what the information tells us. Although the results section summarizes the outcome of data analysis, the methods section often describes in detail how the researchers worked with or analyzed the data. In the article about maternal HIV, the authors describe some of the procedures they used to analyze reports under headings titles "Evaluation of reports" and "Meta-summary and Meta-synthesis." Similarly, the incarcerated women study includes paragraphs under the heading of "Methods" that describe how data were collected and how they were analyzed. The fictional article has a much shorter "Analysis" subsection, in which the author informs the reader that a specific computer program was used to analyze the data that were numbers, and then describes the analysis procedures for the data that were words. Again, the approaches to analyzing quantitative and qualitative data are different and are discussed further in Chapter 4.

Problem

So far, we have reviewed the conclusions, results, and methods sections of research reports: Conclusions discuss the outcomes, decisions, or potential meanings of the study; results summarize what was found; and methods describe how the study was implemented. This brings us to the beginning of a research report, a section often labeled "Problem" or "Introduction." Just as the word suggests, the **problem** section of a research report describes the gap in knowledge that is addressed by the research study. In this section, the researcher explains why the study was needed, why it was carried out in the manner that it was, and, often, what the researcher is specifically asking or predicting.

The introduction or problem section of a research report usually includes a background or **literature review** subsection, which is a focused summary of what has already been published regarding the question or problem. The literature review gives us a picture of what is already known or has already been studied in relation to the problem and identifies where the gaps in knowledge may be. It may report, for example, that studies have only been done with selected types of patients, such as with children but not with adults. Or, it may report that no one has ever tried to ask a particular question before: Perhaps studies have examined occurrence of one or two specific health problems in incarcerated women, but none has examined multiple physical and mental health problems.

The literature review does not necessarily only include published *research* studies. It also may include published reports about issues related to practice or a description of a theory. A **theory** is a written description of how several factors may relate to and affect each other. The factors described in a theory are usually abstract; that is, they are ideas or concepts, such as illness, stress, pain, or fatigue, that cannot be readily observed and immediately defined and recognized. Nursing theories such as Roy's theory of adaptation (1984), Neuman's system model (1982), and Watson's

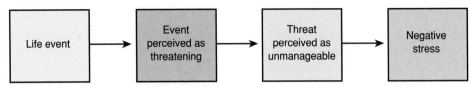

FIGURE 2-3 • Proposed relationships among the four factors in Lazarus's theory of stress and coping (1993).

theory of human caring (1985) are examples of written descriptions of how the four major components of nursing (persons, health, environment, and nursing) may interrelate.

Lazarus's (1993) theory of stress and coping is another example of a theory that most nurses know and that is somewhat simpler than many nursing theories. It proposes relationships among four abstract factors: life events, perceptions of threat, perceptions of ability to manage a threat, and stress. The relationships proposed in the theory are if a life event occurs that is perceived as threatening, and there are no perceived approaches to manage or mitigate that threat, then stress results. Figure 2-3 illustrates the proposed relationships among these four factors.

When a research report discusses a theory in its introduction or problem section, the study usually tests or further explains the relationships proposed in that theory. Therefore, if a study report discussed Lazarus's theory of stress and coping (1993) in the introduction, we expect that the study will be based on, or will examine, some aspect of how life events and perceptions affect stress as described in that theory. If a research study is based on an existing theory, then the researcher often already has an idea of what relationships are expected to be found. These ideas are stated in the form of a **hypothesis**—a prediction regarding the relationships or effects of selected factors on other factors. Not every study will have a hypothesis. For a study to include a hypothesis, there must be some knowledge about a problem of interest so that we can propose or predict that certain relationships or effects will occur. If you remember from earlier in the chapter, qualitative research does not try to predict outcomes, and therefore, a hypothesis is seldom appropriate. Neither the HIV study nor the incarceration study explicitly includes either a theory or a hypothesis. Both studies do describe several factors that may influence the problem of interest, but the problem statements in both studies suggest that the knowledge gap results from not knowing the effects or relationships among these factors. As a result, both studies present purposes or research questions but do not include hypotheses that make predictions. Research questions, purposes, and hypotheses are discussed in Chapter 10.

RESEARCH REPORTS AND THE RESEARCH PROCESS

So far, we have discussed the elements of a published research report. However, in doing so, we have had to at least touch on what a researcher does to conduct a research study. Although this book is not intended to teach you how to be a researcher, it is impossible to use research intelligently if you do not understand the basics of the research process. Just as you do not have to be a cardiac surgeon to understand what open heart surgery entails, you do not have to be a researcher to read and use research in EBN. Fortunately, the research report is written in a manner that closely mirrors the actual research process, so as we focus on understanding and intelligently using research, we also can learn the basics of the process. We overview the steps in that process now and then discuss the different steps further in the following chapters.

Steps in the Research Process

Figure 2-4 illustrates the five steps in the research process and the relationship between them and the sections of a research report. The first step is to define and describe a knowledge gap or problem. Frequently, this step begins with a clinical question or problem, such as the one raised by the RN in the clinical case who wants

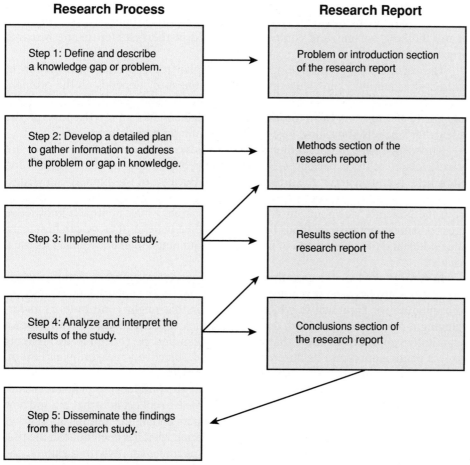

FIGURE 2-4 • The relationship between the research process and the sections of a research report.

to find evidence to guide her care of A.K. A researcher interested in this type of clinical question then performs a literature review to determine what is already known about the problem. Performing a literature review requires using databases, as discussed in Chapter 1, and the researcher should search for and read as many pertinent published articles on the topic as possible. As part of defining and describing the knowledge gap, the researcher also investigates whether anyone has ever implemented a study addressing the clinical question as well as how other people have studied or described aspects of the problem. Although this process may help the researcher to gain a clearer picture of how to construct a study to address the clinical question, it also may make the problem more complicated and confusing. Often, a researcher's question changes as he or she learns about what has already been studied or described. Therefore, the focus of the first step is to narrow and identify something specific for the study, and its culmination is a statement of a problem or purpose. The problem section of a research report partially reflects this step by providing a description of the relevant literature, possibly a theory, and one or more of the following: a research problem, question, or hypothesis. However, the neatly written problem or introduction section of a research report certainly will not reflect all of the thinking, sorting, and comparing involved in the first step of the research process.

The second step is to develop a detailed plan for gathering information to address the identified knowledge gap. Planning the study depends on the problem or question being asked, and the designs of qualitative and quantitative studies differ, partly because of the type of questions asked and partly because of the researcher's beliefs about how best to gain meaningful knowledge.

Qualitative

Knowledge gaps that lend themselves to studies using qualitative methods are usually related to the experiences, beliefs, feelings, or perceptions of individuals, and often, little is known about the area in question. Because of this limited knowledge, qualitative methods provide a broad picture by describing the whole experience from the patient's viewpoint. In addition, a researcher may approach knowledge gaps by using qualitative methods because he or she believes that we can best learn and understand the phenomena of interest by examining the phenomena in its usual context.

Quantitative

In contrast, knowledge gaps that involve a concrete response or action, such as the relationships between psychological distress and social support, lend themselves to a quantitative approach in which each factor that might contribute to understanding a problem is identified, defined, and measured. A researcher who uses a quantitative approach believes that knowledge can best be generated by breaking down a phenomenon into its different pieces and objectively measuring and examining each piece and its relationship to the other pieces.

In this step, the specific methods used to study the problem are planned, including who will participate in the study, what will be done to collect information, and how that information will be analyzed. It requires understanding the various approaches used to systematically gather information, considering what has been done in the past and what kinds of problems have occurred, and planning carefully to maximize the knowledge that will be the product of the study. The methods section of the research report, like the problem section, summarizes the decisions made in this step by specifically describing the sample, procedures, and data analysis used in the study. For example, in the fictional article about nursing students' preferences for first clinical jobs, we are told that the study included junior-year undergraduate nursing students and that, in this program, traditional 4-year, RN-to-BSN and LPN-to-BSN students were included. The report also tells us that a written questionnaire was used to collect the data. The researcher in this study could have decided to study graduating seniors rather than juniors or to conduct in-depth interviews with selected students rather than using a questionnaire. The researcher had reasons for using juniors and having them complete a questionnaire, such as time constraints, student availability, and the researcher's view on meaningful ways to gather knowledge. What we read in the research report usually only reflects the final decisions of the second step of the research process, and the researcher will likely only provide a limited explanation of the methods used.

Because research is a process, a study may not occur as it was designed and planned; therefore, the methods section also may describe any changes made to the study plan as it was implemented. In the maternal HIV study, for example, the authors tell us in the methods section that some studies were excluded from their sample because of clear violations of the rights of human subjects, or the report included no findings (Sandelowski & Barroso, 2003). This change meant that the researchers had fewer studies in their sample. Similarly, the incarcerated women study reports that only 30 of the 107 women who were incarcerated agreed to participate in the study (Kane & DiBartolo, 2002).

The third step in the research process is to implement the study by gathering and analyzing the information in the systematic manner planned in the second step. As mentioned in the discussion of procedures, this may involve numerous different actions, such as tape-recording interviews, performing carefully controlled clinical experiments, or mailing and compiling responses to a questionnaire. In addition to gathering the information, this step involves managing, organizing, and analyzing the information to address the problem being studied. The outcome of this step is reported in the results section of the research report, which is why that section describes the sample and summarizes the answers or outcomes for each measure. Those results may not directly answer the research question, but they do allow the reader to have a better understanding of what happened during the study. For example, the researchers in the incarcerated women study performed physical and mental health assessment on all the incarcerated women and then asked if they would be willing to participate in the study by completing the research questionnaires. It is likely that the researchers did not plan on only having 28% of those incarcerated agree to be in the study. We do not know if one type of incarcerated woman was more likely than another to participate, so as a reader, we have to wonder about the results just a bit. It is important to remember this when reviewing the conclusions because they may not apply equally to all patients.

The fourth step is the detailed analysis and interpretation of the results. In qualitative research methods, this step is woven closely with the third step, with analysis often guiding additional data collection. In quantitative methods, some preliminary analysis and summary of the data usually occur during the implementation step. However, additional analysis and careful interpretation of the meaning of the findings occurs only after all the information from the study is gathered. The researchers will analyze the data, compare their findings to those from previous studies, and decide what they can conclude from the study. At this point, the researcher hopes to answer the question posed, confirm or not confirm the prediction made, or create a meaningful understanding of the phenomena of interest. The actual findings from the study are summarized in the results section of the research report, whereas the implications, or potential meaning of those findings, are included in the conclusions section. As with all the other sections of a report, what is actually included does not reflect everything that the researchers did during this step. They will distill their analysis into a few paragraphs to provide the reader with a succinct summary of what they found and what it may mean for clinical care.

The fifth and final step of the research process is the sharing or dissemination of the findings. Gathering information to gain new knowledge is not a particularly useful activity if no one ever learns about the new knowledge, so an important obligation and commitment of the researcher is to share that research through publications, presentations, posters, and teaching. Research reports, such as the one on maternal HIV, are obviously a major method for disseminating research. However, these reports do not accomplish the goal of disseminating research if the people who need the knowledge cannot understand them. This brings us back to the importance of understanding and intelligently reading and using research in nursing practice.

SUMMARY OF THE RESEARCH PROCESS CONTRASTED TO THE RESEARCH REPORT

The first step of the research process—describing and defining the knowledge gap or problem—is summarized in the background and literature review sections of a research report. These sections give us the context for a research problem and tell us about relevant theory and research regarding aspects of it. The information included in the research report is a synopsis of the much more extensive information that was gathered and synthesized during the first step. The research purpose and specific questions or hypotheses that conclude the first sections reflect the final refinement of the research problem into specific variables and a specific type of research question.

The second step of the research process is reflected in the methods section of a research report. This section tells us the study design, sampling plan, methods of measurement, and procedures. Again, all the previous research, practicalities, and experience that enter into the decisions about settings for a study, the sample, and the measurement are distilled into a few paragraphs describing the final decisions that were reached about the study plan.

The third step of the research process—implementing the study—is usually reflected in the results section of a research report because it is there that we learn who actually participated in the study. We also may see part of the implementation reflected in the methods section if what occurred during the implementation process changed the sampling or measurement approaches taken. In either case, the information included in a report rarely reflects all of the details of a study's implementation.

The fourth step of analysis and interpretation of the results of a study are reflected in both the results and conclusions sections of a research report. Of all the steps of the research process, probably this one is most fully described in the report. However, even with this step, a great deal more goes into the process than is reflected in the results and conclusion sections of most reports.

Finally, the fifth step in the research process is the research report itself. However, developing and publishing a research study report also requires more effort than may be obvious when looking at the final product. Publication depends on several factors. These include the fit between the purpose of the study and the emphasis of journals that publish research, the relevance and quality of the research study, and the ability of the researcher to express clearly and succinctly all the pertinent elements that are needed to fully understand and use the research. The first two factors primarily affect those who will use the research because they affect what research is available through journals and online. Some research journals publish all types of research in each issue; others develop themes for different issues, limiting the types of studies they will publish at any particular time. Other journals reflect specialties, such as obstetric nursing, and are only interested in research that is relevant to that specialty. Some journals do not want to publish research that is highly theoretical because they target readers who want practical and practice-focused information. To disseminate the study findings, a researcher first has to find journals that fit with the purpose of the completed study.

Some research is not published because problems with the quality of the research are identified during the review process that decreases the meaningfulness or validity of the study's results. This does not mean that the research was bad but simply that some flaw or aspect of the study creates enough doubt about the findings or meaning of the results to preclude its warranting publication.

Another factor that affects publication is the ability of the researcher to express in writing adequate information to describe accurately the entire research process. Many of the common errors in research reports that we will discuss throughout this book are errors of omission or lack of complete information. The research process requires much more thought and work than can be described in a research report. The challenge for a researcher, then, and for the reviewers and editors who contribute to the final publication, is to describe clearly and completely all the aspects of the research process that were relevant to their particular study. The goal is to provide the readers with enough information to allow them to understand the study fully and to make intelligent decisions about the usefulness and meaning of the research for practice. One way this is accomplished is by using the language of research to limit the need to fully explain each study aspect. Yet, that very language of research may interfere with using research in practice because the practitioner may not be familiar with or understand the language.

Metasynthesis, Meta-Analysis, Systematic Reviews, and Quality Improvement Reports as Evidence for Nursing Practice

We have been discussing the sections and language in research reports in general; however, there are several unique types of reports we should recognize. These include reports of a single study, reports called metasynthesis, meta-analysis, systematic reviews, and quality improvement. One of the two examples we have been using in this chapter is a report of a single research study. The other article describes a **metasynthesis**, which is a report of a study of a group of single research studies using qualitative methods. There is also a method called **meta-analysis**, which is a quantitative approach to knowledge development that applies statistics to numeric results from different studies that addressed the same research problem to look for combined results that would not happen by chance alone. Both of these methods examine a question or problem about which there have been a number of studies and actually take a sample of studies, rather than a sample of individuals. Metasynthesis and meta-analysis are similar to another special type of research report called a *systematic review*. A **systematic review** addresses a specific clinical question by summarizing multiple research studies, along with other evidence. Systematic reviews differ from metasynthesis and meta-analysis because they by definition will address a clinical question and they do not generally apply statistical procedures to the information collected from individual studies or develop a systematic metasummary of the content of each study.

The sections of reports of metasynthesis, meta-analyses, and systematic reviews resemble those of single studies but may differ in some important ways. Table 2-2 summarizes what you might expect to find in the different sections of reports of a systematic review, metasynthesis, and meta-analysis. All three begin with a section that identifies the problem of interest. In metasynthesis or meta-analysis, the problem identified may be anything that has been addressed in several individual research studies. For example, a recent report of a meta-analysis addressed studies of fall prevention in the elderly (Hill-Westmoreland, Soeken, & Spellbring, 2002), and the metasynthesis of maternal HIV infection addressed the experience of managing both a chronic illness and motherhood (Sandelowski & Barroso, 2003). In contrast, a systematic review addresses a specific patient care or clinical practice question because the intent of the review is to provide evidence for practice.

A systematic review has defined procedures, but they are not always described in the report under a heading titled "Methods." The procedures in a systematic review involve searching and identifying all published reports or primary studies that examine or are related to a particular clinical care problem. The researcher has to define the problem and determine which studies are and are not related to that problem. The researcher also describes the procedures used to search the literature after describing the problem, or perhaps at the end of the report, under a heading such as "Search Strategies."

In contrast, metasynthesis or meta-analysis reports usually have clearly identified methods sections in which the search strategies used, the inclusion and exclusion criteria used for the sample of studies, and the analysis methods applied to the

TABLE 2-2

Components of Reports for Individual Research Studies, Metasynthesis, Meta-analysis, Systematic Reviews, and Quality Improvement Reports

Components of Reports	Traditional Research Study	Metasynthesis	Meta-analysis	Systematic Review	Quality Improvement Study
Problem or Introduction	Review of the literature; theory; statement of a knowledge gap; predictions or hypotheses	Identification of a problem that has been addressed in only a few studies with limited findings	Identification of a problem that has been addressed in several studies with inconsistent results	Statement of a practice problem, including a broad overview of the relevant clinical questions related to the problem	Statement of a standard for patient care that is measurable and specific, usually including a summary of the research basis and clinical basis for the standard
Methods	Description of quantitative or qualitative procedures; sampling methods; data analysis methods	Description of the procedures used to find and select the individual research studies; description of the procedures used to analyze the individual studies	Description of the procedures used to find and select the individual research studies; description of procedures used to code and analyze results from the individual studies; usually includes a table of studies	Description of search strategies and criteria used for including a study in the review	Description of the procedures used to identify selected patient care situations and methods used to collect information about the care in those situations
Results	Description of findings; summary of themes or concepts or results of statistical procedures	Summary of findings, concepts, or themes across the sample of studies	Summary of results of statistical tests on groups of results from individual studies	Summary of research findings categorized and synthesized under clinically meaningful topics; usually includes a table of studies	Summary of the patient care practices that were identified

(continued)

				Quality
Components of Reports	**Traditional Research Study**	**Metasynthesis**	**Meta-analysis**	**Systematic Review**	**Improvement Study**

TABLE 2 - 2

Components of Reports for Individual Research Studies, Metasynthesis, Meta-analysis, Systematic Reviews, and Quality Improvement Reports (*continued*)

Components of Reports	Traditional Research Study	Metasynthesis	Meta-analysis	Systematic Review	Quality Improvement Study
Discussion or Conclusions	Summary of key findings; comparison of results to previous studies; speculation about the meaning of results in relation to theory; description of limitations; recommendations for additional research and final conclusions	Summary of key findings and identification of how these might differ from what is generally accepted understanding; identification of needs for additional research and of limitations in existing studies	Summary of key findings and identification of how these might differ from what is generally accepted understanding; identification of needs for additional research and of limitations in existing studies	Specific identification of practice implications derived from the synthesis of the literature; identification of needs for additional research	Summary of key findings; comparison of findings to established standards; speculation about reasons for differences found; recommendations for changes to remedy any deficits found

sample of studies are all described. Remember that a metasynthesis or meta-analysis examines a sample of research studies rather than a sample of patients.

The results sections of metasynthesis or meta-analysis and systematic reviews differ because the meta-synthesis reports specific integrated concepts extracted from the individual reports, while meta-analysis specifically describes the numeric values from findings of the different studies and the statistical tests used to test those numbers. A systematic review usually summarizes the available studies that address a clinical care question but does not yield new findings in either numerical or written form. A meta-synthesis or meta-analysis may summarize the nature of the studies used, but the core of the findings will be new knowledge in either a numeric or conceptual form. Both systematic reviews and meta-analyses usually provide a table identifying the basic characteristics of the individual research studies that were included, which allows the reader to view the individual studies as needed.

Finally, metasynthesis, meta-analyses, and systematic reviews all have a conclusions section in which the potential meaning of the findings are described. As with single research reports, these types of reports may identify limits to what has been reported and usually recommend areas for future research. A systematic review always addresses implications for clinical practice.

Another important type of written report that describes research is a quality improvement report. A report of a **quality improvement study** resembles a report of a traditional research study, but there are some differences between the two. The problem addressed in a quality improvement study usually concerns whether certain expected clinical care was completed, so the question involves discovering what is being done or what has happened, rather than trying to understand a phenomenon. As with traditional research, a quality improvement study usually examines only a subset of all the occasions when a specified type of care was given. Methods to collect data for a quality improvement study include questionnaires, direct observation, and chart reviews. The report of a quality improvement study describes how information was collected concerning the clinical care and a summary of what was found. This is similar to the methods and results sections of a research report. The conclusions of this type of report include recommendations for improving the quality of care based on what was found regarding the care currently given. The recommendations are similar to the conclusions that are drawn from a research study. (See Table 2-2 for a summary of the sections of quality improvement reports compared with individual research reports, metasynthesis, meta-analyses, and systematic reviews.)

Critically Reading Research for Practice

In Chapter 1, you were introduced to five questions that will be used to organize this text. These questions also provide a broad framework for critically reading reports to evaluate their usefulness as evidence for your EBN practice. As a bachelor's-prepared nurse, you are not expected to critique research reports in depth for their scientific soundness; however, it is important that you are able to critically evaluate research reports to decide whether they can serve as evidence related to your clinical practice question. Therefore, at the end of most of the chapters, we will include a section about common errors in research reports and list a set of questions to ask yourself that will allow you to critically evaluate research reports. Figure 2-5 presents six boxes containing the critical reading questions for the five broad questions that organize this text. Each of these sets of questions will be discussed in detail in the later chapters and are included here primarily to introduce you to them. We will revisit all six sets of questions in Chapter 12 as we discuss research utilization.

PUBLISHED REPORT—WHAT DID YOU CONCLUDE?

We have discussed briefly all of the sections in the published research studies about incarcerated women and maternal HIV. The authors of those studies report directly that mothers with HIV face paradoxes that affect both their experience of their disease and their motherhood, and that incarcerated women need a brief objective screening test for their mental health. If you were the RN in the clinical case, would you now know how to develop a plan of care for A.K.? Why or why not?

One reason it may be difficult to decide how to develop a care plan for A.K. based on the research report is because the nurse may still have questions about the research. What kinds of questions do you think the RN may have about how to proceed in her care of A.K.? One question might be whether she can believe the results of the study about incarcerated women or whether the results are "strong" enough that she is

How to Critically Read the Conclusions Section of a Research Report

Does the report answer the question
"What is the answer to my practice question—what did the study conclude?"

Did the report include a conclusions section?
Did the conclusions section assist me with my clinical problem?
Did the conclusions assist in a general manner or provide specific information about my
  clinical problem?
Did the conclusions section include limitations of the study?
Did the limitations diminish my ability to use the conclusions in practice?
Do the conclusions seem reasonable or warranted based on the results of the study?

How to Critically Read the Results Section of a Research Report

Does the report answer the question
"Why did the authors reach these conclusions—what did they actually find?"

Did the report include a clearly identified results section?
Were the results presented appropriately for the information collected?
Were descriptive versus inferential results identifiable if this is a quantitative study?
Were themes or structure and meaning identifiable if this is a qualitative study?
Were the results presented in a clear and logical manner?
Did the results include information about the final sample for the study?

How to Critically Read the Sample Section of a Research Report

Does the report answer the question
"To what types of patients do these research conclusions apply—who was in the study?"

Did the report include a clearly identified section or paragraphs about sampling?
Did the report give me enough information to understand how and why this sample was chosen?
Is there enough information about the sample to tell me if the research is relevant for my clinical
  population?
Was enough information given for me to understand how rights of human subjects were protected?
Would my patient population have been placed at risk if they had participated in this study?
Can I identify how information was collected about the sample?   *(continued)*

F I G U R E   2 - 5 • Questions for critically reading research reports.

willing to develop her plan of care around that evidence. A second question might
be why the maternal HIV study did not address the experience of testing positive
for HIV when one is pregnant. A third question might pertain to what incarcerated
pregnant women perceive as important to promote the health of themselves and
their baby. You can probably think of other questions. With a further understanding
of the research language and the research process, it is possible to answer most of
the questions posed by reading the published report in more detail. In the next chapter, we look more closely at the conclusions of research reports and what they can
tell us about patient care questions.

How to Critically Read the Methods Section of a Research Report

Does the report answer the question
"How were those people studied—why was the study performed that way?"

Did the report include a clearly identified section describing methods used in this study?
Do the methods make this a quantitative or a qualitative study?
Do I understand what my patient population would be doing if they were in this study or a study using similar methods?
Do the measures and procedures in this study address my clinical problem?
Do I think that the measures used in this study would provide helpful and useful information when used with my patient population?
Do I think what the researcher collected and the method of collection was the best way to address the clinical question?
Do I think that the researcher(s) should have planned the study differently in order to answer my clinical question?

How to Critically Read the Description of Study Design in a Research Report

Does the report answer the question
"How were those people studied—why was the study performed that way?"

Did the report include a clearly identified section describing the research design?
Does the design make this a quantitative, qualitative, or mixed method study?
Does the report address approaches taken to assure study rigor, internal validity, and/or external validity?
Do I think that the researcher(s) should have designed the study differently in order to answer my clinical question?

How to Critically Read the Background Section of a Research Report

Does the report answer the question
"Why ask that question—what do we know?"

Did the report include a clearly identified background and/or literature review section?
Do I think the background discusses aspects of my clinical question?
Does the literature help me understand why the research question is important to nursing?
Is the majority of the literature cited current (less than 5 years old) or very important to understanding the research question?
If a nursing or other theory was presented, does it connect to my clinical question?
Is the specific research question/problem/hypothesis connected logically to the literature and/or theory presented in the background section?
Is the specific research question/problem/hypothesis relevant or related to my clinical question?

FIGURE 2-5 • *(continued)*

SUMMARY

In this chapter, we have examined all the components of a research report and at least have begun to become familiar with the unique language of research. Specifically, we have learned that conclusions are the last section of most research reports and that they identify what was found and complete a report by identifying an outcome. We now understand that the results section of a report contains a summary or condensed version of what the authors believe are the most important findings and that results may be presented as numbers or as words, depending on the data collected for the study. We understand that the methods section of a research report describes the overall process of how the researchers went about implementing the research study, including who was included in the study, how information was collected, and what interventions, if any, were tested. We learned that there are two broad approaches to research: (1) qualitative methods, which focus on understanding the complexity of humans within the context of their lives and attempt to build a whole or complete picture of a phenomenon of interest; and (2) quantitative methods, which focus on understanding and breaking down the different parts of a phenomenon into its parts to see how they do or do not connect as well as involve collecting information that is specific and limited to the particular parts of events or phenomena being studied. Last, we discussed the problem section of a research report, which describes the gap in knowledge addressed by the research study. In this section, the researcher explains why the study was needed, why it was carried out in the manner that it was, and often, what the researcher is specifically asking or predicting.

Besides examining all the components of a research report, we looked at how those sections relate to the actual steps of the research process, and we considered some special types of research reports such as a metasynthesis, meta-analysis, and systematic review. We are now ready to begin looking at each section of a research report in detail in order to assure that you can read and use research as evidence for your professional practice.

OUT-OF-CLASS EXERCISE

Differing Conclusions From the Class Study

The fictional article in Appendix B represents the kind of report that might be written based on a questionnaire that you may have completed in class. In that article, the author suggests that older students may be interested in nonacute settings because they have had more experiences with health care in several settings. In preparation for the next chapter, write a concluding paragraph that could be used to end the fictional article by taking the position that nursing programs must focus on recruiting older students so that more nurses can be obtained for general care and nursing home settings. Then, write a different paragraph taking the opposite position that age should not be considered when recruiting nursing students because it is not clear whether it contributes to choice of nursing practice after graduation. Base your arguments on the findings reported in the fictional article—not solely on your opinions or ideas. Once you complete this exercise, you are ready to read Chapter 3.

References

Hill-Westmoreland, E. E., Soeken, K., & Spellbring, A. M. (2002). A meta-analysis of fall prevention programs for the elderly: How effective are they? *Nursing Research, 51*(1), 1–8.

Kane, M., & DiBartolo, M. (2002). Complex physical and mental health needs of rural incarcerated women. *Issues in Mental Health Nursing, 23,* 209–229.

Lazarus, R. S. (1993). Coping, theory and research: Past, present and future. *Psychosomatic Medicine, 55,* 234–247.

Neuman, B. (1982). *The Neuman system model: Application to nursing education and practice.* East Norwalk, CT: Appleton-Century-Crofts.

Roy, C. (1984). *Introduction to nursing: An adaptation model* (2nd ed.). Englewood Cliffs, NJ: Prentice-Hall.

Sandelowski, M., & Barroso, J. (2003). Motherhood in the context of maternal HIV infection. *Research in Nursing & Health, 26,* 470–482.

Watson, J. (1985). *Human science and human caring: A theory of nursing.* Norwalk, CT: Appleton-Century-Crofts.

Resource

Locke, L. F., Silverman, S. J., & Spirduso, W. W. (1998). *Reading and understanding research.* Thousand Oaks, CA: Sage Publications.

CHAPTER

3

DISCUSSIONS AND CONCLUSIONS
What Is the Answer to My Question—What Did the Study Conclude?

LEARNING OBJECTIVE:

The student will interpret the conclusions of research reports for their potential meaning for evidence-based nursing (EBN) practice.

The End of a Research Report—Discussions and Conclusions

Discussions
    Summary
    Comparison
    Speculation
    Implications for Practice

Conclusions
    Can Conclusions Differ?
    Do We Change Practice?

Common Errors in Research Reports

Critically Reading Discussion and Conclusion Sections of Reports

Published Reports—What Would You Conclude?

KEY TERMS

Conceptualization
Confirmation
Discussion
Generalization
Replication
Speculation
Study design

CLINICAL CASE

C.R. is a 63-year-old elementary school teacher who has had an abdominal aortic aneurysm (AAA) repaired at her community hospital and will be discharged in the next day or so. The standard nursing care plan just prior to discharge for patients from this hospital who have had AAA surgery includes ambulation three times a day with the expected outcome that the patient can walk the length of the corridor three times without assistance. The RN working with C.R. is experienced with post-AAA care and has seen similar patients meet the predischarge ambulation outcome without a problem. C.R. has been encouraged to ambulate; however, she is only walking short distances in her room. The RN reviews conversations with C.R., as well as her chart. She cannot identify any reason why C.R. would not be ambulating more and wonders what else she could assess in order to get C.R. ready for discharge. The RN does a quick search in PubMed using the keywords "AAA" and "ambulation" and does not get any hits. She then tries the keywords "abdominal surgery" and "recovery," which yields numerous hits regarding factors affecting postoperative recovery. One appears particularly relevant, since the patient population in the study is elderly patients who have had major abdominal surgery. The article is titled "Correlates of recovery among older adults after major abdominal surgery" (Zalon, 2004). You can find this article in Appendix A-3. Reading the conclusion or discussion sections of this article will help you to understand the examples discussed in this chapter. In addition, Table 3-1 summarizes the clinical question and the key search words used by the RN in the clinical case. We will include similar tables after clinical cases in later chapters to help you see how a good question for EBN is formed and how you could search for available evidence.

THE END OF A RESEARCH REPORT—DISCUSSIONS AND CONCLUSIONS

In this chapter, we address the first of the five questions that are used to organize this book: What is the answer to my practice question—what did the study conclude? As mentioned in Chapter 1, the major reason a practicing nurse wants to read and understand research is to answer clinical questions, so nurses, such as the one in the clinical case, often go directly to the last section of a research report. That section is sometimes labeled "Discussion," "Conclusions," or both, but its content usually includes both a discussion and conclusions as described here.

TABLE 3-1

Development of a Clinical Question From the Clinical Case

What factors affecting the recovery rate of elderly patients following major abdominal surgery should be considered by the nurse when planning predischarge care?

The *Who*	Elderly patients
The *What*	Rates of recovery from abdominal surgery
The *When*	Postoperative
The *Where*	Inpatient setting
Key search terms useful in finding research-based evidence for this practice question	Abdominal surgery
	Recovery
	Elderly
	Outcomes

When the RN who is interested in the factors that affect the recovery rate of elderly patients following major abdominal surgery reads the discussion section of the report on correlates of recovery from abdominal surgery, she learns that three factors were found to relate to patients' recovery and functional status after surgery, including pain, depression, and fatigue (Zalon, 2004). She also reads that these three factors are related not just to functional status, but also to self-perception of recovery in older patients. Further, the "Discussion and Conclusion" section of the report about recovery after surgery indicates that patients with chronic painful conditions are likely to have subthreshold or major depression. She also learns that since most patients like her elderly patient do not receive home care services, the management of chronic pain needs to be initiated in the acute care setting. Additionally, the RN reads that interventions to address fatigue and depression are important following abdominal surgery. The RN's likely response to reading the discussion and conclusion sections of this report is, "While I now know that these three factors matter, I don't have time before she is discharged to plan and intervene for all three, so which factor matters most?"

The discussion and conclusion sections of research reports initially may not be helpful in clinical questions for several reasons, including:

- The study may not address the question you are asking.
- The researchers may have had problems implementing the study, resulting in an unclear answer.
- The results of the study may have been unexpected or complex and increase, rather than decrease, possible answers to the question.

Later chapters address why research questions may not directly address clinical questions and the many problems that can occur when carrying out a research study. Although this chapter discusses briefly how unexpected results can affect clinical usefulness, understanding results and the results sections of research reports are discussed more completely in Chapter 4. This chapter focuses on a fourth reason why the conclusion of a report may not answer a clinical question: The nurse having inappropriate or unclear expectations about what information can be found in the conclusion of a research report. Just what should we expect to find from the discussion and conclusion sections of research reports?

DISCUSSIONS

This book treats discussions and conclusions as two separate sections, but remember that you often find them combined in published reports. Table 3-2 summarizes the major components of most discussion and conclusion sections. The **discussion** section of a research report summarizes, compares, and speculates about the results of the study. Let us examine these pieces, starting with summarizing.

Summary

The first part of the discussion section in a research report usually includes a summary of the study's key results. This summary usually addresses the results that

TABLE 3-2	

General Components of the Discussion and Conclusion Sections of Research Reports

Section of Report	Major Components of the Section
Discussion	• Summary of key findings • Comparison of results with those of previous studies • Description of whether findings confirm results of similar studies or predictions based on theory • Speculation regarding possible interpretations of results
Conclusion	• Description of the new knowledge that can be accepted based on the study • A conceptualization of the meaning of the results or a generalization of the findings • A description of study limitations

directly relate to the major research question posed by the researcher(s). It also includes the unexpected results and those that stood out as being particularly meaningful. However, this summary usually is brief because it follows a detailed description of the results. It is also likely, unless the study had few findings, that it will not include all of the results from the study. What the brief summary does include are the specific results from the study that the researcher believes are particularly important and meaningful.

For example, the discussion section in the recovery after surgery study (Zalon, 2004) tells us that three factors—pain, depression, and fatigue—"are significantly related to functional status as well as self-perception of recovery in older postoperative abdominal surgery patients" (p. 104). It also states that these three factors taken together are "related to a return to wholeness or functional status" (p. 104). The author specifically identifies the three factors, but does not explain the meaning of the factors in this section of the report.

Comparison

After a brief summary of key or important results, the discussion section of a research report debates the possible meanings of the study results. Questions addressed in research studies are rarely simple or readily answered completely by only one study; therefore, the results provide information that can be explained or understood in several different ways. Hence, the pros and cons of different explanations for the results may be described, forming a written debate. Further, the meaning of the findings usually must be interpreted within the context of existing knowledge, so the discussion section frequently compares the study's results with those of previous studies. The match or lack of match of results of a study to results from previous studies supports the different explanations offered regarding the results. Another important reason for comparing is to provide confirmation of previous findings. **Confirmation** is the verification of results from other studies. Rarely are we comfortable deciding that we are completely certain of the answer to a clinical question based on the findings of only one study. One goal of research is to build knowledge, with each research study adding a new piece to our understanding. However, as with the parts of any building that is going to be stable and strong, the pieces of knowledge must overlap and unite to make a cohesive whole. A study that is a duplication of an earlier study is called a **replication** study, and its major purpose is confirmation. Usually, however, a research study differs from past studies in some ways by, for example, using a different patient group in the study or by using different procedures on the subjects. Whether a study is a replication or a variation on previous studies, the discussion section of the research report describes how the findings do or do not overlap with previous knowledge.

CORE CONCEPT 3-1

The summary of findings in the discussion section of a research report only contains selected results from the study. It does not give the reader a complete picture of the results but does give information about some key or important results.

In addition to discussing how a study's results do or do not confirm those of previous studies, the authors may compare their findings with the predicted results that were based on existing theory. Theory might be considered to be the plans for the knowledge being built about a clinical question: Like the blueprints of a building plan, a theory provides the description of how all the parts of a phenomenon should fit together. Not all research studies are based on a theory or test a prediction from a theory because not enough may be known about a clinical question. However, if the study tests a prediction or hypothesis that was based on a theory and the results show the pieces fitting together as the theory predicted, then the results are considered to confirm that theory. We discuss how theory directs and is built by research in Chapter 10.

Our recovery from surgery article that the RN found did not attempt to specifically test theory, but the discussion section compares the results of the study with the Conservation of Energy Model (Levine, 1991). In addition, the discussion in the article states that "pain and depression contribute to functional loss in older persons" (p. 105) and cites previous studies demonstrating that nursing interventions focusing on these factors improve physical functioning. While in this example the findings of the recovery from surgery article are similar to past studies, it is not uncommon for results from a study to differ from previous studies. This is why we usually need multiple studies to inform our EBN and to make clinical decisions. Results that differ from findings in previous studies require that the author(s) suggest reasons for those differences, which leads us to the third component of most discussion sections.

Speculation

In addition to comparison, the discussion section of a research report speculates regarding the reasons for the results of the study. **Speculation** is the process of reflecting on results and offering some explanation of them. The debate, or speculation, in a discussion generally considers several alternative explanations for the results and provides a rationale for the author's judgments about which is the best explanation.

CORE CONCEPT 3-2

The discussion section of a research report contains a debate about how the results of the study fit with existing knowledge and what those results may mean.

As a Core Concept from Chapter 2 stated, the results section provides the findings of the specific study, whereas the discussion and conclusion sections of a report interpret those findings in light of existing knowledge and theory. This interpretation is appropriately called a *discussion* because it is open to debate. It reflects not fact, but thoughtful informed speculation. Although such speculation is thoughtful and informed and considers alternative possibilities, it is based on the author's knowledge and selection of previous research or theory. Another author might know or select a different theory or body of research to use in his or her discussion.

Why are the meanings of results from almost any study open to debate? The answer lies, in part, in the nature of research. We learned in Chapter 2 that research usually examines a question using a subgroup or sample of people. Although great pains often are taken to include diversity in the people, samples cannot possibly reflect all of the variation that exists in humans. What works with or happens to a few subjects is unlikely to always be exactly what happens with many patients or with everyone.

In fact, qualitative methods assume that experiences are subjectively unique and that although we can increase our understanding regarding a particular question, there may always be individual variations. Returning to our analogy of building knowledge piece by piece, the qualitative research perspective is that the picture of the phenomenon, which is the product in knowledge building, is constantly evolving because our world and our individual experiences are always changing.

Qualitative

Conceptualization is a process of creating a picture of an abstract idea; in the case of nursing research, it is a picture of some aspect of health. Discussions and conclusions of qualitative studies conceptualize some phenomenon related to health as opposed to those of quantitative studies that objectify and isolate parts of the phenomenon. For example, a qualitative study might conceptualize patient satisfaction as a person's overall sense of the quality of the care that is received. A quantitative study may examine patient satisfaction as the total score on a survey of the patient's care experience. If theory is the blueprint or plan for a building, we can view a qualitative study as providing results that are an artist's rendition of how the building

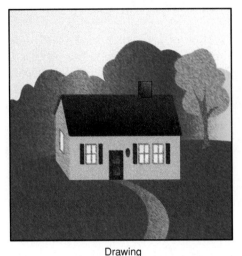
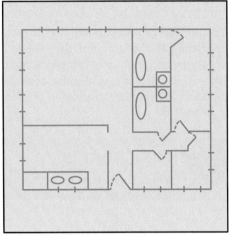

Drawing

Product of qualitative research is like
an artist's rendition.

Blueprint

Product of quantitative research is like a
blueprint, showing details and
how parts go together.

FIGURE 3-1 • Products of qualitative vs. quantitative research.

looks. Similarly, we can view quantitative results as a detailed parts list for constructing the building. The artist's rendition provides a clear sense of how a building might look or even feel and smell, whereas the parts list gives us a sense of how it looks when it is put together and how it might be used, but not of how we will actually experience the building. Figure 3-1 illustrates this concept.

From a qualitative perspective, knowledge is built by creating a "picture album" filled with different "pictures" of a particular aspect of health. Each study result, or picture, gives a sense of the aspect of health at a unique moment in time. As we look at more and more pictures, we get a greater sense of the whole phenomenon. Each qualitative study provides a unique picture that adds to our overall understanding.

Quantitative

Quantitative methods do not assume that knowledge is always changing and evolving; they assume that there are answers to questions and that we can find those answers by reducing, objectifying, and quantifying the components of a phenomenon to understand the relationships among the components. Quantitative methods assume that we get a greater sense of the whole phenomenon by breaking it down to smaller parts, and we get closer and closer to "knowing" the "real" answer to questions when we get the same results in different studies with different groups. The quantitative researcher expects that each study will add more details to the same detailed building plan.

The goal of research is to generalize a study's results. **Generalization** is the ability to apply a particular study's findings to the broader population represented by the sample. The authors of the recovery from surgery study, for example, conclude that standard care approaches to control pain and depression in elderly postoperative patients can be effective with elderly postoperative patients in general. Both qualitative and quantitative research strives to develop knowledge that can be applied to a broader population. However, the term *generalization* is more commonly applied to quantitative research than qualitative research. Nonetheless, a qualitative researcher will often do several procedures to make sure that the findings can also be applied to the population in the area of interest. The value of being able to generalize study findings is an important concept. If the study is conducted well, whether it is a qualitative or quantitative study, then a nurse who reads the study can make better clinical decisions regarding the value of applying the research findings to work with similar populations.

Implications for Practice

The discussion in a nursing research report often includes a debate about the meaning of the study results for nursing practice. For example, the surgery recovery article found that pain, depression, and fatigue were important findings in recovery after surgery. The study then suggests that health care providers need to consider the patient's perspective and the patient's level of involvement in postoperative care. But other clinical interpretations could be made. Because the focus is on elderly patients, health care providers need to consider the patient's family perspective of the elderly patient's capacity to be self-reliant. The author of our article did not choose to discuss any interpretation related to family or spouse care in the discussion of the study results, possibly because it does not fit with the author's philosophy of nursing and health care. However, it is important to realize that choices are made concerning the best clinical interpretation of results, just as choices are made about how the results add to existing knowledge in general. This means that the discussion section needs to be read critically and with an awareness of the different meanings that could be assigned to the study findings.

The RN who reads the discussions in the article about recovery from surgery is reading the author's interpretations of what is believed to be the key findings. The author clearly states that an important finding was that correcting patient misperceptions about the use of pain medication, along with patient teaching about pain medication, would assist patients to recover better. The author interpreted the findings about the use of pain medication to mean that patients had knowledge deficits regarding the use of pain medication. This is a speculation by the author about the meaning of the results and is most likely based on beliefs and past experiences as well as the results of previous research. The author did not specifically test or measure the research participant's knowledge of pain medication. Her interpretation of the clinical implication of her findings is that patients do not understand the correct use of their medications. This is a speculation of meaning based on the finding that "Only 53.2% of participant's took pain medication in the 24 hours before the 3-5 day discharge interview" (Zalon, 2004, p. 105). However, the RN in the clinical case now has one possible answer to her question about what factors to consider in assisting her patient to improve recovery postoperatively. The RN must read previous sections of the report to decide if the author's practice implications drawn from the results match the nurse's beliefs and experiences. We return to the RN's dilemma later in this chapter.

CONCLUSIONS

The conclusions of a research report describe the knowledge that the researcher believes can be gained from the study, given its "fit" with other studies and theories. As stated in Chapter 2 in the discussion of sections of a research report, conclusions from a research study can be powerful because they are used to guide practice. Conclusions move beyond debate or speculation about the results to a statement of what is now "known" about a question or problem. As a result, they generally are worded carefully. Conclusions also may be statements about what we do not know, particularly if the study results do not fit with theory or replicate previous studies. Therefore, it is possible for a conclusion to state that we now know we cannot get the answer for our question using the methods or measures or sample that was used in the study being reported. More often, conclusions include recommendations for building knowledge about a clinical question or health aspect. In either case, the conclusion section almost always describes the limits that must be placed on the knowledge that has been gained from the study.

The recovery from surgery article does not provide concrete answers to the questions it addressed. One reason for this is because when questions are complex, the research results are open to debate and interpretation. Another reason is because almost every study has limitations. Remember from Chapter 2 that limitations are the aspects of a study that create uncertainty about the meaning or decisions that can be derived from it. We suggested that limitations can be viewed as a fence around the results of a research study that confine or limit what we can conclude.

Several aspects of a study may be viewed as limitations, and Figure 3-2 illustrates some of these. We have already alluded to one factor that often limits a study: the sampling—who was included in the study. Although the recovery from surgery

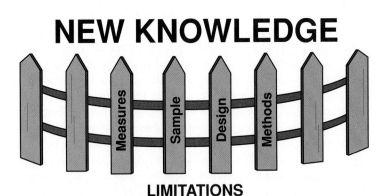

FIGURE 3-2 • Some limitations of the research process, represented by the fence posts.

study included elderly men and women, patients who were viewed as "too sick" or who were not discharged directly to home settings were not included. Additionally, 99.5% of the people in the study were identified as "non-Hispanic white." This aspect of the sample leaves us with uncertainty about the meaning of the results for elderly postoperative patients who live in nursing home settings, who have complex health needs, or who are black, Latino, or Native American. The study aims to produce findings that can be used in various settings, so the limit on the sample indicates that the picture provided by the study results is a picture of only white, non-complex, elderly, postoperative patients who reside in independent living situations. As we will see in Chapters 6 and 7, many other sampling-related aspects can create limits to a research study.

A second factor that may be a limitation is the **study design**—the overall plan or organization of a study. Some study designs create more uncertainty than do others. For example, if the RN in the clinical case read a study that described the cognitive, behavioral, and psychological factors that affect an elderly patient's self-perception of health, she would be uncertain about whether those factors were present before the operative intervention and thus whether they impacted the patient's postoperative recovery. A study that uses a pretest and post-test design, in which measures of self-perceptions of functioning are taken before and after surgery, would remove some of the uncertainty about the clinical use of results because we would know the outcome change that occurred between the beginning and end of the study. Many factors affect a researcher's decision about a study design, including the type of question being asked, the level of existing knowledge, and the availability of resources. Chapter 9 discusses research designs in more detail.

A third factor that may be a limitation involves the measures used in the study. Several problems can occur with study measures. For example, a study's measures may be inconsistent. If blood sugar is measured by using a glucometer that loses calibration halfway through the study, the resulting measures will be inconsistent. Sometimes paper-and-pencil questionnaires are unclear or confusing, causing people to be inconsistent in their understanding of, and therefore answers to, the questions. Another possible problem is that measures may be inaccurate or incomplete. Returning to the study using a glucometer for measuring blood sugars, if the glucometer had gone out of calibration before the study began, the resulting measures would be consistent but inaccurate throughout the study. That is, the measures would consistently be inaccurate. Accuracy and consistency of measures are referred to as *validity, rigor,* and *reliability* in research. The examples given in this paragraph are all reflective of quantitative research, although accuracy and consistency are also a problem in qualitative research. These ideas are the focus of Chapter 8 and will be explored in detail in that chapter.

Finding accurate measures of concepts in quantitative research is a problem in nursing because it is difficult to find ways to quantify some concepts that are important to nurses, such as anger, quality of life, pain, or self-confidence. If measures do not exist, the researcher will either have to make one or not include that factor in the study. Excluding an important factor limits the conclusions that can be drawn. For example, in the conclusion of the recovery from surgery study, one limitation identified was that the author did not measure pain, depression, or fatigue levels in the participants preoperatively. Therefore, the researcher assumed that some of the findings related to surgery, but without baseline measures preoperatively, this is just an assumption. The author did not mention if she did not measure these factors preoperatively because the factors could not be used repeatedly, or she did not anticipate the need for that measurement. The lack of the measurement presents the possibility that pain or fatigue levels as measured postoperatively may actually be better than they were preoperatively and therefore are really not factors impacting elderly patient recovery from surgery.

The methods used in a study are a fourth factor that may limit the conclusions. Not only does a measurement need to be consistent and accurate, it also must be used consistently and accurately. An appropriately calibrated glucometer will still provide results that are inconclusive regarding a person's blood sugar if it is used at different times during the day and with different techniques to acquire blood samples. Similarly, a measure of a person's knowledge about HIV will not be conclusive if one group completed the measure immediately after a patient education program and the other group completed it two weeks after their education program. Therefore, the methods used to conduct a study also may lead to limitations in the conclusions.

The discussion and conclusions section of a research report, then, includes a summary of key results, a comparison of those results with findings from other studies or to existing theory, speculation and debate about the possible explanations for the results and how they fit with current knowledge, and finally, some carefully worded decisions about new knowledge gained in the study. This section includes debate, speculation, and cautious language because research questions are complex, each study contributes only one new piece to the puzzle or one more picture to the phenomenon, and almost every study has some limitations.

Can Conclusions Differ?

At the end of Chapter 2, you were asked to write two concluding paragraphs for the fictional article in Appendix B, taking two different positions regarding who should be recruited for nursing programs based on results reported in the article. Reviewing the results reported in that study, we find that age, type of program, and rating of health affected choice of nursing field. We assume that the goal is to focus recruitment of students on increasing the number of graduates who enter fields that are not considered acute, a goal with which you may not personally agree. One way to interpret the results is to focus on the finding that age was an important factor in choice of field and conclude that older students should be recruited. Therefore, the new knowledge gleaned from the study would be that recruiting older students will increase the numbers of new graduates entering nonacute nursing fields.

However, the finding that health rating was important could mean that the relevant factor is not age and experience, as the author suggests. Rather, the relevant factor may instead be level of health, with students who perceive themselves as less healthy selecting fields of practice that are generally considered less physically strenuous. If this is true, then age is not the relevant factor. Rather, schools of nursing must recruit students who want less physically strenuous positions. This second conclusion would probably be considered relatively implausible, but it illustrates that conclusions can differ based on the interpretation of the results. Because the conclusions drawn from study results can differ as you read discussions and conclusions of research reports, you should carefully consider whether the interpretation provided makes sense to you in terms of your own knowledge and practice.

Do We Change Practice?

We have emphasized that the conclusions of research reports can be powerful because they are used to change practice. We also have pointed out some of the uncertainty that is reflected in most conclusions. Most importantly, we have said that the purpose for nurses to intelligently understand research is for them to use it in practice. Recognizing the limitations of each research study and the complexity of building new knowledge does not imply that research cannot and should not be used in practice. However, it does mean that it is essential to have some understanding of more than just the study conclusions. We must understand why and how much the limitations such as sampling, measures, methods, or design make the results uncertain, and we must look intelligently at the study findings to determine if the author's interpretation is logical.

Each research study reflects only one piece or picture in the process of knowledge building, which is why nurses and other health professionals emphasize the use of systematic reviews. Systematic reviews include the results from many studies as evidence for practice. They compile the results of multiple studies regarding the same clinical question and organize the findings around key aspects related to practice. A systematic review also addresses differences in research studies, such as design, sample, and methods. The end of a systematic review is usually titled "Practice Implications" and summarizes the practice-related points that are most strongly supported by different research studies.

As with individual studies, however, systematic reviews are open to interpretation because the findings of particular studies can be given more or less attention. For example, the author of a systematic review may place less emphasis on negative findings about a procedure and interpret the positive findings to warrant a change in clinical practice. An author may also believe that any negative finding about a procedure questions its use and interpret any negative research to indicate that a procedure should not be adopted in practice. As in individual studies, the conclusions of systematic reviews include some hesitancy or caution and almost always include recommendations for further research. Systematic reviews as evidence for practice can be helpful, but the nurse still must read the review carefully and intelligently to decide how the findings should be used in practice.

COMMON ERRORS IN RESEARCH REPORTS

To be read and used intelligently in practice, the research report must clearly and completely give the reader the needed information. Many nurses assume that if they are not comfortable in their understanding of a research study, it is because they lack knowledge. While this may be the case, it is also possible that part of the problem is a lack of clarity in the research report. While we will summarize below the common ways in which a report can be unclear, we will also discuss common errors that may be found in research reports in later chapters. We do this to help you recognize that sometimes the problem lies not with your knowledge, but with the information provided to you.

As an example of errors in research reports, you may see a failure to include one or more major aspects of a discussion and conclusion. The authors should provide the information discussed in the discussion and conclusions section. As a research reader, you should expect to find a summary of key findings, a comparison of the findings with previous research, and an interpretation of the meaning of the findings within the context of current knowledge. Also, you should find some discussion of the study limitations. The fictional article in Appendix B provides an example of a report that does not include important aspects because it neither compares its results with previous studies nor includes any discussion of study limitations.

A second common error is presenting a confusing summary of key findings or presenting new results. The summary should use language that is consistent with both the common use of terms and how the terms were used throughout the report. It should not include key findings that were not already described in more detail in the results section. Because we are starting at the end of a report, we might not know that information in the discussion was not addressed in the results, but we can quickly find this out if we read the results section. The summary of key findings is a brief, succinct summation. If a result is only provided at the end of a report in this manner, we will likely not have enough information about it to judge intelligently the usefulness of that finding for practice.

A third common error in research reports is overinterpreting the results. Like nurses in practice, researchers want answers to the questions they study. Therefore, it is tempting to overinterpret results by reading into them, generalizing them beyond what was actually found, or discounting the limitations. It is expected that a researcher will understate or be conservative when interpreting study results. However, occasionally, a report presents an interpretation that makes suggestions that are more than what can reasonably be concluded based on the results of the study. For example, if the author of the recovery from surgery article had concluded that negative self-perceptions of recovery potential would predict who will not be able to return to independent living postoperatively, she would have drawn a conclusion that interpreted the results beyond what was indicated—she did not track what factors affected discharge placement, only what affected functional recovery from surgery.

Similarly, occasionally, a research report draws conclusions that are not directly related to the question under study. Suppose, for example, that the author of the surgery recovery article had stated in the conclusion section that discharging elderly patients to any setting other than independent home settings decreased functional recovery postoperatively. This conclusion would not be related to the question the research was studying. Zalon (2004) was attempting to determine whether pain, depression, and fatigue were significant factors in the return of older patients who had major abdominal surgery to functional status. While all of her participants were patients who were discharged to home settings, she was not directly studying discharge setting as part of her research question. It is important to read the conclusions of a study carefully and remember that conclusions are, in part, the speculation of the author. Part of being an RN who uses EBN effectively is to be a careful reader who thinks discriminately about the conclusions drawn from a study.

CRITICALLY READING DISCUSSION AND CONCLUSION SECTIONS OF REPORTS

In Chapter 1, you were introduced to five questions that will be used to organize this text. These questions also provide a broad framework for critically reading reports to evaluate their usefulness as evidence for your EBN practice. Remember, as a bachelor's-prepared nurse, you are not expected to critique research reports in depth for their scientific soundness. However, you are expected to be able to critically evaluate research reports to decide whether they can serve as evidence related to your clinical practice question. Therefore, Box 3-1 presents a set of six questions that you can use to help you in the process of critically reading the discussion and conclusion sections of a report.

The first question to ask yourself is "Did the report include a discussion and/or conclusion section?" While this may seem like a simple question, some reports of research do not present much of a conclusion section, or it is not easy to find and may be buried toward the end of the article. The recovery from surgery article includes a section labeled as "Discussion."

Box 3-1	How to Critically Read the Discussion and Conclusion Sections of a Report

Do the discussion and conclusion sections answer the question "Did the section provide an answer to my practice question—what did the study conclude?"

1. Did the report include a discussion and/or conclusion section?
2. Did the discussion/conclusion section assist me with my clinical problem?
3. Did the discussion/conclusion assist in a general manner or provide specific information about my clinical problem?
4. Did the discussion/conclusion section include limitations of the study?
5. Did the limitations diminish my ability to use the conclusions in practice?
6. Do the discussion/conclusions seem reasonable or warranted based on the results of the study?

A second question to consider when critically reading the discussion and con-clusion sections of a report is "Did the discussion/conclusion section assist me with my clinical problem?" To answer this, one needs to compare the *Who, Where, What,* and *When* contained in the discussion with that of your clinical question. The RN in our clinical case asks the question "What factors affect the recovery rate of elderly patients following major abdominal surgery that should be considered by the nurse when planning predischarge care?" If we look at the discussion section of the recov-ery from surgery article, we find that it discusses elderly patients' rates of postopera-tive recovery from abdominal surgery in the inpatient setting, making it a very good match to our RN's clinical question. The RN in our clinical case would learn about three factors that could be assessed in trying to determine how to best promote recovery in her elderly patient.

The third question to ask yourself as you critically read the discussion and con-clusion sections of reports is "Did the discussion/conclusion assist in a general man-ner or provide specific information about my clinical problem?" The answer is based on the RN's sense of how easily she can change her practice after reading the con-clusions of the recovery from surgery report. While the report assisted the RN in knowing that pain, fatigue, and depression are critical factors affecting recovery, the ways in which these were measured may not easily translate into routine clinical practice and may require more thought and evidence searching to identify potential interventions for these factors.

A fourth question "Did the discussion/conclusion section include limitations of the study?" is answered by examining the discussion section of the report. While not directly labeled, the last few paragraphs of the recovery from surgery report provide limitations of the study. The author discusses the "homogeneity of the patients" as a limitation as well as the fact that the participants were not randomly identified. The importance of this limitation will be discussed in more detail in Chapter 6, which addresses sampling. In addition, the author identifies that some patients were deemed "too sick" to participate, thus limiting participants to healthier elderly patients. Such patients may not be typical and may not closely resemble the patients our RN sees in the clinical case.

Another limitation is identified by the author, who discusses that she did not obtain baseline presurgical levels of pain, depression, and fatigue from the partici-pants. It is important to stop and think about statements such as made by the researcher, which leads us to the next question we need to ask ourselves when crit-ically reading the discussion and conclusion sections of a report: "Did the limitations diminish my ability to use the conclusions in practice?" What do you think it means that the author did not get measures of pain, depression, and fatigue before surgery? How could it influence the interpretation of the findings that are presented? Does it increase, decrease, or not affect the RN's willingness to use these results in resolv-ing her clinical question? This is the process of critically thinking about the evidence for EBN. As you answer these questions, it is important to remember that all stud-ies will have limitations. It is an unavoidable aspect of studying living patients. The question to answer is whether or not the limits are so limiting that the results cannot be generalized to your patients.

The final question to ask when critically reading the discussion and conclusion sections of a report is "Do discussion/conclusions seem reasonable or warranted based on the results of the study?" To answer this, you need to think about what the conclusions seem to say that a nurse should do, and then see if the results section of the report supports this. In the recovery from surgery article, the author tells us that the results section supported the conclusion that "interventions to address pain, depression, and fatigue are important regardless of the reason for hospitalization." To know if this is a logical and clear conclusion, we will need to read the results section carefully. How this should be done is presented in Chapters 4 and 5. We will revisit this question after we learn more about critically reading the results section of research reports.

PUBLISHED REPORTS—WHAT WOULD YOU CONCLUDE?

The discussion and conclusion sections of the report found by the RN in the clinical case tell us several different things. It tells us that pain, depression, and fatigue are important factors that affect recovery of functional status in elderly patients' postabdominal surgery. This confirms the RN's impression that there is something else she can assess and that there are other holistic needs of her patient that she may address to speed recovery. The conclusion also suggests that interventions to address pain, depression, and fatigue in elderly postabdominal surgery patients are important for all patients, regardless of the nature of the major surgery. The discussion did not tell the RN what specific assessments were done to assess pain, depression, or fatigue; she will have to read the results section to answer that question.

The conclusions from this report may contradict another report found by the RN. This is often one of the most confusing and frustrating aspects of EBN. However, it is most often possible to fit the conclusions of apparently contradictory studies together in a meaningful way. For example, the RN might decide from the recovery from surgery article that she must help her staff to recognize and look for depression and fatigue in all patients on the surgical unit. At the same time, another study may suggest that fatigue in postoperative patients is associated with protein deficits. The RN might plan to have her staff assess the protein intake of patients.

The discussion and conclusion section of a research report provides useful information for using research in practice, including a summary of key findings from the study, a comparison of the findings with previous research and theory, and an interpretation of the meaning of the findings. However, although the conclusions begin to answer the RN's clinical question, she will probably want to know more about the assessments that were used in determining fatigue and depression in the elderly. This means that she must read the preceding section of the research report—the results section.

OUT-OF-CLASS EXERCISE

<u>How Do We Organize a Large Amount of Information to Make Sense of It?</u>

Chapters 4 and 5 discuss the results section of research reports. As we mentioned in Chapter 2, these sections often include some of the most complex and confusing language for those readers who are not advanced researchers. We look at some of the key terms in results sections that can readily be understood without having an advanced degree in statistics and discuss how to determine what you need to really understand and intelligently use nursing research in practice.

To prepare for Chapter 4, summarize some of the data from your in-class study exercise in a way that makes it easier to understand or that makes sense of it. When doing this, think about why your method of organizations helps to make it easier to understand. If you did not have an in-class study, your faculty may provide you with some data to use for this out-of-class exercise. Once you have completed this exercise, you are ready to read Chapter 4.

References

Levine, M. E. (1991). The conservation principles: A model for health. In K. M. Schaefer & J. B. Pond (Eds.), *Levine's conservation model: A framework for practice* (pp. 1–11). Philadelphia: F. A. Davis.

Zalon, M. L. (2004). Correlates of recovery among older adults after major abdominal surgery. *Nursing Research*, 53(2), 99–106.

Resources

American Psychological Association. (2001). *Publication manual of the American Psychological Association* (5th ed., pp. 26–27). Washington, DC: Author.

Locke, L. F., Silverman, S. J., & Spirduso, W. W. (1998). *Reading and understanding research.* Thousand Oaks, CA: Sage Publications.

Polit, D. F., & Beck, C. T. (2003). *Nursing research: Principles and methods* (7th ed.). Philadelphia: Lippincott Williams & Wilkins.

DESCRIPTIVE
RESULTS

Why Did the Authors
Reach Their Conclusion—
What Did They Actually Find?

LEARNING OBJECTIVE:

The student will analyze the relationship between the descriptive results of research reports and the selected conclusion of the reports.

Differentiating Description From Inference

Understanding the Language of Results Sections
  Language Describing Results From Qualitative Studies
  Language Describing Results From Quantitative Studies

Connecting Results That Describe to Conclusions

Common Errors in the Reports of Descriptive Results

Critically Reading Results Sections of Research Reports

Published Report—What Would You Conclude?

KEY TERMS

Bivariate analysis	Distribution	Normal curve
Categorization scheme	Frequency distribution	Predictor variables
Coding	Independent variable	Skew
Content analysis	Inference	Standard deviation
Data reduction	Mean	Theme
Data saturation	Measure of central tendency	Univariate analysis
Demographics	Median	Variable
Dependent variable	Mode	Variance

Cඅౢ్Cൠ

CLINICAL **C**ASE

N.B. is a 64-year-old man whose wife experienced a major stroke 6 months ago. Though his wife completed rehabilitation and came home from the hospital 2 weeks ago, she still has difficulty communicating, has an indwelling catheter, and requires assistance to dress and eat. An RN has been assigned to provide home health care to N.B.'s wife, as she needs weekly injections and catheter care. N.B. is very caring with his wife and asks many questions, but after just two home visits, the RN can see that N.B. appears fatigued and has lost weight. The RN wonders what she can do to assist and support N.B. in managing his role as caregiver, recognizing that his health is intertwined with the health of her client. She takes a few minutes at work to search PubMed using the keywords "stroke," "caregiver," and "health" and finds a citation in a journal that appears to be relevant to N.B.'s situation. The article is entitled "Evolution of the caregiving experience in the initial 2 years following stroke" (White, Mayo, Hanley, & Wood-Dauphinee, 2003). This article is presented as Appendix A-4. We will be using the information in the results section of this report as examples throughout this chapter and in Chapter 5. Table 4-1 summarizes the RN's question for this clinical case.

DIFFERENTIATING DESCRIPTION FROM INFERENCE

At the end of Chapter 3, we decided that to base clinical decisions on the conclusions of a research report, we need to have a better understanding of the study results. The results are the specific findings of a study that can provide an answer to the second question we are using to organize this book: Why did the authors reach their conclusion—what did they actually find? This chapter and Chapter 5 address this question.

The results sections of reports summarize findings with two broad goals: (1) to describe or explain the phenomenon of interest and (2) to predict aspects related to that phenomenon. Because qualitative studies approach knowledge development with an expectation of increasing understanding to inform practice, their results use data analysis methods to provide description and explanation. In contrast, quantitative studies may predict, as well as describe and explain, because the assumption behind them is that there is generalized objectivity. Quantitative data analysis aims to not only describe and explain but also allows us to infer what would happen with

TABLE 4-1	
Statement of Clinical Question From the Clinical Case	
What interventions assist and support the caregiver's health and functioning?	
The *Who*	Caregiver
The *What*	Health and functioning
The *When*	While caring for stroke survivor
The *Where*	In home
Key search to find research-based evidence for practice	Stroke
	Caregiver
	Health

other similar groups based on what was found in the present study. **Inference** is the reasoning that goes into the process of drawing a conclusion based on evidence and is common in research work. It refers to the statistical procedures used in most quantitative studies, which therefore are called *inferential statistics.*

It is important to differentiate between results that merely describe what the researcher found and results that are intended to allow inference, because it directly affects what we can conclude from a study. The knowledge we gain from description can assist in the understanding of a situation or phenomenon, and that understanding can help us in our clinical practice. For example, the results in the article about maternal HIV used in Chapters 1 and 2 identify 11 aspects of "mothering work," including surveillance, safety, information, accounting, hope, worry, reconciliation, legacy, redefinition, body, and grief (Sandelowski & Barroso, 2003). The RN working in the prison could use this description of aspects of mothers' work to help her understand and support her HIV-positive pregnant client. What she cannot do, however, is predict that her client will make a successful adaptation to motherhood if she supports and facilitates her in accomplishing these areas of work. The RN cannot make that prediction based on the evidence in the qualitative study because it was a study with descriptive results, not inferential results. Description does not allow us to predict the future or to understand what causes the phenomena that we have described.

To understand cause and effect and to make predictions, we must know not only what is present at a given point in time, but also the order of factors or events and the timing of such events or factors. Why can't description allow us to predict? When we describe the presence of two or more factors, we know that they are present concurrently, but we do not know if one came before the other, if one caused the other, or if some other outside event caused both. Take the simple example of driving a car. If one were to describe the factors involved in driving, one would think of a car, a key, a driver, and a license. However, which factor must come first is not necessarily obvious from that description. Do we need a driver first to get a license? Or do we need a car before we can have a driver? Description does not give us order and timing, so it does not allow us to predict.

CORE CONCEPT 4-1

Results that allow us to predict include information about the order and timing of events or factors.

Only results that allow us to infer provide information that is useful to predict future responses or situations if the same set of circumstances applies. Results that allow us to predict include information about the order of events or factors and the timing of those events or factors. Therefore, results that are intended to allow inference may be used in clinical practice to predict future health-related outcomes under similar circumstances. The article about caregiver experiences found by the RN in the clinical case for this chapter uses inferential statistics in the results section. These results show that almost half of the mental component of the caregivers' health-related quality of life (HRQL) can be explained by the symptoms of the person they cared for as well as by the caregivers' perceptions of burden. These results could be used by the RN in her clinical setting to predict that because N.B.'s wife has a number of symptoms remaining from her stroke, he is likely to experience a lowered mental HRQL.

Not all inferential statistics lead to an understanding of causation, but all are used to infer that what was found in the specific results is also likely to be found in similar cases. Understanding some of the language that is used in the description of results and in inferential statistics is the first step in understanding what results mean for EBN practice. The RN in the clinical case found an article that uses quantitative methods, which we will use in this chapter to gain a better understanding of the language in the results sections of research reports that reflects descriptive data analysis. We will look at the language of inferential statistics in Chapter 5 and will continue to use the fictional article (Appendix B) as an example in both chapters.

CORE CONCEPT 4-2

Research results that only describe or explain cannot be used to predict future outcomes or to directly identify the cause of the findings.

UNDERSTANDING THE LANGUAGE OF RESULTS SECTIONS

To discuss the language in the results section of research reports, we must take a closer look at data and data analysis. As mentioned in Chapter 2, data are the information collected in a study. This information may take several forms—it may be numbers, words, or drawings, and it may be written, spoken, or observed. Once the information is collected, it has to be sorted and organized to be meaningful in answering the questions addressed in the research.

Most research reports' results sections begin by providing a summary of information about individual study variables. A variable is something that varies: It is not the same for everyone in every situation. Therefore, a **variable** is an aspect of the phenomenon of interest or research problem that differs among people or situations. Research aims to understand, explain, or predict those differences or variations. A variable may be some attribute of a person, such as age, health, or beliefs. It may be a test score, such as a score for anxiety level, or a physiological parameter, such as body temperature. It may be an environmental aspect, such as community resources, family support, or employment rates. In all of these examples of variables, we know that there will be differences among people or situations.

Research attempts to gain new knowledge about variables that have been identified as important. In the research articles for Chapters 1 and 2, the major variables studied included maternal experiences in the maternal HIV study, and physical health, mental health, reproductive issues, alcohol and drug use, physical and sexual victimization, family issues, psychological symptoms, and social support in the incarcerated women study (Sandelowski & Barroso, 2003; Kane & DiBartolo, 2002). Think about these for a moment. We can say that these are variables because we expect different people to have different levels of mental health or drug use.

The goal of the maternal HIV study was to understand and describe how the experiences of being HIV positive and being a mother interact and affect each other. In contrast, the purpose of the incarcerated women study was to identify the physical and mental health needs of incarcerated women in order to provide better care to them. The researchers hoped to find key factors or connections that could guide them in the provision of care. The variables for the study found by the RN in the clinical case for this chapter are identified in Table 4-2.

In Chapter 2, we said that multivariate analysis indicates there are more than two variables being discussed, and, in fact, most studies will probably include more than one variable. However, analysis of data at a given point that focuses on only one variable is called **univariate analysis**. When you worked with the data from your in-class study, you were doing univariate analysis—that is, you were organizing data about individual variables.

Another word that you will often see in results sections is *bivariate*. **Bivariate analysis** refers to analysis with only two variables. Notice that the words themselves reveal their meanings: *uni* means "one," and *variate* means "to vary," so univariate is analysis of one variable; bivariate is analysis of two variables; and multivariate is analysis of more than two variables.

Both qualitative and quantitative studies have variables, but information about the variables for studies using these two approaches differs in how data are collected and how they are organized and reported in the results section of a report. The purpose of qualitative studies is to increase our understanding about some aspects of experiences. The results of those studies describe what was found, usually by organizing the data into concepts or themes and then by providing examples of the specific language used by participants to support and clarify the meaning of those concepts. The results describe findings about single variables, usually without using many numbers. Because quantitative studies use numbers to represent variables of

TABLE 4-2	
Identification of Specific Variables in the Caregiver Experience Study	
Dependent Variables	**Independent Variables**
Health-related quality of life—mental	Caregiving
Health-related quality of life—physical	Gender
Overall quality of life	Age
	Symptoms
	Burden
	Level of impairment
	Presence of aphasia
	Vitality
	Health-related quality of life—mental
	Health-related quality of life—physical

interest and then often apply statistical tests to allow inference, we expect to see mostly numbers in the results section of a quantitative report.

CORE CONCEPT 4-3

Both qualitative and quantitative studies have variables, but information about variables for studies using these two approaches differs in how data are collected and how they are organized and reported in the results section of a report.

Qualitative

Language Describing Results From Qualitative Studies

In the Out-of-Class exercise in Chapter 3, you were asked to organize some numerical data so that it would be more informative. If the data had been words instead of numbers, the task of how to create some kind of order would not have been immediately obvious. For example, if you were given written paragraphs from a number of students and were asked to organize this data, you might break down the paragraphs into units that you could organize, such as individual sentences or groups of sentences that address the same idea. You could then organize the sentences according to shared ideas and determine how many different ideas occurred and how much agreement there was about the ideas. The goal of data analysis in a qualitative study is the same as that in a quantitative study: to organize the data and create some kind of an order so that meaning can be found.

Box 4-1 lists excerpts of data that might have been collected in response to "What experiences in your life have led to your anticipated choice for field of nursing practice?," the question identified in the fictional article as the measure used to collect subjective responses to help understand why students chose their fields of practice. Take a moment and read through those responses. Reading data in this form is even less helpful than reading a long list of individuals' ages. For the qualitative researcher, the organizing, ordering, and synthesizing of the data collected represent the heart of the research method. In fact, in most qualitative studies, data are analyzed throughout the process of implementing the study, and the results of this analysis are then used to guide additional data collection. This is in contrast to quantitative studies, in which the researcher usually does not analyze the data until all have been collected because changing the way data are collected, or changing which data are collected, undermines the results of the study.

Another difference between data analysis in qualitative studies and quantitative studies is that no absolute formulas are consistently applied to the data. Qualitative data analysis requires understanding, digesting, synthesizing, conceptualizing, and reconceptualizing descriptions of feelings, behaviors, experiences, and ideas. *Content analysis* is often the term used to describe this process of data analysis. **Content analysis** is the process of understanding, interpreting, and conceptualizing the meanings in qualitative data. To do this, the researcher starts by breaking down the data into units that are meaningful and then develops a categorization scheme. A **categorization scheme** is an orderly combination of categories carefully defined so that no overlap

Box 4-1	Examples of Qualitative Data Collected in Response to the Question, "What Experiences in Your Life Have Led to Your Anticipated Choice for Field of Nursing Practice?"

"I have always loved movies where the nurses save the lives of people during a disaster. I guess, well, it seems like the best place to do that, you know, is, well, the emergency room."

"Nursing is all about caring for people. I mean, I don't know how I would have gotten through my son's illness without the nurses."

"The one thing I remember when I had my tonsils out was the nurse giving me ice cream. It made me feel safe."

"I come from a family of nurses who have all worked in hospitals, mostly the surgical or medical ICU."

"It was the nurse holding my hand when the doctor in the emergency room told me about my brother that made it possible for me to keep going."

"My roommate in college was a nursing student, and she always helped any of us who came to her, whether it was if we were sick or just feeling down."

"Every time I have had to go to the hospital with one of the kids, it was the nurses who really listened to me and made a difference."

"My aunt was a nurse. She always was so strong and sure of herself—I wanted to be just like her."

"The shows I've seen about the flying nurses—that is just such an exciting thing to do, I guess I figured I would never get bored."

"My best friend in high school was in a car accident and I was so scared to go see her. But the nurse, he just really helped me relax and not freak out seeing all the machines and things."

"There was no one like my Grandma Jane—she was the most caring person I ever knew; she nursed about everyone in the family until it was her turn to get sick and die."

occurs. In qualitative analysis, the categorization scheme is developed based on the ideas found in the data; then pieces of data—units that reflect distinct ideas—are put into the categories. This process of breaking down and labeling large amounts of data to identify the category to which they belong is called **coding** or **data reduction**. When this coding or data reduction occurs, the researcher is also refining the categorization scheme and using the categories to guide further data collection.

One might say that there is a spiraling nature to the process of data analysis in qualitative studies, as illustrated in Figure 4-1. The process is not circular because it does not simply return to where it began, but rather evolves to eventually identify key themes or concepts that reflect the meaning of the data. *Theme* is another term

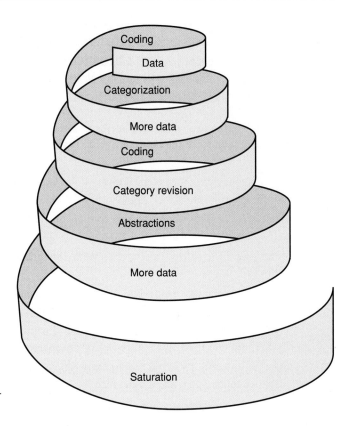

FIGURE 4-1 • Spiraling process of qualitative data analysis.

that often is found in the results section of a qualitative report. A **theme** is an idea or a concept that is implicit in and recurrent throughout the data. Themes are not the concrete, explicit words contained in the data; rather, they are the underlying ideas behind the words. Qualitative data analysis seeks to categorize and understand the data and the relationships among the categories to eventually conceptualize the data into themes. In the maternal HIV article from Chapters 1 and 2 (Sandelowski & Barroso, 2003), the authors used metasynthesis to identify the 11 aspects or themes inherent in mothers' work. The aspects identified in the report were not a direct quote from the participants in the different studies. Rather, they were the themes or ideas that were implicit in the actual statements of participants. The spiral of qualitative data analysis occurs, in part, because as categories are developed through analysis, they are used to collect additional data, which is then coded and categorized. Eventually, data saturation occurs. **Data saturation** in qualitative research is the point at which all new information collected is redundant of information already collected. Data saturation occurs at a time when all new information fits into the newly established coding system so that the new information is saying the same thing as the data already collected. Therefore, no new information is being generated through continued data collection.

Look again at the data in Box 4-1, which have already been broken down into units, mostly sentences—and in a few cases, more than one sentence—that combine to express one idea. Content analysis to develop a categorization scheme might start by using a category for "Caring Experiences" and another for "Television and Movies." As the researcher examines the data and codes them into these two categories, you see that only two of the units fit under the "Television and Movies" category, whereas all the rest belong to "Caring Experiences." The researcher might then notice that, in some cases, the data under "Caring Experiences" suggest a desire to follow in someone's footsteps. This idea can be refined to a category called "Experiences With Nursing Role Models." Once the data that reflect role models are moved into the new category, further analysis of the data that remain suggests that not only caring experiences but also personal caring experiences are being described. Thus, three themes can be derived from the data.

Figure 4-2 shows this process of content analysis in schematic form. This is a simplified example of how a qualitative researcher might analyze data to identify

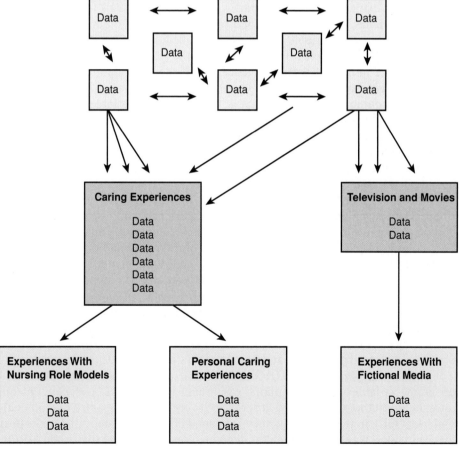

FIGURE 4-2 • Schematic.

themes. Notice that the final three themes identified are never explicitly addressed in the actual data. That is, no piece of data says that it was the nurse role model that led to the choice of field of nursing. The themes identified are implicit; that is, the ideas are repeated differently by different people.

The themes or categories derived from qualitative data analysis are usually reported in the results sections of qualitative research reports. The author of this type of report cannot provide averages or other statistics to describe the data. Rather, the themes or categories are described, often using specific examples from actual data to help make the implicit ideas within the themes clearer.

Quantitative

Language Describing Results From Quantitative Studies

We have said that qualitative research examines at least one variable. Quantitative research differs from qualitative research in that there are two types of variables: dependent and independent (or predictor). Because the purpose of quantitative research is to explain or predict a particular variable, we call that variable the **dependent variable,** which is determined by, or depends on, other variables in the study. It is the outcome variable of interest. In the fictional article about nursing students' preferences for practice, the outcome that the research is trying to explain or predict is choice of field of nursing practice, so it is the dependent variable.

Independent variables are those variables in a study that are used to explain or predict the outcome of interest, that is, the dependent variable. In the fictional article, the independent variables included age, perceived well being, race, and marital status. These were factors that differed among students and that may explain or predict their choice of field, the dependent variable. Independent variables also are called **predictor variables** because they are used to predict the dependent variable.

Notice that Table 4-2 classifies the variables from the caregiver experience study as dependent or independent. The caregiver experience study is quantitative and attempts to explain the caregivers' health-related quality of life and overall quality of life, considering characteristics of both the stroke survivor and the caregiver. You also may notice in the table that the variables "HRQL—mental" and "HRQL—physical" are identified as both a dependent variable and an independent variable. This is an example of a research term being "gray" rather than clearly "black and white." The caregiver experience study sought to "characterize the evolution of the caregiving experience" (White et al., 2003, p. 179). In order to do so, the authors first looked at how HRQL for the caregivers differed from what has been found to be normal for a general population and examined how characteristics of the stroke survivor and the caregiver impact HRQL. Both these analyses looked at HRQL as a dependent variable with the authors' examining what HQRL is dependent on. However, the authors also looked at how caregivers' HRQL impacted overall quality of life (QoL). In these analyses, they examined HRQL as a factor that may affect QoL. Thus, QoL was the variable that depended on HRQL, and that made HRQL an independent variable in those analyses. We discuss types of variables in quantitative research in more detail in Chapter 5.

In preparation for this chapter, you were asked to organize data from your in-class questionnaire to make it easy to understand. What did you do to make the information more understandable? Probably, your first thought was to create some kind of order in the data. The data that you were given consisted of numbers. A logical way to create order is to list the numbers from smallest to largest (or vice versa). Doing so gives a sense of how alike or different people are in the values of the numbers, such as in age or marital status, by showing how many numbers are repeated or are close together and what the smallest and largest numbers are. The next thing you may have done was determine the most common responses. This could be done by simply counting how many times each response was given, by calculating the percentage for each response out of the total responses, or by calculating an average of all the numbers.

Another approach to making sense out of a group of numbers includes using graphs, bar charts, or pie charts. This approach provides a visual representation of the data, which allows us to see the difference between the smallest and largest numbers as well as the most common responses. Figure 4-3 is an example of a histogram

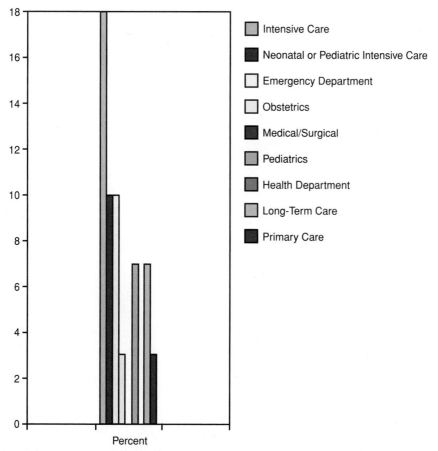

FIGURE 4-3 • Histogram for the frequency distribution of students' choices of field of practice based on results in fictional article.

(a type of bar chart) that could have been included in the fictional article on students' choices for clinical practice.

Hopefully, you found that organizing the data helped you to increase your understanding of what that information meant. Regardless of the approach taken, the product probably helped you to see two things: (1) how much diversity or difference occurred in the data and (2) the most common responses.

Variance, Standard Deviation, and Distribution

In the language of statistics, the diversity in data for a single variable is referred to as the variance, which reflects how the values for a variable are dispersed. The most common or frequent responses in a set of data are statistically described as the measures of central tendency. Each is discussed individually.

Variance is a statistic—a number—that can be used to show how much difference or variety exists in a group of numbers. Table 4-3 lists the ages of nursing students from three different classrooms. With short lists like this, you can look at the numbers and determine that there is more variety in the ages of students in classroom 2 than in classroom 1 or 3. But how do you objectively measure the variety or describe that variety in a way that can be consistently understood and interpreted by anyone? Obviously, just saying that classroom 2 has more variety in age than does classroom 1 or 3 is nonspecific—how much is "more?" You could also say that the ages range from 19 to 21 in classroom 1, compared with ages ranging from 18 to 24 in classroom 2. This is certainly more specific and gives us a better sense of the differences, but the ages of students in classroom 3 also range from 18 to 24 years, yet there is more variety in ages

TABLE 4-3		
Ages of Students in Three Different Classrooms With Variation and Central Tendency		
Classroom 1[*]	**Classroom 2**[*]	**Classroom 3**[*]
20	20	18
21	24	20
20	19	20
20	21	24
19	18	20
21	23	20
20	18	20
20	19	18
19	18	20
20	20	20
$SD = 0.67$	$SD = 2.11$	$SD = 1.63$
$M = 20$	$M = 20$	$M = 20$
Mode = 20	Mode = 18	Mode = 20
Median = 20	Median = 19.5	Median = 20

[*]Age in years.
SD, standard deviation; M, mean.

in classroom 2 than in classroom 3. Therefore, there must be some way to represent the values in between the two numbers that give us the age range.

The variety in a group of numbers is explained statistically by computing a number appropriately called the **variance**, which is the sum of the squared differences between each value in the set of numbers and the mean (average) of those numbers, divided by how many numbers there were in the set minus 1. That can be understood by using the age of students in classroom 1 as an example. The variance is computed by subtracting the average of all 10 students' ages (20) from each student's age and squaring the difference, then adding those squared differences and dividing by 9. We square the differences between the mean to avoid negative and positive differences canceling each other. Therefore, the variance statistic is an average of the squared deviations from the mean. This is a mathematical definition, so you may still be wondering what it is you know when you see a value for a variance.

Whether or not you understand the formula for computing the variance, you can understand that variance tells you how much variety there is within a set of numbers. For example, the variance for the ages in classroom 1 is 0.44 ($s^2 = 0.44$), the variance for the ages in classroom 2 is 4.44 ($s^2 = 4.44$), and the variance in classroom 3 is 2.66 ($s^2 = 2.66$). These statistics reveal that there is more variety in age in classroom 3 than in classroom 1, but less variety in classroom 3 than in classroom 2. Although you can see the variety in the ages by looking at the short list of numbers in Table 4-3, if the list contained 100 numbers or 1000 numbers, it would be much more difficult to get the variety without computing the variance. The variance gives us a specific statistic that represents differences or variety when reporting results for a single variable.

Thus far, we have discussed the variance for a single variable; however, more often the results section of a research report will use a statistic called the **standard deviation** instead of the variance. The standard deviation is simply the square root of the variance, so it also reflects variety among all the numbers. Remember that to compute the variance, we squared differences in values from the mean. This computational process results in the values for the variance being squared units of measurement, such as 4.44 squared years for the variance in classroom 2. The idea of "squared years," however, does not make much sense. If we take the square root of that variance, we get a standard deviation of 2.11 years (not squared years). The standard deviation is, in a sense, the average difference in ages from the overall average age. You can see by looking at the values for the ages in classroom 2 that it makes sense that the variety in ages can be accurately communicated by saying that there is an average of 2 years difference from the overall average. This makes more sense than 4.44 squared years. In contrast, the standard deviation for the ages of students in classroom 1 is 0.67 years (or less than 1 year), and the standard deviation of the ages of the students in classroom 3 is 1.63 years. Standard deviation is usually abbreviated in research reports as *SD*, so a research report giving the standard deviation for classroom 3 would write "*SD* = 1.63." Although classrooms 2 and 3 both have a youngest and oldest student of 18 and 24 years, respectively, the average deviation from the overall average age is clearly greater in classroom 2.

Why do we care about variance and standard deviation? To understand the meaning of results for clinical practice, we must understand how much variety there is in the results. For example, if you were reading a research study that examined the effectiveness of an intervention to relieve pain, and the report tells you that the average rating of pain on a 10-point scale after the intervention was 2, that sounds good. Suppose that two different interventions each led to an average rating of 2, but the first had a standard deviation of 3.5, whereas the second had a standard deviation of 0.7. Although the first intervention led to the same average as the second intervention, the standard deviation tells us there was a great deal more variety in pain ratings with the first intervention. This means that some of the people who received the first intervention had higher scores or more pain as well as possibly lower scores or less pain. Although lower scores may be better, our goal in nursing is to consistently improve pain, and higher scores in some of our patients definitely are not desirable. The second intervention led to much less variety in ratings of pain, which means that most of the subjects scored their pain close to a rating of 2 after the intervention. As a clinician who understands standard deviations, you might decide that the second intervention is more consistent in relieving pain because it has a smaller standard deviation and choose to use that intervention rather than the first one.

A pain intervention study is an example in which we may not want variety because our clinical goal is to consistently decrease our patients' pain levels. In other cases, however, we may want variety to make the information useful clinically. For example, in the caregiver experience article, the authors reported that the mean age of the caregivers in their sample was 56.8, with a standard deviation of 15.3 ($SD =$ 15.3) (White et al., 2003). This means that the average deviation around the age of 56.8 was 15.3 years, telling us that the individuals in the sample had a wide range of ages. Although N.B. is within this age range, the RN in the home health agency works with patients who are mostly over the age of 60, so she must decide if the large range of ages of caregivers in this study will affect the usefulness of this study for her EBN.

Distribution is another term that is used in results sections to indicate the variety or differences found. In research, **distribution** refers to how the findings are dispersed. The variance and standard deviation for a set of numbers give us a clear sense of the spread of those numbers. However, it is not appropriate to compute the statistics of variance and standard deviation for variables that fit into discrete categories, such as type of job preference, rather than variables that are real numbers, such as age. For simplicity, often a researcher will assign numeric values to categories, such as 1 = professional employment, 2 = blue-collar employment. However, the actual numbers "1" and "2" are not a true measure of type of employment, and adding or subtracting the numbers will not tell us the "average" type of employment.

In cases where the variable is a category, we may find distribution described by using a table of percentages, histogram, or pie chart. For example, Table 1 in Appendix B (the fictional article) shows us the frequency distribution of choices of field of nursing. A **frequency distribution** is the spread for how frequently each category occurs or is selected. We see from the table that 60% of students choose intensive care as their preferred field after graduation, and another 10% choose neonatal intensive care and emergency department fields. Figure 4-3 shows the same frequency distribution in a histogram format. Figure 4-4 shows what the frequency distribution would look like in histogram format if none of the students had selected the neonatal and emergency room fields and, instead, had selected the health department and long-term

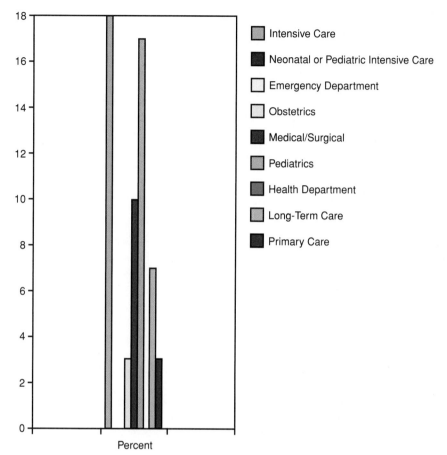

FIGURE 4-4 • Example of histogram for distribution of field of study choices if health department and long-term care were endorsed more frequently.

care fields. You can see that the distribution of choices would have looked different even with 60% still selecting intensive care. Just as the statistic for standard deviation can tell us about the distribution or variety in a numeric variable, a frequency table or histogram can tell us about distribution and variety in a categorical variable.

An important statistical concept that you may remember from your statistics courses is the **normal curve**. A normal curve is a type of distribution that is symmetric and bell-shaped. Figure 4-5 shows two graphs with distribution curves; the one on the left is the familiar normal curve. Many of the variables in life that we are interested in understanding or using in research are distributed similarly to the normal curve. For example, height can range from small, in the case of a neonate, to tall, in the case of a few extraordinary individuals, but most people fall somewhere in the middle, with a relatively even balance on each side of the average height. The normal curve is a theoretical distribution. That means that if we could measure a variable, such as height, for every human on earth and plot all the heights, the result would be this perfectly symmetric bell-shaped curve. One thing that makes the normal curve unique is

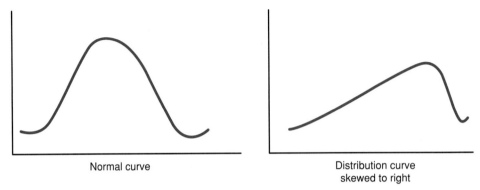

Normal curve   Distribution curve
skewed to right

FIGURE 4-5 • Examples of a normal curve and a curve that skews to the right.

its symmetry; the normal curve can be folded in half at the center, which is the average, and the two sides will match. On the right side of Figure 4-5 is an example of a distribution that has a curved shape but is asymmetric. Much of inferential statistics is based on the assumption that the distribution of a variable would be normal or bell-shaped if all the possible values for the variable were known. This assumption is based on experience with many variables of interest that are normally distributed. Therefore, when reading results, you will find references to a distribution of a variable being "approximately normal."

In summary, one of the important aspects of data that we expect to see described and summarized in the results section of reports is the diversity or variety in the data. This may be described by a univariate statistic called the *standard deviation* (or possibly the *variance*) or a frequency distribution, histogram, or pie chart. In any case, the variety for each study variable is important for us to understand because it affects the clinical decisions we can make based on the study.

Central Tendency

In addition to wanting to know about the diversity in a set of numbers for a variable, we almost always want to know the most common or average response or value for a variable. In quantitative research, a **measure of central tendency** shows common or typical numbers. Central tendency measures reflect the center of a distribution, or the center of the spread. Three univariate statistics, called the *mean*, the *mode*, and the *median*, are the most commonly used measures of central tendency. Table 4-3 shows that the mean value for the ages of the students in each classroom is 20 years. The **mean** is simply the average of all the values for a variable—that is, the sum of all the values divided by the number of values summed. The **mode** is the value that occurs most frequently: In classrooms 1 and 3, the mode is 20 years, but in classroom 2, the mode is 18. Although the mean of the ages in the three classrooms is the same, suggesting that the center of the distributions is the same, the center of the distribution of ages in the three classrooms differs when one looks at the mode.

The **median** is the value that falls in the middle of the distribution when the numbers are in numeric order. Although 20 years is the median age in classrooms 1 and

3, the median age for classroom 2 is 19.5 years (the average of 19 + 20, the two most central values for age in that classroom). Although the mean, mode, and median are all measures of central tendency, comparing the three for a single variable also tells us something about the distribution. Looking at the mean (20 years), mode (18 years), and median (19.5 years) for students' ages in classroom 2, we see that although the average age was 20, more students were younger than age 20 than were older than age 20. The age distribution "leans" toward the younger ages. This leaning is described as **skew** when reporting research results. We have said that the mean, mode, and median are measures of "central" tendency, but if there is a skew in the distribution, these measures will have different values. This tells us that the middle of the distribution is not in the exact center of that distribution; it is off to the left or right of center. The second curve of Figure 4-5 has a skew to the right, which means that the middle of the distribution falls more to the higher range of the possible values. A normal curve does not have a skew. In fact, part of what defines a normal curve is that the mean, median, and mode are all equal.

Now, look at Figure 4-6, which shows curves drawn around the distribution of ages for the three classrooms we have been using as an example. Notice that the curve for classroom 1 is perfectly bell-shaped and symmetric and that the mean, mode, and median are equal. The curve for classroom 2 is skewed to the left, is not symmetric, and the mean, mode, and median are not equal. The curve for classroom 3 looks similar to that for classroom 1, but it is narrower and not symmetric.

Again, why do we care about measures of central tendency? We care because a long list of numbers for a variable, such as a long list of ages or pain ratings, is difficult to make much sense of without some type of organization. A summary of those numbers that tells us the central tendency and distribution also allows us to quickly understand important aspects for the individual variable, such as the most common or frequent value and how much variety there is in the values. This, in turn, allows us to gain more understanding of how the results may or may not apply to real clinical practice.

The data from the in-class study exercise provide an excellent example of how much more we can learn about a variable when the data are summarized to give us the distribution and the central tendency. A second example is shown in Table 2 (White et al., 2003) of Appendix A-4, the caregiver experience report found by the RN from our clinical case. (Had the authors simply given us a list of the scores of the 97 caregivers, it would have been both tedious and frustrating to try to get a sense of their overall health. However, when the author tells us that the range of scores on the Physical Symptom checklist is from 24 to 0 and that the mean and standard deviation for symptoms of caregivers at the first interview is 4.2 (3.5), we have information that immediately tells us the physical health of caregivers in the study. Notice that the mean is provided with the standard deviation inside parentheses. This is a common way to report the mean and standard deviation results. We can then see that, while the mean and standard deviation for physical symptoms increased to 4.5 (4.0) by the last interview, clearly there was not a big increase in symptom scores (White et al., 2003).

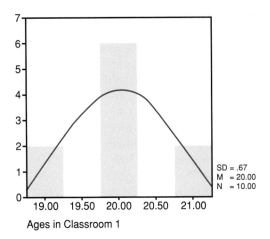

Ages in Classroom 1

SD = .67
M = 20.00
N = 10.00

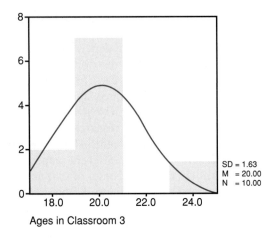

Ages in Classroom 3

SD = 1.63
M = 20.00
N = 10.00

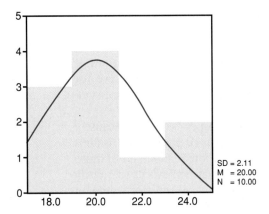

Ages in Classroom 2

SD = 2.11
M = 20.00
N = 10.00

FIGURE 4-6 • Frequency distribution histogram and curves for ages of students in three classrooms. *SD*, standard deviation; *M*, mean; *N*, number in sample.

CORE CONCEPT 4-4

Measures of central tendency and distribution are univariate statistics that summarize information about a variable.

The description of the variables in a study is always an important part of the results section of research reports. Description of data aims to summarize it in a way that makes it understandable and meaningful. Description of only one variable is called *univariate analysis,* and in quantitative research, that description almost always includes information that tells us about the distribution and central tendency for the variables. In reports of qualitative research, the entire results section is descriptive, taking units of data (words, pictures, and sentences) and developing categories and themes to describe that data.

CONNECTING RESULTS THAT DESCRIBE TO CONCLUSIONS

The RN in our clinical case has read the results and discussion sections of the research report about caregivers' experiences. The results started with a description of the caregivers' scores on the measures in this study in the first and second year. These results provide the RN with an understanding of any differences that appear to be present over a two-year period of caregiving for a stroke survivor. The **demographic** data—descriptive information about the characteristics of the people studied—were not included in the results section of this report. Rather, the data were presented earlier in the report in the section on Procedures. So, if the RN read only the results and conclusions sections, she would not know much about the subjects in this study. Both quantitative and qualitative studies almost always include demographic data, although the reports of qualitative studies may not use statistics to describe those characteristics. However, the article found by the RN does include both the mean and the standard deviation for participants' ages, along with percentages for other categorical variables, such as relationship of caregiver to stroke survivor in Table 1 of Appendix A-4 (White et al., 2003).

Checking the descriptive results in Table 1 and Table 2 of the caregiver research report, we find that, in many cases, caregivers' scores on measures of health are similar from initial measurement to a time two years later. Table 2 also compares the caregivers' scores to those of populations of people who were approximately the same age and gender as the caregivers in the study. They are also analyzed using *t* test statistics to look for significant differences. A *t* test is an inferential statistic, and as soon as the authors begin to compare results, they are moving beyond description to inference. Thus, based on the descriptive results alone, there is much that we do not know. Also, when the RN compares these somewhat limited descriptive findings with the content in the discussion section of the report, it is clear that the results of the inferential analysis are being emphasized more than the descriptive results.

The specific results described are the basis for the new knowledge identified in the conclusion. Without reading the results, we would not know what the actual characteristics of the sample were or how the caregivers in the study rated their quality of life, making the clinical implications identified in this study difficult to understand. Having read the results section, however, we find that the conclusions generally are clearer and make more sense.

COMMON ERRORS IN THE REPORTS OF DESCRIPTIVE RESULTS

Two kinds of problems may be found when reading descriptive results in a research report: (1) incomplete information and (2) confusing information. We have emphasized the importance of understanding the distribution and central tendency in variables from quantitative studies to make clinical decisions. One problem that sometimes arises when reading the results is that this descriptive information cannot be found. The authors may fail to provide any univariate statistics about some of the variables in the study, or they may fail to provide all the information needed.

For example, a report may include only a measure of central tendency for an important variable without giving a range of values or the standard deviation. This absence of information about the variation in the variable makes it difficult to know how to interpret the findings related to that variable and can even lead to incorrect conclusions. The previous example of a study that examined two interventions to help pain whose results are a mean pain score of 2 for both interventions is a good example of this. Given the mean scores alone, one might conclude that the two interventions have exactly the same effect. This conclusion would be incorrect, however, because the standard deviations for the mean pain scores in this example (0.7 and 3.5) are different.

Another example of a report with incomplete descriptive results is the fictional article. One of the variables that the author later indicates was important relative to the students' choices of field of practice was their health rating, but the only univariate information provided about the variable is that 20% of the subjects rated their health as fair or poor. We learn neither how the percentages broke down for ratings of "excellent health" or "good health" nor whether most of the 20% of subjects who rated their health at the lower end chose "fair" or "poor." This lack of information affects our ability to interpret the results that are reported later.

Aside from incomplete results, a second problem that may be found in the results section is a confusing presentation of the results. Descriptive results are often reported in tables, and sometimes those tables are not labeled or organized clearly. A table may use titles or identify variables that are inconsistent with the wording used in the text of the report. In fact, sometimes the text of a report fails to refer to the table at all. Another problem is that too much information may be put into the text, rather than used in a table. For example, the information provided in Table 1 in the fictional article would have been confusing and difficult to understand if the author had instead written a paragraph reporting those results as follows:

> Students chose several fields immediately after graduation, with 18 (60%) choosing intensive care, 3 (10%) choosing neonatal or pediatric intensive care, and 3 (10%) choosing emergency departments. One student (3%) chose obstetrics for field of study immediately after graduation, and no students chose either medical/surgical or health department. Two students (7%) chose pediatrics, two students (7%) chose long-term care or nursing home care, and one student (3%) chose primary care.

Although this information could be sorted out by the reader, it is presented much more clearly in the table. A similar problem may occur in a qualitative report if the author does not give us clear descriptions of the categories or themes developed from the study. Look at the fictional article again and at the three themes identified that represented the meaning of experiences students identified as affecting their choice of practice. If the author had simply listed the themes as "personal life experience," "experiences with nursing role models," and "experiences with fictional media," it would be difficult to know how these types of experiences differ. The definitions and examples given in Table 2 make it clear what those themes mean.

CRITICALLY READING RESULTS SECTIONS OF RESEARCH REPORTS

It should be clear from the examples just given that critically reading the descriptive results section of a research report is important. Box 4-2 presents a set of six questions that can be used when critically reading results sections. The first question, "Did the report include a clearly identified results section?," may seem simplistic, but some reports do not present results in a specific section. In fact, the caregiver experience study has placed the results regarding the demographic characteristics of their sample under procedures, rather than results, making it awkward to read and understand the results. The answer to the second question, "Were the results presented appropriately for the information collected?," refers to whether or not descriptions included information about distribution, central tendency, and variation that were appropriate for the study's variables. For example, was information about categories such as marital status presented as percentages, and were both the mean and the standard deviation included in information about variables such as age or scores on a measure? The third question is, "Were descriptive versus inferential results identifiable if this is a quantitative study?". When we consider the results in the caregiver article, we find that it combines descriptive and inferential results in both the written and tabular presentation of results in a way that could be confusing to readers.

If the study that you are reading used a qualitative method, a question to ask yourself in order to critically read the results section is, "Were themes or structure and meaning identifiable if this is a qualitative study?" The maternal HIV study we read for Chapters 1 and 2 is a good example of a qualitative study that clearly identifies the structure and themes found from their metasynthesis in the text and use of figures and tables. Not all reports of qualitative studies will be as clear. This leads us to the next question, "Were the results presented in a clear and logical manner?" For example, the caregiver report organizes the results by using headings that represent the specific objectives established for the study. This is a logical and clear approach to presenting results. The last question to ask yourself as you read the results section of a report is, "Did the results include enough information about the final sample for

---

Box 4-2 **How to Critically Read the Results Section of a Research Report**

Do the results answer the question, "Why did the authors reach these conclusions—what did they actually find?"

1. Did the report include a clearly identified results section?
2. Were the results presented appropriately for the information collected?
3. Were descriptive versus inferential results identifiable if this is a quantitative study?
4. Were themes or structure and meaning identifiable if this is a qualitative study?
5. Were the results presented in a clear and logical manner?
6. Did the results include enough information about the final sample for the study?

the study?" We have already discussed the importance of including demographic information in the report of results of a study, whether it is qualitative or quantitative. We also have identified that the authors of the caregiver experience study did include demographic information but that it was not located in the results section. There does seem to be enough information about demographic characteristics; however, it would have been helpful to know the actual ranges in scores and ages of the participants, as well as the standard deviations, in this study. We will revisit four of the six questions for critically reading results sections of research reports at the end of Chapter 5, after we finish learning a bit about inferential statistics.

PUBLISHED REPORT—WHAT WOULD YOU CONCLUDE?

Understanding what to expect in the reports of descriptive results makes it possible for you to know whether the research is something that might apply to your clinical practice. The RN in our clinical case began her search with an interest in gaining a better understanding of how providing care to a stroke survivor impacts the caregiver. After reading the results and conclusions sections of the caregiver experience article, the RN has an increased understanding of how measures of quality of life may or may not change over time when caregiving. But she does not have much information about how these scores differ from those for people who are not caregivers and whether any differences in quality of life measures found are important. As we said earlier, the descriptive results in this study are relatively limited, and the RN will have to read the inferential results in order to gain a better understanding of the conclusions of the report and what she might do to care for her client and her client's husband. We will continue to look at the language of results sections of research reports in the next chapter, which will add to the RN's knowledge when planning care for N.B. and his wife.

OUT-OF-CLASS EXERCISE

Making Inferences About Well Being and Marriage

Before proceeding to Chapter 5, look at the data collected from your in-class practice study, focusing on two variables: rating of well being and marital status. Complete a univariate analysis of data for each of these variables to summarize distribution and central tendency. To do so, you will need to decide what is appropriate in terms of measure of central tendency (mean, median, or mode) and how to summarize distribution (range, standard deviation, percent). Then, determine what the data tell you in terms of answering the question, "Do married students have higher levels of well being than unmarried students?" Based on the data obtained, answer the question and explain how you arrived at your answer. If you are not using an in-class study, a practice set of data about well being and marital status is provided in Appendix D, which can be used for this exercise. Remember, this is an exercise to motivate you to think more about how results are presented in a research report and what they mean. You will then be ready to begin the next chapter.

References

Kane, M., & DiBartolo, M. (2002). Complex physical and mental health needs of rural incarcerated women. *Issues in Mental Health Nursing, 23,* 209–229.

Sandelowski, M., & Barroso, J. (2003). Motherhood in the context of maternal HIV infection. *Research in Nursing & Health, 26,* 470–482.

White, C. L., Mayo, N., Hanley, J. A., & Wood-Dauphinee, S. (2003). Evolution of the caregiving experience in the initial 2 years following stroke. *Research in Nursing & Health, 26,* 177–189.

Resources

Locke, L. F., Silverman, S. J., & Spirduso, W. W. (1998). *Reading and understanding research.* Thousand Oaks, CA: Sage Publications.

Polit, D. F., & Beck, C. T. (2003). *Nursing research: Principles and methods* (7th ed.). Philadelphia: Lippincott Williams & Wilkins.

Salkind, N. J. (2000). *Statistics for people who (think they) hate statistics.* Thousand Oaks, CA: Sage Publications.

INFERENTIAL RESULTS
Why Did the Authors Reach Their Conclusion— What Did They Actually Find?

LEARNING OBJECTIVE:

The student will interpret inferential statistical results in relationship to their meaning for the conclusions of the study.

The Purpose of Inferential Statistics
Probability and Significance
Parametric and Nonparametric Statistics
Bivariate and Multivariate Tests
    Tests Looking for Differences Between Two Groups
    Tests Looking at Relationships Between Two Variables
    Tests Looking for Differences Among Three or More Groups
    Tests Looking at Relationships Among Three or More Variables
    Tests Looking at the Structure or Components of a Variable
Hypothesis Testing
In-Class Study Data
Connecting Inferential Statistical Results to Conclusions
Common Errors in Results Sections
Critically Reading the Results Section of a Report—Revisited
Published Report—What Would You Conclude?

KEY TERMS

Analysis of variance	Null hypothesis
Beta (β) value	Parametric statistics
Confidence intervals	Probability
Correlation	Regression
Covary	Research hypothesis
Factor analysis	t test
Nonparametric statistics	

CLINICAL CASE

The RN works in a home health agency and has recently started working with N.B.'s wife, who suffered a major stroke 6 months ago. The RN has also taken care of a number of other families where one member of the family has a major role as caregiver. She has noticed that N.B. appears to be experiencing some fatigue and weight loss, which she suspects is secondary to his responsibilities of caring for his wife. She has found an article that seems relevant to her interests in supporting the caregivers of her primary clients and has read it. The article used a quantitative method to examine health-related quality of life and general quality of life for caregivers of stroke survivors (White, Mayo, Hanley, & Wood-Dauphinee, 2003). This article used several statistical terms in the results section, which the RN must interpret to decide what the results mean for her as she considers whether she can use the study as evidence to guide her practice. Since the article used in this chapter is the same as that used in Chapter 4, the box describing keywords and the clinical question will not be repeated in this chapter.

THE PURPOSE OF INFERENTIAL STATISTICS

Chapter 4 discussed the meaning of the language used in research reports when descriptive results—those that describe or explain a variable or variables—are presented. This chapter continues the discussion of how to understand the results sections of research reports but focuses on inferential results—those intended to explain or predict a variable or variables. Notice that the word *explain* is included in both of these definitions. This is because there is an overlap between simple description—a description that explains—and explanation that can be used for prediction. We are looking at a continuum of statistics that build from simple knowing, to understanding and explaining, and finally to predicting, as shown in Figure 5-1.

Let us look at a simple example using the results about the ages, gender, and degree status of students in a nursing class shown in Table 5-1. The mean ($M = 27$) and standard deviation ($SD = 6$) for the age of the students is an example of simple description. Notice in Figure 5-1 that the mean is followed by the standard deviation in parentheses. This is often the form used to report a mean and standard deviation in the results of a research report. This example of descriptive univariate statistics tells us that the students are relatively old and that there is a fair amount of variation in the ages, but we have no idea why the variation exists. To have some explanation of the variation, descriptive statistics might be used to give us information about the age of the men versus the age of the women in the class. In the example,

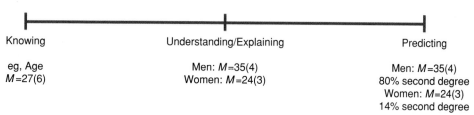

Knowing

eg, Age
$M=27(6)$

Understanding/Explaining

Men: $M=35(4)$
Women: $M=24(3)$

Predicting

Men: $M=35(4)$
80% second degree
Women: $M=24(3)$
14% second degree

FIGURE 5-1 • A continuum for the purposes of data analysis.

TABLE 5-1

Fictional Data for Ages, Gender, and Degree Status of a Nursing Student Class

Subject Number	Age (in years)	Gender	Degree Status
1	20	F	1st
2	23	F	1st
3	33	M	1st
4	21	F	1st
5	25	F	1st
6	40	M	2nd
7	32	F	2nd
8	20	F	1st
9	26	F	1st
10	25	F	1st
11	37	M	2nd
12	26	F	1st
13	23	F	1st
14	22	F	1st
15	24	F	2nd
16	30	M	2nd
17	35	M	2nd
18	21	F	1st
19	25	F	1st

the mean age for the male students is 35 ($SD = 4$), whereas the mean age of the female students is 24 ($SD = 3$). We now have a partial explanation of the variation in ages: There are both men and women in the class, and the men in the class are older than the women. The variation in age is explained to some extent, but we do not assume that we can use students' gender distribution to predict the age of students. However, if we discover that 80% of the male students are second-degree students , whereas only 14% of the females are second-degree students, this additional information can potentially be used for prediction. We can speculate that men may be more likely to pursue nursing as a second career and that the more second-degree students there are in a class, the older the students will be. To test whether we can use the number of second-degree students to predict age of students in a classroom, we must use inferential statistics.

Why use inferential statistics instead of just descriptive statistics? Because at this point, we do not know if the differences and relationships among variables found in this classroom occurred by chance alone. We know that there are differences in this particular classroom, but we cannot know whether, in general, second-degree students are more likely to be men and older. Descriptive statistical results allow us to know and explain variables that we are interested in understanding, but we have to go a step further to use that explanation to predict or infer how those variables may occur in the future. This can be done through the use of inferential statistics, which are based on the concepts of probability and statistical significance. Therefore, to understand results that use inferential statistics, we must understand these terms.

PROBABILITY AND SIGNIFICANCE

As the RN in our clinical case starts to read the section of the report titled "Caregiver characteristics in first and second years following stroke," she encounters the language of inferential statistics in the statement at the end of the section that states "the measure of HRQL did not change with the exception of the 'social function' subscale of the SF-36, which increased significantly between the first and second years of caregiving (p < .01)" (White et al., 2003, p. 183). In Chapter 2, we defined *significance* as a low likelihood that any relationship or difference found in a statistical test occurred by chance alone. Quantitative research often attempts to take what has been found in a specific situation, that is, one study, and infer that similar results would occur in other similar situations. The RN in the clinical case not only is interested in what happened in the study by White et al., but also wants to predict that the same thing will happen in her practice setting if she uses the information from the study to guide her practice.

In inferential statistics, we test for relationships, associations, and differences among variables that are statistically significant. We do this by creating distributions of test statistics that reflect variables having no connection between them, are unrelated, or are not different. In Chapter 4, we said that a distribution refers to how the findings are dispersed. A distribution of test statistics shows how the statistics from hundreds of samples would look if plotted on a graft. Then, we compute a test statistic for the results in our particular study and compare what we found in our sample or specific situation to what would be predicted to be found if there were not a relationship or difference in the variables. By convention, researchers say that if the test statistic falls into the range where we would expect 95% of all statistics to fall, given that there is no relationship or connection, then it is a nonsignificant statistic. Stated in the opposite way, if a test statistic falls *out of the range* of values that we would expect to occur 95% of the time, if there were no relationship among the variables, then we say it is a statistically significant value.

To illustrate this idea, we will use the statistic reported in the fictional article from Appendix B about the difference in ages of nursing students who choose acute settings versus nonacute settings. The article states that there was a significant difference in age and gives a test statistic of "$t = 2.1, p < .05$." The "t" value is a test statistic for differences in means between two groups, which we will discuss later in this chapter. In this case, the statistic was computed for the differences in the average ages of students who did and did not select an acute care setting for field of practice. Now look at Figure 5-2, which shows a distribution that is a normal curve, in this case a t distribution. Notice that for the t distribution, zero is at the center, and the possible values for the t test become larger at either end. A t distribution shows how the t tests for hundreds of different samples of two variables *that did not differ from each other in the "real" world* would be distributed. Now, returning to age as a variable of interest, if in the real world the ages of two groups are *not* different, then most of the time we would not get a big difference for the ages in any particular sample, and the t test statistic would be a small number. However, occasionally, by chance alone, we get a large difference in age between groups in a sample (perhaps because a 12-year-old genius is in a particular sample).

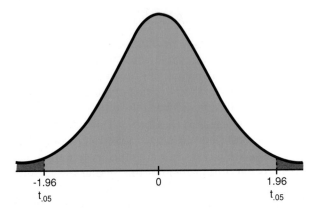

FIGURE 5-2 • *t*-Distribution for differences in two means in a sample when there is really no difference in the "real" world; green zone shows where 95% of values will fall, and two red zones show where 2.5% of the values will fall.

Using the example from the fictional article, if students in the real world who did and did not pick acute settings were approximately the same age, then most of the time, if we took a sample of ages of students, choosing the two types of setting and computed a *t* test, the value would be plotted on the distribution somewhere toward the middle, in the green zone. In fact, the green zone marks where a *t* test value will fall 95% of the time if the two variables tested are not different. The red zones at either end of the normal curve are the areas where the *t* values will fall by chance alone 2.5% of the time if, in the real world, the two variables tested are not different. When we say that a test statistic is significant, we are saying that we will achieve that statistic only a small percentage of the time if there is no difference or connection between the variables.

When the RN in the clinical case reads that the scores on the "social function" subscale of the SF-36 increased significantly, she knows that what was found in this study probably did not happen by chance. How much "probably" means, or what the probability is that whatever was found happened by chance is reported by a *p* value. The *p* value represents the **probability** and is defined as the percentage of the time the result found would have happened by chance alone. In the caregiver experience study, the authors indicate that the *p* value to the significant increase in social function scores was .01, which translates to 1%. This means that the statistic computed for the difference in social function scores from the first to last interview would only happen 1 out of 100 times by chance alone. If the *p* value were .05, then the statistic would only occur by chance 5 out of 100 times (5%), and if the *p* value were .001, the statistic would only occur by chance 1 out of 1000 times (1/10 of 1%). Statistical significance, no matter what test has been used, means that the results are unlikely to have happened by chance alone. Therefore, we infer from the finding of statistical significance that the difference, association, or relationship that we tested statistically is one that exists in the real world because we were unlikely to get our statistic by chance alone. Remember that inferential statistics are only used in quantitative methods because only in quantitative studies do we assume that the absolute truth can be found.

Statistical significance is also sometimes described in the results sections of research reports in the form of confidence intervals. **Confidence intervals** state the range of actual values for the statistic we are computing (such as the difference in the mean ages of nursing students who do and do not choose acute care settings), in which 95 out of 100 values would fall. A confidence interval for the differences in ages between nursing students choosing the two types of settings might be 0.8 to 6.2, and a research report might state that the differences in the means of ages for the two groups was 4.2, with a 95% confidence interval (0.8, 6.2). This means that given the difference found in the study, 95 out of 100 times, the difference in ages between the two groups of students will fall between 0.8 years and 6.2 years. Notice that this range does not include zero, so there is a low likelihood that there is zero or no difference. The caregiver experience study from Appendix A-4 reports confidence intervals in Table 3 of the results sections for results of a regression analysis. We will briefly discuss regression analysis later in this chapter, but for now, simply note that "95% CI" refers to a 95% confidence interval. Confidence intervals are almost always stated for the 95% range, whereas the probability of getting the result reported if there really were no difference or relationship is usually reported as one of three possible percents, 5% ($p < .05$), 1% ($p < .01$), and 0.1% ($p < .001$). Table 5-2 summarizes the differences between p values and confidence intervals.

CORE CONCEPT 5-1

Inferential statistics are used to report whether the results found in the specific study are likely to have happened by chance alone. Statistical significance is not an absolute guarantee that the values are really different or related in the real world. Rather, statistical significance means that there is less than a 5% chance that the amount of relationship or difference found happened by chance.

TABLE 5-2

Comparison of *p* Values and Confidence Intervals

	p Value	Confidence Interval
Assumption	The relationship or difference tested is zero	The relationship or difference is that found in the data
Meaning	Gives the percentage of the time that we would get the test statistic by chance alone	Gives the range of values (biggest and smallest numbers) that would occur 95% of the time for the relationship or difference found
Interpretation	The smaller the value, the less likely that the test result occurred by chance alone	The smaller the range, without zero in it, the more confident we can be that the test statistic reflects the "real" world

Returning to the caregiver experience article and the report of a significant increase in social function scores, we now know that whatever the test statistic was, it was unlikely to have happened by chance. In this case, the authors probably used a *t* test. We will discuss more about that test shortly.

CORE CONCEPT 5-2

Whether the report includes p *values or confidence intervals, the authors are telling you how likely it is that the results from the study were due to chance and, therefore, how likely it is that these results can be used to infer that there would be similar results in similar future situations.*

PARAMETRIC AND NONPARAMETRIC STATISTICS

Before we begin to discuss some of the specific statistical tests that you are likely to find reported in the results sections, you must understand the difference between *parametric* and *nonparametric statistics*. These terms refer to the two broad classes of inferential statistical procedures that can be applied to numeric results from studies. **Parametric statistics** can be applied to numbers that meet two key criteria: (1) the numbers must generally be normally distributed—that is, the frequency distribution of the numbers is roughly bell-shaped; and (2) the numbers must be interval or ratio numbers, such as age or intelligence score—that is, the numbers must have an order, and there must be an equal distance between each value. **Nonparametric statistics** are used for numbers that do not have a bell-shaped distribution and are categoric or ordinal. Categoric or ordinal numbers represent variables for which there is no established equal distance between each category, such as numbers used to represent gender or rating of preference for car color.

Understanding that there is a difference between parametric and nonparametric statistics is important for two reasons. First, although it is the researcher's responsibility to decide which type of inferential statistics should be used, as an intelligent reader of research, you should understand that the decision is not always clear-cut. In fact, whole books are written about which types of statistics should or should not be used with selected data. Therefore, the author of a research report may include a sentence or two stating that either parametric or nonparametric statistics were used and the rationale for that decision. Second, types of statistical tests used in research differ depending on the kind of numbers in the results. Thus, more than one type of statistical procedure is needed to look for the same kind of relationship. For example, often research is looking for differences between two groups. If the variable that we expect to be different in the two groups has interval or ratio numeric values (and is distributed roughly normally or bell-shaped), such as age, then the researcher can use a *t* test. But if the variable that we expect to be different for the two groups is a category, such as choice between red or green cars, then the researcher cannot use a *t* test and may use something called a Kruskal-Wallis one-way analysis of variance (ANOVA) test. The *t* test is a parametric statistical test, and the Kruskal-Wallis is a nonparametric test, but both help us to look for differences between groups. As we discuss some of the more common statistical tests that may be described in the results section of a research report, we will identify parametric and nonparametric statistics so that you will recognize and understand some of each class of statistical procedures.

CORE CONCEPT 5-3

Researchers use different types of statistics to test for the same kind of relationship, depending on the form of data collected. The research report may tell you why a particular type of statistical test was applied.

BIVARIATE AND MULTIVARIATE TESTS

The RN in our clinical case is not interested in becoming a statistician, but she does want to know how and perhaps why the quality of life changes for caregivers of stroke survivors. The section of the caregiver experience report titled "Caregiver HRQL compared to population norms" includes a number of statements about significant differences on the quality of life measures of the caregivers compared with those known to be the normal scores for populations in general. These statements of significantly different scores such as "caregivers scored significantly higher on the PCS [physical component summary] and significantly lower on the mental subscales and the MCS [mental component summary]" (White et al., 2003, p. 183) indicate that the authors found something that was not likely to be a chance occurrence and that might be useful in understanding or predicting the quality of life of stroke survivor caregivers. Table 5-3 summarizes some of the most common statistical tests used in nursing research by three general purposes for tests. In general, we use statistical tests to (1) look at differences between groups for one or more variables, (2) look at relationships among two or more variables, or (3) look at relationships of factors within a variable itself. Each of these general purposes addresses a different type of question. When we perform statistical tests to look at differences, we are asking some version of the question "Are groups unlike one another on a given variable or variables?" When we perform tests to look at relationships among variables, we might ask "Is there some natural connection between two or more variables?" Finally, when we look at relationships within a variable, this question might come to mind, "What are the natural components that make up a variable?" The statistical tests used when we are only looking at two variables or two groups are different from those we use with three or more variables or groups. We will first look at bivariate statistics—that is, statistical tests that are used with just two variables.

TABLE 5-3

Common Statistical Procedures Categorized by Type of Relationship Tested and Number of Variables Included

Type of Relationship Tested	Two Variables— Bivariate	Three or More Variables— Multivariate
1. Differences—are groups unlike one another on a given variable or variables?		
Independent groups	■ *t* test (parametric) ■ Sign test or median test (nonparametric) ■ Mann-Whitney *U* (nonparametric) ■ Wilcoxon rank test (nonparametric) ■ Fisher Exact test (nonparametric)	■ ANOVA (parametric) ■ ANCOVA, MANOVA, One-way ANOVA (parametric) ■ Kruskal-Wallis one-way ANOVA (nonparametric) ■ Chi-square for independent samples
Related groups usually over time	■ Paired *t* test (parametric) ■ McNemar change test (nonparametric)	■ Repeated measures ANOVA (parametric) ■ Friedman two-way ANOVA (nonparametric)
2. Relationships between variables—is there a natural connection between two or more variables?	■ Pearson *r* (parametric) ■ Spearman rho (nonparametric) ■ Kenndall tau (nonparametric) ■ Contingency coefficient (nonparametric)	■ Multiple regression (parametric) ■ Canonical correlation (parametric) ■ Path analysis (parametric) ■ Structural equation modeling (parametric) ■ Discriminant analysis (parametric) ■ Logistic regression (nonparametric)
3. Relationships within a variable—is there a structure within a variable?		■ Factor analysis (parametric) ■ Cluster analysis (nonparametric)

ANOVA, analysis of variance; ANCOVA, analysis of covariance; MANOVA, multiple analysis of variance.

Tests Looking for Differences Between Two Groups

In our discussion of significance and probability, we used an example from the fictional article from Appendix B in which the author wanted to explain or predict choice of field of practice. To do so, the author divided the students into two groups: those who chose an acute care setting and those who did not. The author then looked for variables that were significantly different between the groups, hoping that they might help to understand and predict which students would select nonacute practice settings. A *t* test was used to test for significant differences. A **_t_ test** computes a statistic that reflects the differences in the means of a variable for two different groups or at two different times for one group. The two groups being tested might consist of anything of interest to nursing, such as men and women, single-parent families and two-parent families, those who quit smoking and those who did not, or hospitals with level-one trauma centers and hospitals without them. In all of these examples, one variable differentiates the two groups. Alternately, the "groups" might be the same unit at different points in time, such as families before and after a divorce, smokers before and after a smoking cessation program, or hospitals before and after a level-one trauma center is added. The variable tested can be anything that can be measured as a continuous number, such as age, family functioning, self-efficacy, or cost per patient visit.

The fictional article reports the results of two *t* tests. The two groups for both of these tests were the same: those who chose an acute setting and those who did not choose an acute setting. However, the tests looked for differences in two different variables. In the first test, the researcher tested to see if age differed between the groups, and in the second test, the researcher tested to see if health rating differed. In both cases, there was a statistically significant difference between the groups in the variables. The author also tells the reader that "there was no significant . . . differences in number of years of post-secondary education and field of study." Because the test was not statistically significant, no test statistic is reported here, but the author believes it is important to tell you that the possibility of this difference was tested and was found not to be present. When using research in clinical practice, it is equally important to understand whether or not a difference or relationship is significant. Findings that there are no significant differences or relationships help us to rule out factors that will affect our clinical care.

The caregiver experience study in Appendix A-4 also reports the results of *t* tests in Table 2 and in the text of the results sections. However, the authors do not explicitly say that the statistical test they are reporting is a *t* test in the results sections. They simply state that "caregivers scored significantly higher on the PCS and significantly lower on the mental subscales and the MCS" (White et al., 2003, p. 183). If the RN in the clinical case reads the methods section earlier in this research report, she would see that under a heading titled "Data Analysis," the authors do indicate that they used *t* tests to compare mean scores for variables. However, now that we understand about statistics to compare two groups, we can look at the means for a variable, such as PCS, and see that subjects in the study had a mean score of 52, while individuals not caregiving but who were matched in age and gender to those in the study, had an average score of 49. And we can recognize that a *t* test was used when the authors indicate that this was a statistically significant difference.

Other statistical tests that examine differences between two groups are mostly nonparametric and include the Fisher exact test, Mann-Whitney test, Wilcoxon signed rank test, McNemar test, and sign or median test (Table 5-3). It is not necessary to understand exactly how these tests are chosen and applied, but it is important to understand that whenever one of these tests is reported in the results section, it is being used to examine differences between two groups. If the *p* value that is reported with the test is less than .05, then there was a difference between the groups that probably did not occur by chance alone.

Tests Looking at Relationships Between Two Variables

In nursing research, we often look for relationships or connections between two variables. When two variables are connected in some way, they are said to covary. Two variables **covary** when changes in one are connected to consistent changes in the other. For example, height and weight covary in healthy growing children. As the height of a child increases, the weight usually increases as well. Another example of covariance is found between the amount of practice of a procedure, such as urinary catheterization, and the number of errors. In this case, as the variable "amount of practice" increases, the variable "number of errors" consistently decreases. The statistical test used to examine how much two variables covary is called a **correlation**.

Two things are important to notice about a correlation statistic, also called a *correlation coefficient*. First, it is important to notice whether the number is negative or positive. In the example of the correlation between height and weight in children, the number for the correlation will be positive because the two variables move in the same direction; that is, they both increase. In the second example, the correlation between practice and errors will be negative because the two variables move in opposite directions. Figure 5-3 shows two graphs that can represent the two examples. Notice that in the first graph, the points all fall along a line that moves diagonally from the bottom to the top. This shows that there is a positive connection or relationship between these two variables because as one goes up, the other goes up. In contrast, on the second graph, the points fall along a line that moves diagonally from the top and down toward the opposite end. This shows that there is a negative connection or relationship between the two variables because as one goes up, the other goes down.

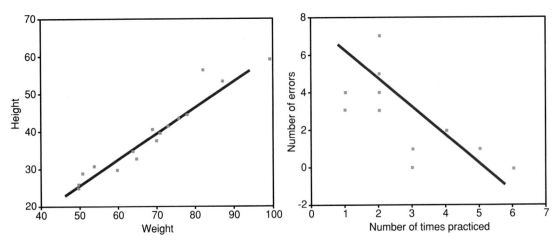

FIGURE 5-3 • Scatter plots showing a positive relationship between height and weight in children and a negative relationship between practicing a procedure and number of errors.

Second, it is important to notice the magnitude of the number for a correlation coefficient. Because of the way a correlation coefficient is calculated, it can only have a range of values from –1 to +1. A relationship between two variables that is "perfect"—as one goes up, the other goes up or down in exactly the same amount—will have a value of either –1 or +1. The lines drawn in the middle of the two graphs in Figure 5-3 show what perfect correlations look like. In real life, there is almost never a perfect correlation. Returning to the example of height and weight in children, we can observe that some children will become taller and not gain very much weight, and others will become only a little taller and gain more weight. Therefore, there will not be a consistent increase in weight each time there is an increase in height, as is shown in the scatter plot in Figure 5-3, where each spot represents one child, and the spots do not all fall along a perfectly straight line. However, the bigger the value of the correlation coefficient, the more consistent and stronger the relationship is between the two variables.

To test whether or not two variables covary, a correlation statistic is computed and tested to see if the computed value is likely to have occurred by chance. The caregiver experience report does not include any correlation statistics; however, the recovery after surgery article discussed in Chapter 3 (and shown in Appendix A-3) does provide a list of correlation values in Table 2, titled "Correlation Matrix for Study Variables at Each Time Interval" (Zalon, 2004, p. 103) and is copied for your convenience in Table 5-4. You can see that the statistics in the table show the covariation between different study variables. For example, pain at time of hospitalization covaried with depression with a statistical test value of .37. From what we have just learned about correlation statistics, we know this means that pain and depression were connected to each other and, as one increased, the other did as well. We now have a greater understanding of the sentence in the results section of the recovery after surgery report that states "The correlation between pain and depression was significant at each time point . . . " (Zalon, 2004, p. 102). We know that a *correlation* is a statistic looking at covariance or relationships between two variables.

If two variables covary, then they are connected to each other in some way. However, correlation does not tell us how the two variables are connected or whether one of the variables causes the change in the other. For example, if we had no other information besides the correlation statistic for height and weight of children, we would be left wondering whether weight causes growth in height, height causes increased weight, or both tend to increase because of some other factor we have not considered, such as age or nutrition. Therefore, correlations are inferential statistics that explain about relationships but cannot be used to predict because they do not tell us anything about which variable "causes" the other variable to change.

CORE CONCEPT 5-4

A correlation between two variables only tells us that they are connected in some way, not the cause of that connection.

TABLE 5-4

Correlation Matrix for Study Variables at Each Time Interval From Recovery From Surgery Report

	1	2	3	4	5
Initial (Hospitalization)					
1. Pain	—	.37*	.52*	—	−.20*
2. Depression		—	.53*	—	−.09
3. Fatigue			—	—	−.20*
4. Functional status				—	—
5. Self-perception of recovery					—
3–5 Days Post-Discharge					
1. Pain	—	.27*	.39*	.12	−.25*
2. Depression		—	.60*	.36*	−.28*
3. Fatigue			—	.26*	−.13*
4. Functional status				—	−.09
5. Self-perception of recovery					—
One Month Post-Discharge					
1. Pain	—	.33*	.22*	.33*	−.44*
2. Depression		—	.51*	.50*	−.50*
3. Fatigue			—	.42*	−.32*
4. Functional status				—	−.50*
5. Self-perception of recovery					—
Three Months Post-Discharge					
1. Pain	—	.26*	.50*	.39*	−.24*
2. Depression		—	.54*	.43*	−.35*
3. Fatigue			—	.46*	−.34*
4. Functional status				—	−.53*
5. Self-perception of recovery					—

*$p < .01$
Source: Adapted from Zalon, M. L. (2004). Correlates of recovery among older adults after major abdominal surgery. *Nursing Research, 53*(2), 103.

If we look at Table 5-4 again (Table 2 from the article), we see a matrix of numbers that shows the correlation statistics for each of the possible relationships between different pairs of variables. If we want to know whether there was a relationship between depression and fatigue one month post-discharge we look under the heading "One Month Post-Discharge," at the correlation coefficient in the row titled "Depression" and the column numbered 3 (for Fatigue). There we see the statistical value of .51*. The asterisk next to the statistic is decoded at the bottom of the table and indicates that this statistic had a *p* value of .01. This means that in only 1 out of 100 chances would we get a statistic of 0.51 for the relationship between depression and fatigue in surgery patients one month after discharge. Therefore, we decide that there is a relationship between depression and fatigue and will expect to find such a relationship in other groups of post-surgical patients a month after they have their surgery. We also learn from this number that the connection or relationship between depression and fatigue is positive, meaning that as depression goes up, an individual's fatigue goes up as well. Finally, we know that the strength of the connection is moderate because .51 falls approximately halfway between zero, which indicates no connection at all, and one, which indicates a perfect connection.

Numerous types of correlation statistics can be computed between two variables, but the one you will probably find most frequently is the Pearson product-moment correlation, which uses the symbol "r" to represent the value of the bivariate relationship. Besides the Pearson product-moment correlation, other types of correlation statistics include the Spearman rho, the Kendall tau, and the phi. In all cases, the statistic gives the strength of the covariance between two variables.

The results section of the recovery from surgery article presents a number of correlation coefficients in the table, and we see that not all of the correlations reported were positive; in fact, the correlations between self-perception of recovery (item 5 in the table) and the other four variables are all negative. We know from these negative correlations that the connection between self-perception of recovery and factors such as pain, depression, and fatigue is one where as one goes up, the other goes down. If you think about this concept, it makes sense. We would expect that the more pain or depression patients are experiencing, the less likely they are to see themselves as recovered from their surgery.

Because the size of the correlation coefficient reflects how strong the connection was between the two variables, we see that there was a moderate relationship between the variable "pain" and the variable "fatigue" ($r = .52, p < .01$). This is in contrast to the correlation between pain and perception of recovery ($r = -.20, p < .01$). Although both of these connections are statistically significant, the strength of the relationships is different. What we understand from these statistics is that although as pain goes up and perception of recovery goes down, the connection between the two variables is not that strong, whereas there is a moderately strong connection between both pain and fatigue going up.

Tests Looking for Differences Among Three or More Groups

Frequently, nursing research addresses questions about more than just two groups. For example, we might be interested in comparing patients who smoke, patients who have never smoked, and patients who have quit smoking for their rates of respiratory complications after cardiac surgery. We can perform three different t tests to examine differences in complication rates between smokers and those who have never smoked, then between smokers and former smokers, and then between those who have never smoked and former smokers. Keeping up with these comparisons makes one's head whirl, and obviously, the number of comparisons required would become more complicated with the more groups we have. In addition, each time we get a result that is statistically significant, a small chance remains that we are wrong in our decision that the result did not happen by chance. These chances of being wrong add up when we do multiple statistical tests to answer just one question, making our chance of an error in our decision much larger when we do three or more tests on the same set of variables. The alternative is to use a different type of statistical test called an *analysis of variance* (ANOVA).

An **analysis of variance** tests for differences in the means for three or more groups. Although it is not necessary that you do the calculations for an ANOVA, it may be helpful to know what the test does, which is reflected in its name. The ANOVA compares how much members of a group differ or vary among one another with how much the members of the group differ or vary from the members of other groups. In other words, the test analyzes variance, comparing the variance *within* a group with the variance *between* groups. For example, an ANOVA test of respiratory complications in three groups of patients categorized by smoking status calculates how much variation there is in respiratory complications within the patient group that smokes, the patient group that never smoked, and the patient group that formerly smoked. It then calculates the amount of variation in respiratory rate between the smoking patients, the patients who never smoked, and the former smokers. Finally, the test compares the variation inside the groups with the variation between the groups to see their differences or similarities. The test statistic in ANOVA is usually an "F ratio" value, and like other statistical tests, the final test statistic is then compared with a set of statistics one would get if there were no differences between the groups. The F ratio compares the variation between groups with that within groups, and the larger the F ratio, the more variation between groups. However, the value of F ratios differs depending on the number of groups compared and the number of people studied, so it is not possible to make general statements about the meaning of the F ratio, except within the context of significance testing. If the F ratio value for a particular study falls into the area of statistics that have less than a 5% chance of occurring by chance, then we decide there is a statistically significant difference between the groups. In the example of respiratory complications, if the F ratio were significant, we would be able to decide that smoking and smoking history affect the rate of those complications.

Neither the fictional article nor the caregiver experience article used an ANOVA because neither study needed to compare the means of three or more groups. However, in reading nursing research results, you often find this statistical test, or a variation of it, reported in the results section. Other versions of the ANOVA allow the addition of more variables and various interconnections among variables into the ANOVA. Some of the most common are analysis of covariance (ANCOVA), multiple analysis of variance (MANOVA), and one-way ANOVA. For each of these, the basic purpose of the test is to compare means of an independent variable among three or more groups. Some of the most common nonparametric statistical tests that also test for differences among three or more groups are the Kruskal-Wallis and the Chi square test (Table 5-3).

In addition to comparing three or more groups, we often want to look for differences within groups during three or more points in time. Continuing with the example of patients who smoke and their respiratory complication rates, suppose that instead of comparing them to patients who never smoked, we compared smoking patients' respiratory complication rates before and after pulmonary toilet care over a 3-day period. In this case, we are not comparing different groups, but the same group over time. The statistical test used in this type of situation is a repeated measures ANOVA. Like the other ANOVA tests, it calculates differences in variance within the group at each time point but compares those variances to the variances between the time points. Commonly used nonparametric tests for differences within groups at three or more points in time include Friedman tests and the Cochran Q.

Tests Looking at Relationships Among Three or More Variables

Just as we are often interested in differences among three or more groups, we also are interested in how a group of more than two variables covaries. For example, in the caregiver experience article, the authors are interested in how a set of variables, such as caregiver's age, gender, symptoms and perceived burden, all covary in relation to an individual's mental health-related quality of life (HRQL:MCS). If each of these variables is connected to the HRQL:MCS but is also connected to each other somewhat, how much does each variable independently contribute to the variation occurring in the mental health-related quality of life? Our goal is to understand what factors or variables connect to the different HRQL:MCS scores and in what direction and to what extent so that we can use our knowledge of those connections to increase the potential that we can impact the mental health-related quality of life of our patients who are caregivers. If caregivers' scores reflecting their HRQL:MCS were a big pie, each of the factors studied might be a piece of that pie, although those pieces will overlap somewhat, as shown in Figure 5-4. We are interested in seeing not just how much each factor by itself connects, but how the factors overlap so that we know which of the many factors might be the most useful to focus on when planning our EBN care. The statistical procedure that we use to look at connections among three or more variables is called *regression*. **Regression** measures how much two or more independent variables explain the variation in a dependent variable. The regression procedure allows us to predict future values for the dependent variable based on values of the independent variables.

Let us apply this to the study being read by the RN in our clinical case. The researchers in the caregiver experience study know that caregivers' HRQL:MCS differed depending on their gender and their age. They also think that physical symptoms and perceptions of burden are likely to affect HRQL:MCS. While nurses cannot change the age or gender of an individual, they might be able to impact physical symptoms and burden. But how much do these factors covary with HRQL:MCS versus simply varying with age?

Knowing that four variables are connected to mental health-related quality of life is helpful, but it will be more useful for the RN to know the factor that makes the biggest difference so that she knows where to focus her efforts. A regression analysis gives the information needed to know how much different factors independently contribute or connect to a dependent variable. Table 3 in the article from Appendix A-4 reports the results of the regression analysis performed by the authors in order to examine how much of an effect each of the four factors that they had identified contributed to variation in HRQL:MCS. The table has several columns, but we are going to focus on only two of them: the columns labeled "sβ"

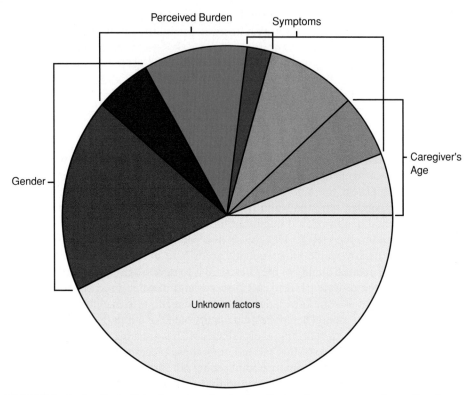

FIGURE 5-4 • Illustration of overlapping factors that make up a person's quality of mental health. *Purple* shows overlap between caregiver's age and symptoms, *blue* shows overlap between symptoms and perceived burden, and *dark violet* shows overlap between perceived burden and gender.

and "R^2 95% CI." Under the column labeled sβ, the statistical value for relative contribution of each of the factors is listed. A **beta** (β) value tells us the relative contribution or connection of an independent variable to the dependent variable. The "s" indicates that the beta given is a standardized value, meaning that the betas for the factors can be compared with one another. Therefore, we can see that, as caregivers' ages rise, their HRQL:MCS scores increase and that as their physical symptoms and burden go up, their HRQL:MCS scores go down. In addition we see that the "Symptoms" factor—that is, the caregiver's physical symptoms—has the biggest number, so symptoms have the biggest effect on mental health quality of life.

The R^2 refers to how much of the variation in HRQL:MCS scores the factor studied explains. The 95% CI refers to what we would expect the beta value to be 95% of the time, given the results that we found in the study. Notice that "Caregiver gender" does not have a value in either column for the first interview time period because it did not covary independently with HRQL:MCS scores at the time of the first interview. Also, notice that the 95% CI is relatively large for the beta value for caregiver age. This tells us that the independent effect of age on HRQL:MCS could range from almost zero to changing the scores by almost 4 points. In contrast, the 95% CI for the physical symptoms ranges from –8.05 to –3.93, telling us that in 95% of samples, we would expect the scores on physical symptoms to decrease mental health-related quality of life scores anywhere from 4 to 8 points. In summary, what you should understand is that each variable in a regression analysis is tested to determine whether it is independently connected with the dependent variable. If it is connected, a test of how much or to what extent it is connected is provided. Knowing this, the RN in our clinical case can see from this result that physical symptoms of caregivers is the biggest contributor for HRQL:MCS and, therefore it may be an important factor to target if she is trying to improve the mental health-related quality of life of N.B. In addition to regression analysis, numerous statistical procedures examine relationships among three or more variables. The names of some of the most common types of procedures used in nursing research are listed in Table 5-3 and include canonical correlation, path analysis, structural equation modeling, and discriminate analysis.

Tests Looking at the Structure or Components of a Variable

We have discussed bivariate statistical tests that look for differences between two variables and tests that look at relationships between two variables. We also have discussed multivariate tests that look at differences or relationships among three or more variables, and we have identified several parametric and nonparametric statistical tests for each purpose. The last general purpose for statistical procedures is to look at the structure or components within a variable of interest. These types of statistical tests are used when the variable of interest is complex and not easily measured using a single item or question. The researcher may collect information about the complex variable using several different questions or measures and then want to determine the connections among the questions or measures. For example, a nurse researcher might be interested in studying patient satisfaction associated with care. Several aspects of care may influence satisfaction, such as availability, communication with providers, cost, and whether expectations for care are met. The researcher might develop 60 statements for a survey, each of which affect some aspect of satisfaction. Responses to the survey may be scores on a scale to indicate the respondents' level of agreement with each of the statements. Scores to all 60 statements can be added together to produce a single score for satisfaction, but this does not help us to understand the important components of satisfaction that make up that score. Statistical procedures, called **factor analysis**, can be used to look for discrete groups of statements that are more closely connected to each other than to the other statements. Factors are the components or discrete groups of measures or statements that covary closely. In our example, the researcher might find that statements about paying bills, insurance, and difficulty getting referrals all covary more closely then statements about communication. These statements might be said to reflect a factor that could be called *barriers to satisfaction*. Factor analysis will identify groups of measures of a single variable that are connected closely enough that the connections are not likely to happen by chance. In clinical practice, a study that uses a factor analysis procedure has the potential to provide knowledge about some of the components or parts that comprise a health-related concept, such as fear, pain, or denial. The nonparametric statistical test that may be used to look at structure within a variable is called *cluster analysis*.

To summarize, several specific statistical procedures are used to test for differences and relationships. The types of tests differ depending on the type of data and whether two, or more than two, variables are to be tested. When any of these tests are applied to specific data, they produce a test statistic that will be symbolized in a unique manner, such as a "*t*" statistic, "*F*" statistic, or "*r*" statistic. The specific statistic from the study is compared with a distribution of statistics that would have occurred in similar data by chance alone if there were really no relationship or difference. If the statistic from the study falls into the range of values that occur less than 5% of the time, it is likely that there was a relationship or difference, and the result is statistically significant. Often, the level of statistical significance is specifically stated in the form of a *p* value or confidence interval.

HYPOTHESIS TESTING

In Chapter 2, we defined *hypotheses* as predictions regarding the relationships or effects of selected factors on other factors. Inferential statistics are used to test whether the predictions in hypotheses are "accurate," so hypotheses direct which statistical procedures are used with the data. The results for two types of hypotheses may be described in a research report. The first type, a **research hypothesis**, is a prediction of the relationships or differences that will be found for selected variables in a study. None of the reports of research that we have read to date have used hypotheses. However, if the caregiver experience article had used a research hypothesis, it might have stated, "Increases in caregiver age, physical symptoms and perceived burden will all negatively impact their health-related quality of life." This hypothesis predicts that as age, symptoms and burden go up, that quality of life goes down. This is a clear prediction that not only will there be a relationship, but also that it will be negative. The authors of the caregiver experience study did not give us predictions in the form of hypotheses; they used research objectives instead. Their objectives are identified at the beginning of their report, and we will discuss these further in Chapter 10.

The second type of hypothesis that may be tested and reported about in the results section of a research report is a statistical hypothesis that is often called the *null hypothesis*. A **null hypothesis** always predicts that there will be no relationship or difference in selected variables. Remember that, in general, researchers want to be cautious about jumping to conclusions based on the results of a particular study. This is why researchers agree that statistical test results are acceptable only when they would occur by chance less than 5% of the time. Otherwise, even if we find a difference or relationship in the data, we decide that it was just a chance happening, and we cannot prove that there was a "real" relationship. The null hypothesis reflects this same thinking by stating our prediction about relationships or differences in the negative, predicting no relationship or difference. The researcher must then find enough evidence to reject that prediction, a statistically significant test result being the evidence that is required.

In summary, a research hypothesis is stated in the positive and predicts the nature and strength of a relationship or difference among variables. It is the researcher's hope that the results of a study support the prediction. A statistical hypothesis is stated in the negative, and it is the researcher's desire for statistical tests to be significant so that the null hypothesis can be rejected. Not all quantitative research studies use hypotheses, but if there are one or more hypotheses, they are usually identified in the section of the report that describes the research problem. Chapter 10 discusses hypotheses in more detail.

IN-CLASS STUDY DATA

To illustrate the use of inferential statistics, let us look at the data that were collected in your in-class study. If you are not using an in-class study, you can refer to a sample set of data in Appendix D that could have been collected in a nursing class. Suppose that before this data were collected, you had observed that your fellow students who were married were generally healthier than those who were not married. You wonder whether this is true and realize that the data from your in-class study could be used to test this idea because a question about marital status and a question about overall health is included. This means there are two variables of interest: (1) marital status and (2) rating of health. The question of interest concerns differences between two groups and might be stated as "Is there a difference in health rating between married and unmarried nursing students?"

To use the in-class data to answer this question, you must first divide the health ratings into two groups: the health ratings of students who indicated that they were married and those who indicated that they were single, divorced, or widowed. Once this is done, it is easy to get an average health rating for the two groups and to see if they are different. If they are exactly the same, or close, you probably do not have to look any further for a tentative answer to your question based on this data. If there is a difference, the next question is whether the difference is in the direction you predicted and whether it is big enough that you can believe that it did not happen by chance alone. Looking at the average health ratings will tell you whether single students seemed to have higher or lower health ratings. However, you cannot judge whether the findings prove or disprove your hypothesis because the ratings may have been simply chance findings. This is the place where inferential statistics come in because if this information is entered into a statistical computer program, you can run a t test to calculate differences in the means for rating of health of married and unmarried students.

If you are using an in-class study, predict whether some difference found in your class data will be significant before your professor runs an independent t test to determine the t value for your in-class data. For the fictional data in Appendix D, the computer calculates that the mean health rating for single students is 3.1 and the mean rating of health for married students is 2.3. These ratings look different and are opposite from what was predicted before data were collected. When we do a t test, we get a t value of 2.7 ($p = .011$), so there is a significant difference in health ratings between single and married students. However, from this data, we can conclude that the evidence does not support the hypothesis that married students are healthier; instead, it supports the opposite idea. In this fictional study, single nursing students had significantly higher ratings of their health than did married nursing students. That it was a statistically significant difference tells us that we can be sure that the difference did not happen by chance alone.

CONNECTING INFERENTIAL STATISTICAL RESULTS TO CONCLUSIONS

There are several important connections between results and conclusions of reports that have used inferential statistics. If inferential statistics were used, we know that the goal of the researcher is to predict that the findings of the study apply to similar situations or groups in the future. Therefore, we expect to find in the discussion and conclusions statement both how the results can be applied to similar situations or groups in the future and what aspects of the study may limit our ability to draw conclusions about future situations or groups. In the fictional article, for example, the author summarizes the findings and then concludes that "Nursing programs that are particularly concerned about shortages in non-acute settings may be able to expand this work force by focusing their recruitment efforts on older students and by further developing or expanding RN to BSN and LPN to BSN programs." The author is saying that in the future, age and type of program of study are likely to be connected with choice of field of study, just as they were in the article. Although the author fails to give any statement of the limitations of the conclusion, the size of the sample—one class of 30 nursing students—might be a reason to consider limiting it.

If the results of a report included hypothesis testing, we should also expect a statement in the conclusions of the report about whether the hypotheses were rejected or accepted. Most important, the meaningfulness of statistically significant results should be discussed in the discussion and conclusions section. Throughout this chapter, we have talked about statistical significance; however, the presence of statistical significance does not necessarily indicate that the results are meaningful for clinical practice. Conversely, lack of statistical significance does not necessarily mean that there is no clinical significance in the results. The presence of statistical significance depends on several factors, one of which is the number of cases in the study. This is logical, given that we are trying to use probability to help us to infer connections or differences in the real world. If the study only includes a few cases or subjects, then the chances of a "weird" or unusual case affecting the average result is pretty high. The test distribution for a study with only a few cases results in a large "green" zone and a small "red" zone because there is a good chance that a single odd case will change the actual test statistic (Fig. 5-2).

CORE CONCEPT 5-5

The size of the sample, or number of cases, in a study affect the likelihood that a statistical significance will be found.

A study that has a large number of cases has a high likelihood of finding statistically significant findings, simply because whatever is found is not going to be affected easily by the chance that an odd case fell into the sample. However, the difference or connection that is found may not be large enough to have meaning for clinical practice. The author of the fictional article, for example, does not give the average ages of students who selected acute and nonacute settings. It is possible that the difference in age was only 1 or 2 years. A difference of this size may be statistically significant but may also be too small to have any meaning when one is trying to recruit individuals to nursing.

A clinical example of the difference between statistically significant and clinically meaningful findings might be a study of ratings of pain, such as the one discussed in Chapter 4. Suppose that this study has 500 subjects and that after one group receives an intervention, the mean ratings of pain are 2.5 (1.3) for patients getting the intervention and 2 (1.5) for patients not getting the intervention. In Chapter 4, we used an example where the standard deviations were different, although the means were the same. In this example, the means are different, whereas the standard deviations are similar. The researcher might report that there was a statistically significant difference in pain ratings between the group that did and did not get the intervention. This means that the difference in ratings was not likely to happen by chance. However, if you look at the difference, it is not large and may not, in fact, be clinically meaningful. You must decide whether a difference of only one half of a point is large enough to warrant implementation of the intervention, even though you may believe that this difference is unlikely to have occurred by chance. Thus, statistical significance does not necessarily imply clinical significance.

We would expect, therefore, that the conclusions of a research study that used inferential statistics would address whether the statistically significant findings were also meaningful findings. We also would expect that the conclusions would address whether findings that were *not* statistically significant might still warrant further consideration because they appear to be clinically meaningful.

CORE CONCEPT 5-6

Statistical significance does not directly equate with clinical meaningfulness.

COMMON ERRORS IN RESULTS SECTIONS

As with the reports of descriptive results, two kinds of problems may be found when reading inferential statistic results in a research report: (1) incomplete information and (2) confusing information. Incomplete information occurs when the results section of reports gives us the statistical test results, including the *p* value or confidence interval, but does not give us the descriptive results needed to interpret the statistically significant result. For example, suppose that the author of the fictional article from Appendix B had told us that there was a significant difference in health rating ($t = 2.1, p < .05$) among students who chose acute versus nonacute fields of practice. The test statistic alone does not tell us which group had the higher health rating, so it is impossible to interpret the meaning of this statistically significant difference.

Another example of incomplete information might be a research report that includes a statement that there was a statistically significant finding but does not provide the test statistic. Because some of the statistics tell us a great deal, the lack of the statistic can limit our understanding of the results. If the author of the recovery from surgery report in Appendix A-3 had told us only that there was a significant relationship between pain and depression, we would have no idea about the direction of that relationship or its strength. It would be conceivable that those who had greater pain had less depression, which would be a negative relationship with the value for "r" being negative. Of course, the author does give us all of the correlation coefficients, so we know that the r value was .37 at the time of initial hospitalization, which tells us that there was a positive relationship and that it was weak to moderate.

A third type of incomplete information is a failure to test for relationships or differences that might be meaningful for understanding the results of the study. The fictional article reports in the results section that age and health rating were both different in students who chose acute versus nonacute fields of practice. One might wonder whether age and rating of health are related. This is a logical question, given what we know about aging and health, and the answer would help us better understand the meaning of the results of this study. However, the author does not test for a relationship between these two variables, so we are left wondering about the possibility of this relationship.

In addition to incomplete information, research reports may present results in a manner that is unclear or unnecessarily confusing. The titles of tables should clearly identify the table's content and should be referenced within the text of the results section. Labels for columns should be consistent with the use of language in the text and with accepted language for reporting statistical results that may be tested and reported about in the results section. The authors of the caregiver experience report might have provided a bit more explanation in Table 3 (Appendix A-4), for example, by telling us specifically what is meant by a "standardized regression coefficient." The third column in Table 3 also is confusing because it is labeled R^2 and 95% CI. We are not sure, however, if the 95% CI is for the R^2 statistic or for the standardized beta that is reported in the row below the R^2 value. Since the authors report 95% CIs for each of the other beta values, we can guess that is their application. Nonetheless, this is a confusing presentation of results.

Lastly, sometimes a researcher may overinterpret or overgeneralize about results from a study. For example, if the author of the recovery from surgery article had taken the finding of a relationship between pain and depression, concluding that all patients who have abdominal surgery will be depressed because they will have pain, that would be an overgeneralization. There was a relationship between pain and depression in that study, but that does not mean that all patients who have pain will be depressed. Similarly, sometimes a researcher actually incorrectly interprets a statistical result. Taking the same example, suppose that an author interpreted the correlation between pain and depression to mean that pain *causes* depression. A correlation means that there is a connection, but it does not tell us that one of the two connected variables caused the other. These last types of errors are not likely to appear in research reports published in peer-reviewed journals because those types of errors will be found and corrected. However, occasionally, research results in the public sector are overinterpreted or incorrectly interpreted.

CRITICALLY READING THE RESULTS SECTION OF A REPORT—REVISITED

In Chapter 4, we looked at six questions that can help you to read critically the results section of a research report. These questions are shown again in Box 5-1. Let us revisit some of these questions now that we have talked about inferential statistics. The second question to consider asks, "Were the results presented appropriately for the information collected?" As we discussed in the previous section, at times, the results presented are either incomplete or confusing. For example, we stated earlier that the caregiver experience results section from Appendix A-4 does not tell us directly that the statistical test results for which they are reporting *p* values in Table 2 are derived from *t* tests. To provide notation indicating *p* values without clearly identifying the statistical test used is inappropriate and can confuse a reader. The third question listed for critically reading results also addresses a concern with Table 2 in the caregiver experience report. That question asks about clear identification of descriptive versus inferential results. This table presents descriptive results for each of the measures in the study, but also reflects inferential results by indicating that there is statistical significance in some cases. The authors probably would have improved our ability to use their research if they had provided descriptive findings, and then had given the results of the *t* tests.

Box 5-1	How to Critically Read the Results Sections of Research Reports

Do the results answer the question "Why did the authors reach these conclusions—what did they actually find?"

1. Did the report include a clearly identified results section?
2. Were the results presented appropriately for the information collected?
3. Were descriptive versus inferential results identifiable if this is a quantitative study?
4. Were themes or structure and meaning identifiable if this is a qualitative study?
5. Were the results presented in a clear and logical manner?
6. Did the results include enough information about the final sample for the study?

As we indicated in Chapter 4, this study was quantitative, so we cannot use it as an example for answering the fourth question for critically reading results sections. However, we can decide about the fifth question, which asks how clearly and logically the results were presented. In general, although the tables in this report were a bit confusing, the authors did use their research objectives to organize the presentation of their results and to clearly indicate this at the beginning of each section. Therefore, we might decide that the results are presented clearly and logically. Finally, the last question refers to information about the sample. The caregiver experience report does provide a table about the characteristics of the final sample in the study, although it is not included within the results section. This table does appear to give us the details about the sample that we might need, such as age and gender. We will have to evaluate this aspect of the results further after learning more about samples and sampling.

PUBLISHED REPORT—WHAT WOULD YOU CONCLUDE?

The RN in our clinical case now has an increased understanding of the results and conclusions of the study examining caregiver experiences in providing care to stroke survivors. She knows that there were several statistically significant differences in how caregivers and noncaregivers score on health-related quality of life measures. She also knows that selected factors, including caregiver burden and physical symptoms, appear to explain partially the mental health quality of life in caregivers. The authors also have indicated that they found only one statistically significant difference in caregiver scores on the quality of life measures from the first to the second year of their study. They state a limitation of the study is the sample because all the caregivers in the study were caring for individuals with major functional disability. The RN must decide whether she can use the evidence from this study to guide her practice with N.B. as well as with other caregivers in the future. However, she does notice that the majority of caregivers in the study were female and wonders if some aspect of the approach to sampling led to more female than male caregivers being included. Since the caregiver that she was initially concerned about is a man, the RN needs to know more about how this sample was selected before she can decide how useful this evidence is for her practice. Chapter 6 addresses samples and how they affect the conclusions we can draw from research.

The RN in our clinical case has learned from the results section of the report that physical symptoms and perceived burden affect a caregiver's mental health quality of life. She does not know, however, exactly what is meant by "mental health quality of life" and the types of physical symptoms that may affect that quality of life. In order to answer those questions, the RN will have to read the methods section of the report, which we will discuss in Chapter 8.

OUT-OF-CLASS EXERCISE

What Do You Want to Know About Samples?

The next two chapters focus on the process of sampling and the meanings of different types of samples. In preparation for reading the next chapter, think about your in-class study sample. Write a list of information that you would like to have about the characteristics of the sample for this study, including a rationale for why you would like that information next to each item. Then, think about what you know about the composition of your class, and assume that an interesting result that has implications for nursing education was found in the in-class data. If you were writing the conclusions of a report about this finding, how would you describe the group of individuals to whom the results might be applied in the future? Write a short paragraph describing this group, including to whom the results probably apply and to whom they probably do not apply. If your class did not use an in-class study, you can do this exercise by pretending that a study was conducted using your class group. List what you would want to know about the people in the study and why. Then, given what you do know about those in your course group, write a short paragraph describing to whom the results of a study with this course group probably would apply and to whom they probably would not apply. After you complete one of these exercises, you are ready to begin Chapter 6.

References

White, C. L., Mayo, N., Hanley, J. A., & Wood-Dauphinee, S. (2003). Evolution of the caregiving experience in the initial 2 years following stroke. *Research in Nursing & Health, 26,* 177–189.

Zalon, M. L. (2004). Correlates of recovery among older adults after major abdominal surgery. *Nursing Research, 53*(2), 99–106.

Resources

Field, A. (2000). *Discovering statistics using SPSS for Windows.* London: Sage Publications.

Locke, L. F., Silverman, S. J., & Spirduso, W. W. (1998). *Reading and understanding research.* Thousand Oaks, CA: Sage Publications.

Pedhazur, E. J., & Schmelkin, L. P. (1991). *Measurement, design, and analysis: An integrated approach.* Hillsdale, NJ: Lawrence Erlbaum Associates.

Polit, D. F., & Beck, C. T. (2003). *Nursing research: Principles and methods* (7th ed.). Philadelphia: Lippincott Williams & Wilkins.

Salkind, N. J. (2000). *Statistics for people who (think they) hate statistics.* Thousand Oaks, CA: Sage Publications.

Talbot, L. A. (1995). *Principles and practice of nursing research.* St. Louis: Mosby.

SAMPLES
To What Types of Patients Do These Research Conclusions Apply—Who Was in the Study?

Samples Versus Populations
  Does the Population for This Study Reflect the Types of Patients or Situations of Interest?
  Does the Sample in the Study Reflect the Population of Interest?
  Does the Approach for Choosing the Sample Limit the Usefulness of the Study Results?

Sampling in Qualitative Research
  Strengths and Weaknesses of Qualitative Sampling Approaches
  Sample Size in Qualitative Research
  Summary of Qualitative Sampling

Sampling in Quantitative Research
  Strengths and Weaknesses of Quantitative Sampling Approaches
  Sample Size in Quantitative Research
  Summary of Quantitative Sampling

Differences in Qualitative and Quantitative Sampling

Problems With the Sampling Process

Problems With Sampling Outcomes

Common Errors in Reports of Samples

Connecting Sampling to the Study Results and Conclusions

Critically Reading the Sample Section of Research Reports

Published Reports—Would You Change Your Practice?

KEY TERMS

Bias	Power analysis	Sampling frame
Cluster sampling	Probability sampling	Sampling unit
Convenience sample	Purposive sampling	Saturation
Criteria for participation	Quota sampling	Selectivity
Generalizability	Random assignment	Simple random sampling
Matched sample	Randomly selected	Snowball sampling
Nonprobability sampling	Response rate	Stratified random sampling
Population	Sample	Systematic sampling

Each of the RNs in the clinical cases discussed in previous chapters had an EBN clinical question and sought an answer through evidence in research-related publications. As we reviewed what each could conclude regarding their questions, we had to wonder whether the results and conclusions of the study could be applied to the patient or patients of concern to the RN. Specifically, we wondered:

1. What are the most effective interventions to meet the complex needs of a woman who is pregnant, is about to become a mother for the first time, is in jail, and is suffering from HIV?
2. What factors affect the recovery rate of elderly patients following major abdominal surgery that should be considered by the nurse when planning predischarge care?
3. What interventions assist and support the health and function of caregivers of stroke patients?

In exploring the topic of research samples, we will use a new clinical case, revisiting the four previous clinical cases as well as the research found by our RNs.

CLINICAL CASE

S.P. is 45-year-old married insurance salesman who suffered a traumatic brain injury (TBI) while skiing last year. He collided with a tree and was in a coma for two weeks. He has had substantial recovery of functioning but requires a considerable amount of care to meet daily needs, and he is still wheelchair bound. Although he has recently gone home from a rehabilitation hospital, he has not returned to work and is on disability. The RN works for the hospital and has been assigned to see S.P. and his wife in the home setting. The RN has been impressed by how difficult all of this has been on S.P.'s wife.

The RN is active in her professional nursing organization, and about a month after she started caring for this family, she attended a local district nursing meeting. While networking at the meeting, she spoke with a colleague who works in intensive care. They discovered that they had a shared interest in the needs of family members of clients with TBI and decided to develop a protocol that addresses family caregiver needs from the moment of hospitalization through the return to the community. They agreed to do a literature search, and the RN from the ICU found an article entitled "Needs of family members of patients with severe traumatic brain injury: Implications for evidence-based practice" (Bond, Draeger, Mandleco, & Donnelly, 2003) (Appendix A-5). Table 6-1 identifies the clinical question of the RN and the key search terms used in her search.

TABLE 6-1

Development of a Clinical Question From the Clinical Case Study

What are the ongoing needs of family members of patients with severe TBI that should be included in a family support program that follows the family from injury until community discharge?

The *Who*	Family members of patients with TBI
The *What*	Needs related to family member injury
The *When*	Immediate postinjury until community discharge
The *Where*	Inpatient setting
Key search terms useful in finding research-based evidence for this practice question	Acute injury
	Caregiver needs
	Family support
	TBI

Regardless of whether we are using EBN strategies to answer questions related to using research to guide discharge planning or to direct the planning of care, education, or programs, it is important to answer the question "To what types of patients do these research conclusions apply?" We must consider this question because a study may address a clinical problem of interest to you, but it may not have used a sample that reflects your patients. As an RN, you will need to understand the implications of different sample types to your ability to use study results as evidence in EBN to address clinical practice effectively. One of the first things that you will need to understand is the difference between a sample and a population.

SAMPLES VERSUS POPULATIONS

As discussed, research is rarely able to include in one study all the cases that might be affected by the research question. A study of cardiovascular risk factors in children with insulin-dependent diabetes mellitus (IDDM), for example, could not possibly study every child with diabetes. A study of female patients with HIV who are pregnant is a smaller group, but it is still impossible to include all of these women in one study. All of the studies discussed so far were interested in understanding something about a larger group of patients than those included in their actual studies. The larger group, called the study **population**, is all of the individuals that the researchers are interested in studying. The population for any particular study is defined by specific common characteristics. For example, the population of interest in the "Motherhood in the context of maternal HIV infection" (Sandelowski & Barroso, 2003) study (Appendix A-1) had three common characteristics; they (1) were mothers, (2) were HIV positive, and (3) were female. The population of interest in the Zalon (2004) study, "Correlates of recovery among older adults after major abdominal surgery" (Appendix A-3), shared characteristics of (1) being elderly, (2) having post-major abdominal surgery, (3) being discharged to home care setting, and (4) being identified as not too sick. In the "Evolution of the caregiving experience in the initial 2 years following stroke" study (White, Mayo, Hanley, & Wood-Dauphinee, 2003) (Appendix A-4), the population shared characteristics of (1) being caregivers, (2) having been in the caregiver role for a 2-year period, and (3) caring for a person who experienced a stroke. Notice that it is possible to clearly identify the common characteristics that comprise each population.

Of course, none of these studies included every member of the population of interest. There are thousands of caregivers for stroke patients. There are thousands of elderly who have abdominal surgery every year, so the research will select a smaller, more workable group for conducting their study. This subset of the overall population that is included in a study is called a **sample**. To understand whether a study applies to your clinical situation, you can start by considering three general questions about the study sample and the related population: (1) does the population for this study reflect the types of patients or situations that I am interested in understanding?, (2) does the sample in the study reflect or fit with the population of interest?, and (3) does the approach taken to choosing the sample limit how much I can use the results of the study?

Most of this chapter addresses the third question, but the first and second questions are also essential to answer in order to understand and use research in clinical practice.

Does the Population for This Study Reflect the Types of Patients or Situations of Interest?

As we have discussed many times, EBN is a process of decision making regarding clinical questions that looks at available evidence to answer a clinical question. If research-based evidence is to be meaningfully considered in your EBN strategy, you will need to decide whether a study addresses a population that is relevant or clinically similar to the patient group you are interested in understanding. To do this, you will need to identify the common characteristics of your patient population. One of the ways to identify clearly the population that fits your clinical question is to use the *Who, What, When, Where* approach to forming an EBN clinical question. As you use this approach, you are, in essence, listing characteristics of the population in which you are interested. This will then give you a comparison of those characteristics of the identified sample within a research report.

Nurses occasionally have a problem using research because they look for studies that exactly fit the specific patients with whom they are working. In the clinical case in Chapter 3, if the RN caring for C.R., the 63-year-old woman who is post-AAA, had searched the Cumulative Index to Nursing & Allied Health (CINAHL) for a study that specifically addressed needs of 60-year-old patients, she would have had difficulty finding studies matched to such a narrow population. In another example, if the RN in the clinical case in Chapter 1 who is caring for A.K., the incarcerated pregnant woman with HIV, had searched for a single study that included all of those characteristics, she would have likely found little or nothing. The combination of gender, pregnancy, HIV diagnosis, incarceration, and adjustment to motherhood as patient characteristics is so specific that no one may have implemented a study focusing on that narrow a population. By broadening the characteristics that define the population to only pregnant women with HIV or to incarcerated women with HIV, however, the RN found two studies. When these two studies are taken together, they cover all of the characteristics that could potentially apply to the RN's specific patient care situation. Yet, too broad a definition of the population might have found studies with populations that were too different from A.K., making them useless in planning care for her. For example, a literature search that used only the term *HIV* would yield a large number of studies, many without any attention to pregnancy or incarceration. Although there may be some overlap between the concerns of the population of women with HIV and women who are in jails, clearly there are some important differences that affect how useful these studies will be to understanding A.K.'s case.

How do you learn what the population of a study may be? Several places in a research report should identify the population for the study, but in this chapter, we focus on the section of most reports that is labeled "Sample," "Sampling Methods," or something similar. In this section of the report, the author identifies how individuals were selected for the study and lists its **criteria for participation**. Remember our definition of a sample—that it is a subset of the population; therefore, the criteria for participation in the study should be the common characteristics that define the population of interest. In the study report used in Chapter 1 from Appendix A-2 on the complex needs of incarcerated women (Kane & DiBartolo, 2002), the authors state that their study included "30 women … who were incarcerated … and who were asked to participate" (p. 215). This tells us that the target population was incarcerated women who were willing to participate, but does not tell us what their legal charges were or for how long they were incarcerated. The RN caring for A.K. might have preferred to find a study with a population that consisted of patients arrested for shoplifting or women sentenced to 10 months of jail time, but a study about adult women who are in jail does match some of A.K.'s characteristics. In contrast, the study used in Chapter 1 from Appendix A-1 on motherhood and maternal HIV infection (Sandelowski & Barroso, 2003) is a metasynthesis study. Here, the findings of several studies were examined, and the actual identification of the sample is more difficult to find. The report did not have a specific section called *sample*, but under the heading "Focus on Motherhood" (p. 472), the authors tell us that "sample size ranged from 3 to 159, with a total sample size of 1,141." The section also tells us that "all of the women were of reproductive age, and most were mothers or were pregnant." These types of statements supply us with sample characteristics that we can compare with the population of interest to the RNs in our clinical cases. In summary, it is important to identify the criteria for study participation in order to understand the targeted research study population and to decide on its applicability to your clinical practice.

Does the Sample in the Study Reflect the Population of Interest?

At first glance, this question may appear to be the same as the first question, but it is not. Once a study defines the population of interest—that is, the larger group we are interested in gaining knowledge about—the researcher must find a way to recruit or get a sample of individuals who are members of that population. This is sometimes more difficult than it might seem. Occasionally, it is not ethical to ask members of the population to submit to the study, and it might be difficult to get members of the population to agree to be in a study. As well, there occasionally may be limits inherent to a setting that make it difficult to get members from the population of interest. We discuss each of these potential problems in getting study samples later in this chapter. For now, it is important to realize that a researcher may define the population of interest for a study one way and end up with a sample that does not fit that planned population.

We discovered an example of lack of fit when we discussed the limitations of the recovery from surgery study. The population of interest for that study was elderly adults who were recovering from major abdominal surgery, but the sample ended up comprising only those elderly who were not considered very sick. The study author acknowledged that this was most likely not the common type of elderly person who had major abdominal surgery. This probably occurred because it was considered too strenuous to enroll very ill patients into the research study, and often it was impractical because the elderly sick patient was too ill to participate in answering the questions the researcher asked. Fortunately for the RN, C.R. was a fairly healthy schoolteacher, so the limitation in the sample-to-population in this case was less of a concern. To read intelligently and to use research, it is important to identify (1) the population of interest, (2) the population for a particular research study, and (3) whether the sample reflects that population of interest.

CORE CONCEPT 6-1

A researcher may define the population of interest in one way but end up with a sample that differs from that defined population.

Does the Approach for Choosing the Sample Limit the Usefulness of the Study Results?

Our third broad question considers how the researcher obtained his or her sample and whether that approach limits how you can use the study conclusions in clinical practice. To address this, we first must discuss some of the unique language used in research to describe samples.

The language used differs between qualitative and quantitative studies because the general purposes of the two types of research differ in two broad areas: (1) constraining versus enriching the complexity of samples and (2) rigidity or flexibility in sampling. In general, qualitative research neither tries to predict future occurrences of the phenomena nor attempts to control any aspects of the phenomena as it is studied. Therefore, samples in qualitative research try to derive what is called *rich samples*. These samples contain as many of the complex aspects of the phenomena as possible. Qualitative research samples are also flexible. As researchers begin to understand more about what they are studying, the sample may change. These approaches to sampling can be contrasted to quantitative research, where the researcher will often attempt to constrain aspects of the phenomena when studying it and the sample is generally rigid, not changing after it is selected. We will now discuss these significant differences between qualitative and quantitative research in more detail.

SAMPLING IN QUALITATIVE RESEARCH

Qualitative

When reading qualitative research, understanding whether the sample fits the population of interest is essential because the subjective experiences of the sample are at the heart of the study. Suppose that a researcher studies homeless patients' satisfaction with health care. The population of interest in such a study would have the characteristics of (1) being homeless, and (2) having had experiences with health care. If the researcher enrolls subjects who have been homeless in the past but are now in some type of housing, even temporary housing, this might alter the fit. The meaning of the experiences for formerly homeless individuals is likely to be different from the meanings for those who are currently homeless. Because the goal of this hypothetical research would be to inform our practice by increasing our knowledge about the overall satisfaction with the experience of receiving primary health care as a homeless person, a sample of formerly homeless individuals would not have been appropriate and would have entirely changed the population for the study.

In our clinical case, the RN is interested in developing a support program for caregivers of TBI patients. In looking for research-based evidence to support her EBN practice, the RN finds the "Needs of family members of patients with severe traumatic brain injury" report (Bond et al., 2003) (Appendix A-5). A qualitative study such as this has a goal of broadly increasing our understanding of the population of interest, recognizing that each piece of the picture that we collect gives us a better sense of the whole phenomenon. In order to accomplish this, the sample must then be composed of individuals who have knowledge of the phenomena. In our example of the researcher looking at homeless patients' satisfaction with primary health care, the phenomena of interest to the research is satisfaction with care. So, to find a sample of this population, she would need to select individuals who are homeless and who, while homeless, had received primary care services.

As the researcher plans to find such a group of individuals, we will notice one of the first obvious things that differentiate a qualitative sample from a quantitative sample. In qualitative research, the individuals who comprise a sample are most often called *participants, volunteers, members,* or *informants* rather than being called *subjects*. Use of these terms reflect the perspective seen in qualitative research that the individuals are an active part of the research process and are sharing their knowledge and experiences with the researcher.

The qualitative researcher is looking for the most content and the most contextually rich sources of data available to understand the meaning of the experiences of interest. Immersion in the experience with as much complexity as possible is critical in understanding these realities and experiences. Therefore, the qualitative researcher wants each participant or informant to be different so as to lend additional insight, or richness, about a particular phenomenon. The researcher will intentionally seek ways to find individuals who are deeply involved and a part of the phenomenon being studied. In the study of family members of patients with severe TBI (Bond et al., 2003), the researcher searched for family members of patients admitted to a neurological level I trauma ICU. In this sense, they could be assured that they were finding severely ill patients, and thus, family members who were deeply involved in the phenomena of interest, supporting patients with traumatic brain injury. Think about how the sample would have been less rich if they used a small community hospital ICU or family members of a patient who had TBI in the past year. Under the "Methods: Setting and Participant" heading (p. 65), the authors list the inclusion criteria for obtaining their sample. This criteria identifies the characteristics of the sample, and, therefore, of the population. They identify (1) that participants were family members of a patient with a diagnosis of TBI who was at least 18 years or older, (2) that the patient had a Glasgow Coma Scale (GCS) score of 8 or less, and (3) that the patient was hospitalized in the ICU for at least 24 hours. In reading this, we then know that the participant sample was composed of family members of someone who is very ill (based on the GCS score) and who has been in the hospital long enough for the family to have had experience with a loved one in an ICU setting. There was no attempt to limit the sample to one type of family or to one type of role such as parent or spouse; rather, acquiring a sample that reflected diversity was the goal. The type of sample used in this study is called a **convenience sample** because it includes members of the population who can be readily found and recruited and are "convenient" for the researcher to recruit.

Qualitative research may also use an approach called **snowball sampling**. A snowball sample is just as the name implies. The researcher will start with one participant or member of the population and will then use that member's contacts to identify other potential participants for the study. The next few participants will share other contacts who may have experiences of interest, thus ever increasing the sample. Snowball sampling is most commonly used when the researcher would have difficulty in finding participants who might otherwise not be identified easily. Snowball sampling often allows the inclusion of several views or experiences.

Another type of sampling used in qualitative research is **purposive sampling**. A purposive sample consists of participants who are intentionally or purposefully selected because they have certain characteristics related to the purpose of the research. The characteristics sought in the sample will vary, depending on the approach taken by the researcher. Occasionally, a researcher's goal is to obtain as much diversity as possible in the sample, but sometimes the goal is to focus intently on a particular aspect of the phenomenon under study. If researchers are interested in understanding smoking cessation, they may wish to look at a purposive sample of individuals who have quit smoking in the last month. In this approach, they will purposefully not recruit individuals who are still smoking or who have been tobacco free for over a year. But the researchers may also take a different approach and purposefully recruit individuals who have tried three or more times to quit but who are still smoking. From these examples, we can see that different experiences with a phenomenon may be used by researchers to select the sample purposefully.

Strengths and Weaknesses of Qualitative Sampling Approaches

A convenience sample for a qualitative study has the advantages of being relatively easy and inexpensive to acquire, but may have the disadvantage of yielding a group of participants that is not as diverse and cannot provide as rich a detail about the phenomenon of interest. For example, a convenience sample of homeless people from just one shelter may yield individuals who have been homeless for only a short time because of the location of the shelter or the type of services offered at that shelter.

Similarly, purposive sampling has its advantages and disadvantages. A purposive sample in a qualitative study actively seeks to enrich the data by including participants who have a particular type of experience, characteristic, or understanding to share. The potential disadvantage to this type of sampling is the possibility of prematurely focusing the data collection on one experience or understanding and missing the broader range of data that may come from a convenience sample.

Sample Size in Qualitative Research

Qualitative sampling strategies are fluid and flexible and are intentionally and thoughtfully revised as the data analysis suggests new avenues to explore or aspects that need additional focus. These strategies are used to seek a detailed and rich understanding of the aspect under study. This process continues until the information shared by participants has become redundant and no new information is being added; at this point, the researcher identifies that **saturation** has occurred. Saturation of data is the point in data collection at which the data become repetitive and no new information or participants is being added.

Sample size is usually dictated by the process of data analysis in qualitative research; data saturation is an example. The size of the sample in a qualitative study is dictated by the method of study and the complexity of the phenomenon of interest. Because the data collection methods in qualitative research yield much data from each participant, the sample sizes in this type of research are usually smaller than in quantitative research. The composition and richness of the setting and participants, rather than the sample size, tell us how useful the results of a qualitative study may be with our own patients. In general, qualitative samples tend to use fewer than 50 participants. Some methods might only require two to five participants. The sampling strategy and the complexity of the phenomenon of interest also dictate sample size in qualitative research.

Summary of Qualitative Sampling

In general, sampling strategies in qualitative research seek to identify participants who have experience with the phenomenon of interest to the researcher and who will bring detail and complexity to the study. Even when a researcher uses a purposive sample to focus on a particular type of experience, the goal remains to have as much depth and detail as possible. As a result, sampling in qualitative research is usually driven by the data being collected and may change as the study progresses. In our above example of smoking cessation research, if the researcher used purposive sampling, he or she might have a sample of participants who have quit smoking in the last 6 months. In collecting data from this sample, the researcher begins to understand that all of the participants had a significant stressor in their lives in the month before they quit. The researcher at this point may begin to seek out new participants who are smokers who have experienced a significant stress in the last week so that the process of making the decision to quit can be more fully examined. The example highlights how qualitative researchers collect data and analyze it concurrently as well as how they can use insights from the data to guide further participant recruitment.

SAMPLING IN QUANTITATIVE RESEARCH

Quantitative

The sampling approaches in quantitative research focus on acquiring subjects who match the population of interest as closely as possible. To accomplish this goal, sampling strategies in quantitative research either attempt to remove extraneous variation from the study subjects or to use strategies that prevent the sample from being limited to any particular group or characteristic. In general, quantitative studies that seek to describe and understand some aspect related to health and health care use sampling strategies that lead to a sample that closely resembles the target population. Studies that seek to predict or to test predictions use sampling strategies focused on eliminating factors that might confuse the results of the study. For example, a quantitative descriptive study of the process of smoking cessation should include subjects who have the different economic, educational, racial, and gender backgrounds found in the community of interest. We saw in the qualitative section above that these were not issues of concern to the qualitative researcher. In contrast, a study of the effectiveness of a smoking-cessation program that compares a group using the intervention to a group not using it should ensure that the groups are similar in factors such as race or education. If these factors differ, they might affect quitting success and make it difficult to determine whether the intervention itself made a difference.

In either case, one of the goals in sampling is to avoid bias. **Bias** occurs when some unintended factor confuses or changes the results in a way that can lead to incorrect conclusions. We say that a bias distorts or confounds the findings, making it difficult or impossible to interpret the results.

The goal of limiting or avoiding the introduction of bias into the study sample is reflected in the consistent use of the term *subjects* to describe the members of the quantitative sample. By using this term, it conveys that the researcher is separate and as removed as possible from those in the sample. The distance and impersonal tone implied by using *subject* is intended to help the researcher to avoid introducing any of the researcher's expectations or interests into the study findings. Just as we saw several different approaches to selecting the qualitative sample, there are many ways to select the quantitative sample. Next, we will look a few of these approaches.

Nonprobability Sampling

Quantitative studies usually use nonprobability samples. **Nonprobability sampling** uses approaches that do not necessarily ensure that everyone in the population of interest has an equal chance of being included in the study. These types of sampling strategies usually are used because they are easier or less costly or because it is not possible to identify everyone in the population. Some of the types of nonprobability samples may sound familiar, as they include convenience samples, purposive sampling, quota sampling, and matched samples.

The same processes are used to obtain a convenience sample in quantitative research as in qualitative research. This type of sample consists of subjects who meet the participation criteria and who can be readily identified and recruited into the study. For example, the study used in Chapter 1 (Appendix A-2) that examined the complex physical and mental health needs of rural incarcerated women (Kane & DiBartolo, 2002) used a convenience sample of 30 women who were in a jail setting. The criteria for participation in the study were (1) being an incarcerated female, (2) having the willingness to volunteer, and (3) having the ability to read and sign the consent form. Any woman in the jail was in the pool and could have been in the study. The pool of all potential subjects for a study is also called a **sampling frame**—that is, the pool of all individuals who meet the criteria for the study and, therefore, can be included in the sample. When the study tells us that the sample was one of convenience, we know that subjects from the sampling frame were included because they could be conveniently accessed, often on a first-come, first-served basis. This means that those who heard about the study first, or were most open to being in a study or happened to be nearby when the researcher came to recruit the subjects, were the ones in the study. Because there was not an equal chance for every woman in the jail to participate in the study, the sample was a nonprobability sample.

Purposive sampling is used in quantitative research as well, particularly when the population of interest is unusual or difficult to access. Remember that purposive sampling is the careful and intentional selection of subjects for a study based on specified characteristics. Although purposive sampling is used frequently in qualitative research, it is used less often in quantitative research because the potential for introducing unintended bias into the sample can be high. None of the quantitative studies discussed so far has used a purposive sample. This type of sample might be used in quantitative research if the researcher were interested in describing family adaptation when a member survives a lethal health problem. The researcher might intentionally seek out the families of individuals who have survived ovarian and pancreatic cancers because they are two of the most lethal types of cancer. Clearly, other lethal conditions occur in health care, but the categories of ovarian and pancreatic cancer are readily identifiable and consistently have low survival odds. Therefore, the researcher might purposely select families with survivors of these two conditions.

Quota sampling is another type of nonprobability sampling in which every member of the population does not have an equal chance of being included in the study. In a quota sample, one or more characteristics are identified that are important to the study, and they are used to establish limits on or quotas for the number of subjects who will be included. The goal is to make the sample more representative of the population in a situation where all members of the population cannot be identified. For example, the researcher studying nursing students' choices of field of practice might have decided that gender would be an important factor to consider. After discerning that the known percentage of male nursing students in her state was 16%, she might have used quota sampling to ensure that her sample would have a similar gender composition. She may have done that by setting a goal of recruiting 21 female nursing students and 4 male nursing students so that 16% of the sample would be male.

The last type of nonprobability sample often used is a **matched sample**. In a matched sample, the researcher plans to compare two groups to explain or understand something that differentiates them but knows that some other important characteristics could confuse or bias understanding. To prevent the other important characteristic(s) from making comparison difficult, the researcher intentionally selects subjects whose important characteristics are the same, or matched. An example of this approach might be found in a study of urinary retention care. Suppose the researcher indicates that the original sample for the study comprised 102 long-term care patients who had a permanent indwelling urinary catheter and 102 long-term residents who were intermittently catheterized. The researcher wants to compare indwelling and episodic catheter patients in terms of how often the patients developed infections and did not want the groups to differ on their risk for bed sores, which can also cause infection. Therefore, the specific factors that put a patient at risk for bed sores such as decreased mobilization, poor nutrition, and the presence of skin tears were identified before the study, and subjects were recruited who were similar on those characteristics but differed on whether they had indwelling catheters or were episodically catheterized. This matched the subjects—that is, they had the same risk factors for infections within each group. Again, all acutely ill patients did not have an equal chance of being in the study because they were included only if they had risk factors for urinary infections that were similar to those of other subjects who differed from them in terms of catheter status. Thus, at the beginning of the study, for each subject in the indwelling catheter group, there was a subject who matched him or her in risks for infection in the noncatheterized group.

Probability Sampling

Quantitative studies that intentionally try to predict some aspect of health are more likely to use probability-sampling strategies than nonprobability strategies. **Probability-sampling** strategies ensure that every member of a population has an equal opportunity to be in the study. The most common types of probability-sampling strategies are simple random sampling and several variations on that sampling: stratified random sampling, cluster sampling, and systematic sampling.

Although **simple random sampling** is familiar to most people, the principles involved in this type of sampling are important to understand. Here, all the members of a population of interest must be identified and listed, and each member of the population is assigned a number. Therefore, to select a random sample, all members of the population must be part of the sampling frame. After deciding how many members of the population will be in the study, the researcher uses some device, such as a random number table (Fig. 6-1) or a computer program, to select who will be in the study. Box 6-1 discusses the use of a random number table to identify a random sample. Researchers arbitrarily pick a number from a random number table, which consists of rows and columns of numbers, and then continues in any direction in the table to select numbers. Because all possible numbers are represented in the table, it is by chance alone that the number of any particular member of the population is chosen.

In **stratified random sampling**, the population of interest is first divided into two or more groups based on characteristics that are important to the study, and then members within each group are **randomly selected**. If a researcher were interested in studying some aspect of nursing students in Wyoming that may be significantly

79	75	64	48	5	70	28	68	79	66	64	40	6	59	30	11	42	29	97	9
65	25	22	58	19	27	80	36	63	16	25	20	12	93	47	1	38	42	19	79
58	13	92	29	56	10	51	38	16	0	97	76	65	40	67	34	20	39	86	79
18	97	73	96	28	54	85	80	9	77	43	47	89	13	24	61	6	63	86	99
91	70	17	84	26	21	82	24	42	32	51	94	89	35	93	10	15	28	71	98
81	78	61	93	75	27	17	39	20	18	66	98	12	73	96	88	31	3	57	72
9	7	49	77	38	53	87	86	52	42	12	14	37	5	50	68	80	4	90	15
50	28	27	49	31	67	53	91	15	48	23	83	90	65	25	69	31	14	79	82
72	66	0	83	52	25	93	26	39	23	10	73	44	58	13	85	21	24	22	79
59	27	90	21	52	41	73	40	83	49	93	97	81	40	49	51	7	44	56	39

FIGURE 6-1 • Random number table of 200 numbers between 0 and 99.

different for undergraduate and graduate students, the population of all nursing students could be stratified—that is, divided according to level of study. Then, the students in each stratum would be listed and assigned a number, and the selection of a random sample would be carried out twice, first with the undergraduate students and then with the graduate students. This strategy is similar to the nonprobability sampling strategy of quota sampling, except that in stratified sampling, members in each stratum have an equal opportunity to be in the sample.

Cluster sampling is a third type of probability sampling that can make it easier to acquire a random sample. This type of sample occurs in stages, starting with selecting groups of subjects who are part of a larger element that relates to the population and then sampling smaller groups until eventually individual subjects are selected. A cluster sample of nursing students in Wyoming might start by listing every National League for Nursing (NLN)-accredited undergraduate and graduate program in Wyoming. A random sample of ten of these programs might be selected, and then a random sample of 200 students might be chosen from a list of every nursing student in those ten programs. Every student in Wyoming had an equal opportunity to be selected for the sample, but the researcher did not have to identify and list every student to select that sample. Instead, the larger element of colleges and

Box 6-1	Using a Random Number Table to Identify a Random Sample

In order to identify a random sample, the researcher must enumerate the entire population. Then, the researcher arbitrarily picks a number from a random number table, which consists of rows and columns of numbers, and continues in any direction in the table to select numbers. Because all possible numbers are represented in the table, it is by chance alone that the number of any particular member of the population is chosen. Therefore, to obtain a random sample of nursing students in Wyoming, a researcher must identify and list all nursing students in the state. If the researcher wants a sample size of 100 nursing students, he or she will assign numbers to each student; pick a number in the random number table; and continue to read off numbers going down, up, or diagonally through the table, until the numbers of 100 students have been picked. Because the goal of quantitative research is to generalize and to avoid bias, a simple random sample is considered the best type of sample because the only factors that should bias the sample would be present by chance alone, making it highly likely that the sample will be similar to the population of interest.

universities with accredited nursing programs was sampled, followed by sampling from those colleges and universities.

The last type of probability sample that may be used in nursing research is a **systematic sample**. This strategy is similar to the random sample because the members of the population are identified and listed. However, rather than using a random digit table to select members of the population, the members are selected at a fixed interval from the list. The selected interval may be every tenth member, every fifth member, or any other interval that will lead to a sample of the size desired. When using a systematic sample, it is important to ensure that the members are not listed in some order that creates bias in the sample. For example, the students from every NLN program of nursing in Wyoming might always be listed starting with undergraduate students followed by graduate students. If the researcher were using systematic sampling, taking every fifth student for a total of five subjects from each program, the students selected might all be undergraduates because only the top part of each list would be included in the sample. If, on the other hand, the students in each program were listed alphabetically, selecting the fifth student for up to five subjects would lead to a sample that was likely to consist of undergraduate and graduate students in the proportion that exists in the population as a whole. Table 6-2 summarizes the types of samples used in qualitative and quantitative research. The same strategy is described using slightly different language, depending on whether it is used in a qualitative or quantitative study.

Strengths and Weaknesses of Quantitative Sampling Approaches

As with qualitative methods, a convenience sample for a quantitative study also has the advantages of being easy and inexpensive, but it has the disadvantage of not having

---

TABLE 6-2

Sampling Strategies for Qualitative and Quantitative Research

Qualitative Research	Quantitative Research
Convenience sample: Participants who are readily available and represent the phenomenon of interest are included in the sample.	**Convenience sample:** Members of the population who are easily identified and readily available are included in the sample; a nonprobability sample.
Snowball sample: Participants who are known to and recommended by current participants are identified and included, building the sample from a few participants to as many as are needed.	**Quota sample:** One or more criteria are used to ensure that a previously established number of subjects who fit those criteria are included in the sample; a nonprobability sample.
Purposive sample: Participants who are intentionally selected because they have certain characteristics that are related to the purpose of the research are included in the sample.	**Purposive sample:** Subjects in the sample are limited to those who have certain characteristics that are related to the purpose of the research; a nonprobability sample.
	Simple random sample: Subjects are selected by enumerating all members of the population, and a completely random process is used to identify who will be included; a probability sample.
	Stratified random sample: Members of the population are grouped by one or more characteristics, and subjects are selected from each group using a completely random process; a probability sample.
	Cluster sample: Groups of the population are enumerated and selected by a completely random process, then individual subjects from within these groups are randomly selected; a probability sample.
	Systematic sample: The members of a population are enumerated and every k^{th} member at a fixed interval is selected as a subject; a probability sample.

control over factors that may prejudice the study. A convenience sample consists of those subjects who happen to be at the right place at the right time to be included in the sample. What brings those people to the "right" place and time may have to do with their age, economic status, education, illness, or history—factors that may then prejudice the results of the study. In addition, because a convenience sample takes those who are readily available, often on a first-come basis, participants who willingly and readily volunteer may differ in significant ways from those people who would be more reluctant to participate.

In quantitative research, purposive sampling is used to identify a sample that has certain characteristics relevant to the population of interest. The advantage is that selected factors are clearly defined and identified in the sample, but the disadvantage is that the greater a sample is limited and defined by selected characteristics, the less likely it is to reflect the population at large. In the example of a purposive sampling of families with a member who has survived ovarian or pancreatic cancer, for example, both of these cancers occur in relatively young individuals, leading to their families being relatively young and making the results less applicable to older families. A second bias that may be introduced in this sample is that cancer may make unique demands on families that other highly lethal conditions, such as a severe closed head injury or acute pancreatitis, do not.

In quantitative research, nonprobability sampling strategies are usually more likely to allow bias to enter a sample and make it less likely to be representative of the population of interest. This is because all nonprobability samples have the potential for some outside unidentified factor directing who is and who is not included in the study. By definition, probability samples eliminate the potential of some outside factor systematically entering into the sample because all of the members of the population have an equal chance of being included. However, probability-sampling strategies have the disadvantage of being complex, costly, or not feasible, given the population of interest. For example, it would not be possible to enumerate all of the homeless individuals in any particular state as one might enumerate all of the nursing students, making a probability sample more difficult. However, it might be possible to enumerate all homeless shelters in a state, use cluster sampling to randomly select shelters, and then randomly select residents of these shelters. This would yield a probability sample of homeless people who are housed in shelters within the state—but not of all homeless people because many homeless individuals do not use traditional shelters.

One approach that is taken to decrease the potential for a bias in a sample using quantitative methods is to assign subjects randomly to different groups. This is not truly a sampling strategy, but more of a research method that is used to offset a potential problem that can occur from nonprobability sampling. **Random assignment** ensures that all subjects have an equal chance of being in any particular group within the study. The sample may be one of convenience or purposive, so there may be some bias influencing the results. However, because that bias is evenly distributed among the different groups, the bias will not unduly affect the outcomes of the study.

Obviously, random assignment is only an option when a study is going to include more than one group of subjects because the process requires giving each subject in the sample an equal chance to be in any particular group. If a researcher were interested in studying HIV prevention for homeless individuals, he or she might use random assignment of different shelters to try to decrease any bias rather than using a convenience sample of one homeless women's shelter. Often random assignment is desirable but not feasible. In our example, if the researcher wanted to test the usefulness of an HIV prevention program for homeless women, there might be great difficulty in creating two groups and in giving such an intervention to some women in a shelter and not to others. Table 6-3 summarizes the advantages and disadvantages of different sampling strategies.

Not all samples consist of individuals. A **sampling unit** is the element of the population that will be selected and analyzed in the study. The unit depends on the population of interest and can comprise individuals, but it can also be hospitals, families, communities, or outpatient prenatal care programs. Occasionally, samples consist of more than one sampling unit. If we continue with our example of a

TABLE 6-3

Advantages and Disadvantages of Sampling Strategies in Qualitative and Quantitative Research

Sampling Strategy	Qualitative Research		Quantitative Research	
	Advantages	*Disadvantages*	*Advantages*	*Disadvantages*
Convenience sample	Easier to identify participants; often provides a breadth of information	May "miss" a source of information that is not readily available	Inexpensive; easier to recruit subjects	Most likely to include biases that make it difficult to generalize
Purposive sample	Focuses research on the potentially richest sources of information	Only likely to become a disadvantage if the sampling becomes too narrowed	Locates a sample that is hard to recruit or identify	Likely to include many unique characteristics that limit the ability to generalize
Snowball sample	Allows the researcher to locate sources of information that might otherwise not be identified or available	Could lead to focusing the research and understanding prematurely		
Quota sample			Allows the researcher to control the sample on selected characteristics, so that it more closely resembles the population of interest	Open to systematic variations that can bias the sample
Simple random sample and stratified random sample			Eliminates likelihood of a systematic bias in the sample, so that results are more readily generalized	Time-consuming; costly; may not be feasible to enumerate the population
Cluster sample			Same advantages as a simple random sample, but more efficient	Population of interest may not be readily grouped or the groups identified may narrow the population
Systematic sample			Can be easy to implement	May introduce a bias if there is some systematic factor embedded into the list that occurs at regular intervals

researcher interested in HIV prevention in homeless women, the researcher might use shelters as the sampling unit and compare two or more types of shelters. Then, the researcher might move to the level of individuals in the shelters. When the sampling unit is shelters, there may be only six or eight in the sample; whereas when the unit becomes the individual residents of the shelters, there may be 75 to 100 in the sample.

Sample Size in Quantitative Research

In addition to understanding how the approach taken to sampling will affect to which patients the results of the study will apply, it is important to understand how the sample size affects the ability to draw conclusions from a study. In quantitative research, the goal of **generalizability** drives the sample size. Probability samples often can be smaller than nonprobability samples because probability samples control for bias through the random selection process. Nonprobability samples must be larger in general so that any unusual or systematic factors that could bias the study will be canceled out by the number of subjects. For example, if the study "Evolution of the caregiving experience in the initial 2 years following stroke" (White et al., 2003) (Appendix A-4) had only included nine caregiver/stroke survivor pairs instead of the 97 used, there would be a good chance that some of those dyad pairs would have unusual circumstances, such as having had significant personal problems prior to the stroke or having been estranged from each other before the stroke, that might bias the results. Even one or two of the nine pairs having unusual circumstances or characteristics could have had a significant impact on the study's results. However, with 194 in the sample (97 pairs), the impact of only one or two individuals with unusual circumstances will not be as great. Therefore, in general, the larger the sample size in a quantitative study, the more likely the sample will be representative of the population of interest, and the more likely the study will apply to our clinical situations.

In addition to the logic inherent in obtaining larger samples to eliminate the effects of odd or unique cases, sample sizes in quantitative research are determined by the goal of having a reasonable likelihood that the inferential statistics applied to the data will yield statistical significance. Remember that inferential statistics are used to calculate a test statistic that is then compared with a distribution for test statistics occurring by chance alone for that particular sample size. The larger the sample size, the more likely we are to get results that are statistically significant—that is, that did not happen by chance alone. However, it is always costly to recruit and implement a study with many subjects, so it is useful for the researcher to know how large a sample is likely to be needed to be able to apply inferential statistics accurately to the data. Quantitative researchers often use a process called **power analysis** to determine how large a sample they will need. This allows the researcher to compute the sample size needed to detect a real relationship or difference in the phenomenon under study, if it exists. You may see a written statement of power analysis indicating that a specified sample size was adequate. In this way, the authors are telling you why they used the selected sample size.

Summary of Quantitative Sampling

The goal of quantitative sampling strategies is to acquire a sample that is as representative as possible of the population of interest so that the findings from the study can be generalized. To accomplish this, quantitative studies control and limit differences in the sample that may bias or distort the results. Quantitative research does not necessarily want everyone in the study to be exactly alike, only that the sample is similar to the population of interest.

Nonprobability approaches, such as quota sampling and matched sampling, limit variations that may bias a study. For example, it is generally recognized that the people who are most likely to agree to participate in research studies are white and educated. There are several social and historical reasons for this, but as a result, researchers may implement sampling strategies that specifically target under-represented groups using a quota or matched sample approach.

The goal of probability sampling is to ensure that every member of a population can be in the study so that no systematic factor defines the sample and makes it different from the population.

Quantitative sampling often limits or controls the variety that qualitative sampling seeks. Researchers in quantitative studies remove themselves from the selection of subjects to eliminate personal bias. Therefore, in quantitative research, a sampling plan is identified and strictly followed, and analysis of data usually is not started until the entire sample is identified and recruited. If the sampling plan includes stratifying or matching, then selected characteristics of the sample are identified and analyzed throughout the selection process, but the findings regarding the variables of interest are not examined until the entire sample is in place. While qualitative studies will thoughtfully change sampling strategies in response to data analysis, a quantitative study will usually follow a clearly identified plan that is determined before sampling has started and that is not modified during the sampling process.

DIFFERENCES IN QUALITATIVE AND QUANTITATIVE SAMPLING

Earlier, we stated that qualitative and quantitative sampling differ in overall goal and approach. Because these goals are different, the strengths and weaknesses of the different strategies for each approach differ as well. This is important to understand because it allows you to understand better how a sample and the approach taken to obtain that sample affect the usefulness of the research for your EBN practice. A summary of the differences in sampling approaches between qualitative and quantitative research is provided in Table 6-4.

CORE CONCEPT 6-2

Sampling strategies in qualitative and quantitative research differ in their goals and approaches, even when they are using a similar strategy.

TABLE 6-4		
Differences in Sampling Approaches Between Quantitative and Qualitative Research		
Sampling Approach	**Qualitative Research**	**Quantitative Research**
General goal of sampling	To include as many sources as possible that add to the richness, depth, and variety of the data	To ensure that only the variables of interest influence the results of the study by limiting extraneous variations in the sample
Approach to sampling	Usually driven by the data as it is collected; therefore, flexible and evolving as the study develops	Established before beginning the process of sampling and followed strictly to avoid introducing bias into the sample
Language for those in the sample	Participants, volunteers, and informants	Subjects

PROBLEMS WITH THE SAMPLING PROCESS

As we discussed sampling, it may have crossed your mind that many patients are intimidated by or distrustful of the research process and may decline to participate. This reluctance is a hard reality of research with human subjects: The goal of finding a representative sample might jeopardize the goal of maintaining the rights of individuals. Chapter 7 will discuss in detail the rights of human subjects, but we will mention here that researchers know that the process of seeking informed consent can bias a sample because of some systematic characteristic that causes certain individuals to decline to be in a study. Studies that examine who generally agrees to participate in research studies show that those who are more educated are more likely to participate than those who are less educated. Thus, in research, the sample may have more highly educated patients than those with less education simply because the consent process is intimidating or because research is not viewed as valuable by those with less education. Clearly, the obligation to ensure that the basic human rights of potential subjects are protected supersedes the concern that consent processes may limit study enrollment, but researchers must consider this factor as they examine the results of their studies.

An associated problem that can occur in sampling is the withdrawal of subjects partway through a study. Individuals who agree to participate may withdraw for a number of reasons, such as personal problems, lack of time, or even physically moving out of an area. A researcher will usually plan for subject withdrawal by attempting to include more subjects in a research study than are actually needed. However, if there is some consistent reason why subjects withdraw, then the ability to generalize results of the study is limited. For example, if subjects in the caregiver experience study who found the process of caregiving extremely stressful decided to drop from the study to relieve one burden, then the final sample in the study would not reflect the general population of caregivers, only the population of caregivers who were not severely stressed. In fact, you will notice that the authors indicate that they started with 181 caregivers but have only included 97 caregivers in their study. They do tell us the variety of reasons why caregivers dropped from the study, including 52 subjects who "refused follow-up after the initial interview" (White et al., 2003, p. 179) (Appendix A-4). The RN from the clinical case in Chapter 4 who was caring for N.B. will have to consider this potential problem with the sample in the study in order to decide whether or not the results can serve as evidence for nursing practice.

Withdrawal from a study is an active statement of a decision to no longer participate in that study. Sometimes subjects do not formally withdraw but simply drop out without notification or are lost to follow-up. In this case, the subject simply cannot be found to complete a study or does not return study materials. For example, in studies of smoking cessation, there is always a concern that the subjects who do not succeed in quitting may drop out of the study due to discouragement. This can lead to the final sample including a higher proportion of successful quitters than is really the case, biasing the results by yielding an artificially inflated success rate.

Whether a potential subject declined to be in a study, withdrew, or was lost to follow-up, it is important to know as much as possible about what happened during the sampling process in order to make informed decisions about the use of the results in clinical practice. Therefore, as an intelligent user of research, you should expect that the sampling section of a research report will tell you enough about the process of acquiring the sample so that you can judge how that process affected the results. Often, that information includes a statement about the number of potential subjects who declined to be in a study, withdrew, or dropped out. When subjects withdraw or drop out of a study, some information is usually given about them. Researchers can use this information to compare the subjects who stayed in the study with those who did not, and they may be able to tell us whether there is some important difference between those who did and did not stay in a study. The caregiver experience article does just that, comparing the caregivers who dropped out of the study with those who stayed in the study on their initial data collection. They report that "there were no significant differences on baseline characteristics (age, gender, living arrangements, education, kin relationship to person with stroke)" (White et al., 2003, p. 180) (Appendix A-4) between those who dropped out and those who stayed in. The authors do not tell us if there were any differences in the characteristics of the family members to whom caregivers provided care.

In addition to concern about who agrees to be in a study and who stays in a study, another problem that can affect the sampling process is the exclusion and inclusion criteria. As discussed earlier, sample criteria define a study's population. A criterion for exclusion is a characteristic that makes the potential subject ineligible for the study, and a criterion for inclusion is a characteristic that makes the subject eligible for the study. Researchers choose to focus on inclusion or exclusion, depending on the nature of the desired sample. In a convenience sample in which numerous subjects are being sought, a researcher will generally discuss exclusion because most individuals will be eligible to participate, and only a few will be excluded. A study that aims for a tightly controlled sample will more likely describe criteria for inclusion because the focus is on who can enter the study.

In either case, these criteria define the study's population and may limit how the results can be used in practice. For example, an RN working on a surgical unit in a large, multicultural city would certainly find the recovery after surgery study relevant to practice. However, the study on recovery from surgery excluded subjects who were unable to read or write English, thus excluding a large number of the population of interest in this RN's situation. To use the results of the recovery from surgery article in practice, an RN on an urban surgical unit would need to decide if results with subjects who do speak and write English are likely to be meaningful for those who do not.

The last problem with the sampling process is having incomplete data. This is a problem of data collection, but it is closely linked to how a sample may be changed or limited, which affects how useful it is for clinical practice. *Incomplete data* refers to partial information about the variables in a study. Although the specific problems that can lead to incomplete data are addressed in Chapter 8, the effect of this is that the researcher may drop data about selected subjects from the analysis of the results. This raises the question of whether those subjects had some characteristic or characteristics that led to their incomplete data. If so, then a systematic bias will be introduced into the final sample.

Suppose, for example, that some of the subjects in a smoking cessation study completed only part of a questionnaire used by the researcher and did not answer questions about how much they were smoking after they completed a smoking-cessation program. If the researcher drops these subjects from the analysis (because the amount of smoking after the program is a major variable in the study, and there are no data available for these subjects), then it is likely that the sample is biased in the direction of subjects who were successful and, therefore, willing to report their smoking status. We do not know why the data were incomplete, but we must be concerned that the reason is connected to the variables under study.

In summary, several aspects of the sampling process can lead to problems with the final study sample. The criteria used to identify who will be included or excluded from a study may narrow the sample to the point that the population represented no longer reflects the characteristics of real patient populations. Subjects may withdraw or fail to follow up for some consistent reason that is related to the purposes of the study itself, thus limiting what we can learn from the study. Incomplete information may be collected because of some factor that relates to the study, causing some data about subjects to be dropped from the data analysis and changing the actual sample. As intelligent readers and users of research, nurses must understand not only the strengths and weaknesses of different sampling strategies discussed in this chapter, but also what can go wrong with the sampling process and how that affects the meaning of the study. Table 6-5 summarizes the problems discussed. Other factors that can lead to problems with samples are discussed in the next section.

PROBLEMS WITH SAMPLING OUTCOMES

In addition to problems with the sampling process, some problems can occur with the sampling outcomes—that is, the final sample—that are only indirectly related to

TABLE 6-5

Potential Problems with the Process of Sampling

Problem	Example
Subject withdrawal from study	After starting in a study, subjects may decide that they do not want to continue to participate. If some aspect related to the study leads to withdrawal, it can bias the sample.
Lost to follow-up	After agreeing to be in a study, subjects become unavailable to be in it. This may include not returning questionnaires, missing appointments, moving, or having a change in telephone number. If the subjects lost to follow-up represent a particular characteristic related to the study (perhaps high income), then the final sample may have a bias.
Exclusion/inclusion criteria applicability of the sample	If a sample is tightly controlled or restricted to make the research successful, it may lead to the population being so specific that clinical meaningfulness is limited.
Incomplete data	Data are not provided, are skipped, or are missed, causing the researcher to drop subjects from the analysis of the results. If there is some systematic reason for the data being incomplete, dropping subjects can bias the results.

the strategy used and problems that can occur in the sampling process. Previously, we discussed the importance of avoiding bias, an unintended factor that confounds the findings of a study, in a sample. Some sampling strategies, such as nonprobability sampling, are more open to a bias, whereas others, such as probability sampling, are less open to it. When a researcher uses a nonprobability sampling strategy, the process may be implemented correctly, but the resulting sample may still be biased.

One type of bias that can be introduced in a nonprobability sample occurs when a researcher fails to recognize or consider subjective factors or approaches that could influence participation in the study. For example, a researcher may be more comfortable approaching either men or women when trying to recruit subjects, thus unconsciously biasing a study in the direction of one gender. In addition, a researcher may collect data only at a certain time of the day, such as Monday through Friday, between 8 AM and 5 PM, preventing anyone who works 12-hour shifts or night shifts from being in the study. If type of work and hours worked are related in some way to what is under study, then a bias has been introduced.

Another kind of bias may occur as a result of the unique characteristics or perspectives of the person who is actually recruiting subjects. For example, because an RN's main role is to provide care for patients, he or she may not be particularly motivated to provide a patient with information about the potential to participate in a study or may conclude that a patient does not need to be bothered with a study. An example of this introduction of bias into a sample might be a study that is conducted in a clinic that cares for both physical and mental health problems. If the person recruiting subjects primarily works with the mental health patients and recruits familiar patients, then the subjects in the study are more likely to have mental illness than the overall population of the clinic.

A second problem that can occur with samples is **selectivity**. Selectivity is the tendency of certain population segments to agree to participate in studies. In this case, the bias is not introduced by the researcher but by those people who are willing and interested in being in a study. We have already discussed one kind of general selectivity that occurs in all research: the tendency of more educated individuals to agree to participate compared with less educated individuals. However, selectivity can occur that is more specific to the purposes of a particular study. A particular study may attract people who are worried about the problem under study or those who are lonely and want someone with whom they can talk. It may be that mostly women are willing to participate in a particular study or, perhaps, only people with family members who have experienced a particular problem will return a mailed questionnaire. The difficulty for the researcher and for the user of research is to determine whether some aspect of the study may have led to selectivity in the sample and how this, in turn, affects the knowledge gained from the study.

Limited response rates can be another problem with samples. **Response rate** is the proportion of individuals who participate in a study divided by the number who agreed to be in a study but did not participate in it. Response rate is not a significant problem when the study occurs in a controlled setting, such as a hospital, because those who agree to participate are essentially a captive group. However, in almost any research survey in which subjects are recruited and asked to return a questionnaire or provide data by appointment, some individuals do not return the questionnaire or keep the appointment. As with the other problems that affect samples, we need to know who the nonresponders are and why they did not respond. Their lack of a response caused by a factor related in some way to the study could bias the sample. In these types of situations, the research report should tell you the response rate so that you have an idea of whether a large or small number of possible subjects did not participate in the study. Withdrawal and dropping out of a study are two reasons why response rates can be low.

All of the problems in samples that we have discussed occur in recruiting subjects for any type of study, but they will cause more problems in nonprobability samples than in probability samples. Although the potential bias of a low response rate can affect a random sample, the effects of selectivity and researcher bias are mostly offset in a random sample because the entire population is enumerated, and all members of the population have a chance of being included in the study. Therefore, it is common to find more detail describing the sampling process and the final sample when nonprobability sampling is used because the researcher wants to ensure to the reader that steps were taken to prevent the potential biases that may be present in the final sample.

In summary, three factors are related to both sampling strategy and the sampling process that can lead to problems in samples. The first is bias *introduced by the*

TABLE 6-6	
General Potential Problems with Samples	
Problem	**Example**
Bias in subject recruitment	Some aspect of the recruitment process allows an unidentified factor to enter into the identification of subjects requested to participate in the study. Examples include time of day of sampling or recruiter comfort level with selected subjects. *Selectivity:* Certain subjects volunteer to be in the study due to some characteristic that could relate to the problem being studied. Examples include subjects who are older and lonely being more available or subjects who care about a particular problem volunteering. This can lead to over-representation of one segment of the population in the sample.
Response rate	Many potential subjects or actual subjects do not participate in the study. If a study has a low response rate, then the ability to generalize the results of the study to the entire population of interest is limited.

researcher or the individual recruiting the sample that reflects the beliefs or characteristics of that researcher or recruiter. The second is *self-selection by individuals* within the population that can lead to a bias. The third is a *limited response rate* that makes us wonder about the characteristics of those who did not respond and how they differ from those who did. Table 6-6 summarizes these three types of problems with samples.

COMMON ERRORS IN REPORTS OF SAMPLES

The most common error that occurs in study reports of sampling is a lack of adequate detail, leading to the inability to decide whether the types of subjects or participants allow us to apply the results of the study to our clinical situation. In qualitative research, this error will most likely take the form of an inadequate description of the study setting and participants. We have been using the example of a researcher examining a study pertaining to homeless individuals' satisfaction with health care. In order to determine if the results of such a study are useful to our clinical practice, we must have information about the environment of the participants. If this research had only used participants who were housed in substance-free shelters, the understanding gained from the study would be less complete than the understanding gained from a study of participants from several settings, including a clinic, a soup kitchen, and different shelters. The qualitative study of motherhood in context of maternal HIV infection (Appendix A-1) provides some useful information about looking at the setting for a study. The Sandelowski and Barroso study (2003) was a metasynthesis study. As such, it examined results from 114 published studies or reports. While the authors do not specifically state it, a logical conclusion would be to assume that this many studies were conducted in somewhat different settings. The authors do tell us that the included studies were conducted with women living with HIV-positive status in the United States. However, more information about the composition of the communities, the living arrangements of the participants, and the length of time that the different women have been HIV positive would have further increased our understanding about to whom the results of this study may relate.

In quantitative studies, the information that may be missing or inadequate in a research report usually involves the process of acquiring the sample. To judge either the representativeness of a sample or whether the sample reflects the clinical population of interest requires knowing the sampling strategy and the sampling criteria as well as how the strategy was implemented. For example, a convenience sample of nursing students exiting a college of nursing building at lunchtime is more likely to be representative of the nursing students in that college than a convenience sample of students from any one particular classroom. This is because students who exit the building are more likely to reflect a range of levels of study, whereas a single class will mostly consist of students at the same level.

Similarly, a random sample of homeless shelters that then takes a convenience sample of homeless individuals is less likely to yield a representative sample of homeless persons than a random sample of those staying at all shelters on a particular night. To use information about sampling intelligently, we must know the setting where the study occurred and the process of implementing the sampling plan. We also must be given the descriptive statistics that relate the characteristics of the final sample acquired. For example, consider the sample for the recovery from surgery article (Zalon, 2004) (Appendix A-3). Nothing in the sampling plan for that study indicates an intention to limit the study to Caucasians, yet the sample was 99.5% non-Hispanic whites. The author tells us in the report section called "Sample" that "Patients 60 years of age or older who had undergone abdominal surgery were recruited from three community hospitals" (p. 101). She does not mention the geographical location of those hospitals. Only by reading carefully later in the report do we see that the sample was almost all white and, therefore, that the results of the study only reflected Caucasians.

CONNECTING SAMPLING TO THE STUDY RESULTS AND CONCLUSIONS

We started this chapter by asking whether the results and conclusions from the five different studies used so far could be used to guide practice in the different clinical situations described in previous clinical cases. Sampling strategies connect to the results of a study in several ways. In both qualitative and quantitative studies, the characteristics of the sample affect the meaning of the results. The appropriateness and focus of sampling in a qualitative study both are driven by and drive data collection, and the detail and complexity of the resulting themes or theory will reflect that sampling. In quantitative studies, the sampling strategy dictates how certain we can be that the results found represent what exists in the real population. Along with sample strategy, sample size also affects the believability of study results. In the clearest connection between sampling and the potential results, some studies require a certain sample size to use certain inferential statistical procedures.

Sampling should also be connected to the conclusions of a study. The nature of the sample and the sampling strategies used may be either a limitation of the study or an aspect that needs further evaluation. For example, let us take the study we introduced in this chapter, "Needs of family members of patients with severe traumatic brain injury" (Bond et al., 2003) (Appendix A-5). In this study, the authors identified the setting as a level I neurological ICU unit. In the conclusions section, the authors state, "Results of studies on the need of families of patients with traumatic brain injury may indicate nurses have overlooked an important concept, namely empowerment of patients and patient's families" (p. 71). This conclusion fits with the sample used. If the authors had stated that their conclusion applied to families of patients with any kind of traumatic injury, we would have had to question the connection made. To determine whether this is a correct conclusion, another study may be needed that tests empowerment strategies in a similar population.

CRITICALLY READING THE SAMPLE SECTION OF RESEARCH REPORTS

Box 6-2 provides us with questions to ask when critically reading the sample section of a research report. The first question is "Did the report include a clearly identified section or paragraphs about sampling?" This is fairly straightforward, yet it is surprising that sometimes we have to hunt to find the information about sampling. In the report "Needs of family members of patients with severe traumatic brain injury" (Bond et al., 2003) (Appendix A-5), we can easily find the sample information

---

Box 6-2 **How to Critically Read the Sample Section of a Research Report**

Does the report answer the question "To what types of patients do these research conclusions apply—who was in the study?"

1. Did the report include a clearly identified section or paragraphs about sampling?
2. Did the report give me enough information to understand how and why this sample was chosen?
3. Is there enough information about the sample to tell me if the research is relevant for my clinical population?
4. Was enough information given for me to understand how rights of human subjects were protected?
5. Would my patient population have been placed at risk if they had participated in this study?
6. Can I identify how information was collected about the sample?

on page 65 under the heading "Method: Setting and Participants." However, in the article "Motherhood in the context of maternal HIV infection" (Sandelowski & Barroso, 2003) (Appendix A-1), it is more difficult to find information on the sample. Part of this is reflective of the different types of research methods used, and some may be the style of the authors' writing or the format of the journal in which the report is published.

Our second question is "Did the report give me enough information to understand how and why this sample was chosen?" The report found by the RN in the clinical case for this chapter, "Needs of family members of patients with severe traumatic brain injury" (Bond et al., 2003) (Appendix A-5), is a good example to look at to answer this question. It gives us a sense of who the sample represented—family members of patients admitted to an 11-bed neurological ICU unit in a level I trauma center—and identifies further inclusion criteria. The article gives a clear sense of who were included in the sample, but do we know why they were chosen? This is less clear, and in order to understand this, we will need to read the review of the literature section, which will be discussed in Chapter 10.

Our third question is "Is there enough information about the sample to tell me if the research is relevant for my clinical population?" This is an important topic in EBN practice. If you plan to use research-based evidence in order to answer clinical questions, you need to critically examine if the sample is similar to the population in which you are interested. The first part of answering this is based on how well you have formed your clinical question. As you remember from Chapter 1, your question gives a "Who, What, Where, When" that establishes who and what makes up your clinical population. Once you know whom you are interested in, you then need to see what the report tells you about the sample. The clinical case for this chapter yielded a clinical question of "What are the ongoing needs of family members of patients with severe TBI that should be included in a family support program to follow family from injury until community discharge?" This clinical question tells the RN in our case that the researchers are looking for evidence about a population that includes (1) family members of TBI patients, (2) family members who can describe their needs, and (3) family members whose TBI patient ranges from a newly injured patient to a patient moving to community placement. If we then check the report, we see that there is a nice match between the RN's clinical population of interest and the sample.

As we continue to critically read the sample section of a research report, we come to our fourth question, "Was enough information given for me to understand how rights of human subjects were protected?" The issue of using human subjects will be discussed in detail in Chapter 7, but we probably have some awareness now that sample subjects can be vulnerable and have rights even if they agree to participate in research. All subjects need to know the risks of any research and to have the right not to be coerced into participation. In the "Needs of family members of patients with severe traumatic brain injury" report (Bond et al., 2003) (Appendix A-5), the authors tell us clearly on page 65 about the rights of human subjects. They state that consent forms were signed by all participants and that all participants were given an explanation of the research study including "the risks, the benefits, the time commitment, measures taken to ensure anonymity and confidentiality, and the voluntary nature of the study." We will see in Chapter 7 that this is a good, clear statement regarding the protections of subjects' rights. We see similar but perhaps less clear statements in other reports that we have read. For example, in the Kane and DiBartolo report of "Complex physical and mental health needs of rural incarcerated women" (Appendix A-2) used in Chapters 1 and 2, we see a statement in the sample section on page 215 that "Participants who declined to participate were not asked the reason why, as this was thought to be a form of coercion; moreover, it was feared that such questioning would interfere with requests for future health care." Here, the researchers are identifying to their readers that they were aware of the need to protect the rights of the sample and that they took steps to do so.

The fifth question we can ask is "Would my patient population have been placed at risk if they had participated in this study?" In order to answer this, you need to be clear of who your patient population is. Much like we stated in addressing the third question, a strong clinical question needs to be formed with a clear *Who, What, Where,* and *When* in order to answer this. In our clinical case, our RN is interested in the ongoing needs of family members of patients with severe TBI that should be included in a family support program to follow family from injury until community discharge. As she reads "Needs of family members of patients with severe traumatic brain injury" (Bond et al., 2003) (Appendix A-5), the RN will need to think about what the sample was asked to do while they were participating in the study. In the same study, the family members were asked to participate in interviews to discuss their needs. As we think about it, there is usually not much risk to the sample when participating in interviews. But what if the researcher had decided to take blood specimens to measure serum cortisol and track the stress level of family members in that manner? We can now see a little more risk is present. The subject may bleed from the site of the blood draw, or the site might become infected. While unlikely, it is not risk free. Finally, what if the researcher in this study had decided to include brain scans using the injection of a contrast dye prior to the scan in order to measure activity in the stress-related areas of the family members' brains as they experienced having a family member in the ICU? We can now see a considerable increase in the risk to the sample. The injection of a dye prior to the brain scan will give the best results, but the dye can be dangerous, people can be allergic to it, and the injection might be the source of significant complications. Thus, to answer our fifth critical question, we need to look at what our sample was asked to do and then decide if our population could, and would, be willing to do the same procedure.

Our final question is "Can I identify how information was collected about the sample?" This is very important because it begins to speak to your ability to implement an evidence-based change in patient care based on the study. The RN in our clinical case about meeting the needs of family members of patients with severe traumatic brain injury is interested in helping the families of her patients. If she is to make changes, she will want to see if the information collected during the study could reasonably be collected in her population. The authors of traumatic brain injury study (Bond et al., 2003) report that they collected information in the form of interviews. They also state that the interviews were conducted in private areas of the waiting room.

What is not as clear is how often the interviews were collected and whether the time frame and number of interviews were the same for every participant or if they varied based on the status and length of stay in the ICU of the family member.

PUBLISHED REPORTS—WOULD YOU CHANGE YOUR PRACTICE?

The importance of being able to critically read something like the sample section of a report is to allow you to become comfortable in deciding which evidence you should use in EBN. As your skill at reading research-based evidence improves, the overarching question becomes, "Should I change my practice based on this published report?"

In this chapter, we have concentrated on critically reading the sample section as part of reaching a conclusion about EBN. We have seen thus far that sampling strategies discussed in a report are directly connected to results and conclusions and that understanding the language and meaning of sampling in research adds one more piece to the puzzle of reading and comprehending research for use in EBN practice. Once you have decided whether the population for the study reflects the type of patients or situations that are of interest to you, the subjects' rights were protected, the sample reflects your population, and the approach taken to choosing the sample limits the meaning of the study, you are well on your way to knowing whether the study results can be applied to your clinical question.

As we review the reports that we have examined so far, you may be starting to see that the RNs in our clinical cases have not so much changed their minds about practice as much as they have acquired a better sense of how useful these research studies will be for their practice. They have received insight into other issues to consider, and they have raised other questions. EBN provides information, but it will never directly tell you what to do. As the RN, you will always need to think through the evidence and apply it to your practice in the best way.

In summary, information about the sampling strategy and the actual sample are important in understanding which results of a study may apply to your clinical question. Unique language is associated with the sampling process for both qualitative and quantitative research. Sampling in qualitative research gathers as rich and complete a set of data as possible, and sampling strategies are guided by and may change based on the concurrent data analysis. Sampling in quantitative research eliminates potential bias and gathers information from a subset of the population that closely resembles the actual population. Sampling strategies in this type of research are carefully planned, with important characteristics defined and used to limit or control the subjects. Probability samples are considered to be better than nonprobability samples in quantitative research because these types of samples eliminate systematic bias, but they are also more difficult and costly than nonprobability sampling. Sample size depends on the strategy and methods used, with qualitative samples generally being smaller than samples for quantitative studies.

Understanding the language of sampling and the meaning of the sampling strategies helps to make the relationship clear between the sample and the results and conclusions of the study. This chapter focused entirely on the language and process of sampling in quantitative and qualitative research. What we have not discussed is the important subject of the rights of individuals who participate in research. This topic is discussed in the next chapter.

OUT-OF-CLASS EXERCISE

Free Write

Before you move on to the next chapter, take a moment to think about the in-class questionnaire that you may have completed or about some past occasion when you were asked to participate in some type of research. Write a paragraph describing how the study or questionnaire was explained to you and what you were told with regard to filling it out. Then, write your thoughts about whether your rights, safety, and privacy were protected. Finally, write down types of individuals or situations that you feel should be excluded from participating in research . What makes you believe that these individuals or situations should or should not be included in research? Refer to these paragraphs as you read Chapter 7.

References

Bond, A. E., Draeger, C. R. L., Mandleco, B., & Donnelly, M. (2003). Needs of family members of patients with severe traumatic brain injury: Implications for evidence-based practice. *Critical Care Nurse, 23*(4), 63–72.

Kane, M., & DiBartolo, M. (2002). Complex physical and mental health needs of rural incarcerated women. *Issues in Mental Health Nursing, 23,* 209–229.

Sandelowski, M., & Barroso, J. (2003). Motherhood in the context of maternal HIV infection. *Research in Nursing & Health, 26,* 470–482.

White, C. L., Mayo, N., Hanley, J. A., & Wood-Dauphinee, S. (2003). Evolution of the caregiving experience in the initial 2 years following stroke. *Research in Nursing & Health, 26,* 177–189.

Zalon, M. L. (2004). Correlates of recovery among older adults after major abdominal surgery. *Nursing Research, 53*(2), 99–106.

Resources

LoBiondo-Wood, G., Haber, J., & Krainovich-Miller, B. (2002). Overview of the research process. In G. LoBiondo-Wood & J. Haber (Eds.), *Nursing research: Methods, critical appraisal, and utilization* (5th ed.). St. Louis: Mosby.

Locke, L. F., Silverman, S. J., & Spirduso, W. W. (1998). *Reading and understanding research.* Thousand Oaks, CA: Sage Publications.

Pedhazur, E. J., & Schmelkin, L. P. (1991). *Measurement, design, and analysis: An integrated approach.* Hillsdale, NJ: Lawrence Erlbaum & Associates.

Polit, D. F., & Beck, C. T. (2003). *Nursing research: Principles and methods* (7th ed.). Philadelphia: Lippincott Williams & Wilkins.

SAMPLING ERRORS AND ETHICS: WHAT CAN GO WRONG?

LEARNING OBJECTIVE:

The student will evaluate the sampling process, considering legal and ethical principles and potential problems inherent in that process.

Which Nursing Actions Are Research and Require Special Ethical Consideration?

Informed Consent

Critically Reading Reports of Sampling and Recognizing Common Errors

Published Reports—What Do They Say About Consent and the Sampling Process?

KEY TERMS

Anonymous	Five human rights in research	Practice
Assent	Informed consent	Risk:benefit ratio
Coercion	Institutional review board	Withdrawal
Confidentiality	(IRB)	

CLINICAL CASE

We have thus far looked at several aspects of the process of research as we have followed our RNs in the four clinical cases discussed in earlier chapters. As you can see, there is much to consider as a nurse draws conclusions about clinical questions that are based on research studies. For example, in Chapter 6, we saw the importance of considering the sampling approaches used in studies. In Chapters 4 and 5, we saw the importance of considering inferential and descriptive statistics, or in Chapter 3, the importance of carefully critiquing the discussion and conclusions sections of studies. However, in addition to knowing about the sampling approach, statistics used, or the conclusions reached, we must also understand the legal and ethical principles that guide the conduct of the researcher in today's world. Ethical and legal considerations are important because they help us understand who can be recruited into research studies, how the research can recruit these people, and how the studies are to be conducted. Understanding the ethical and legal issues surrounding research also helps us to understand why we often do not find studies on the specific populations with which we are working, or those that we are interested in knowing more about.

To better understand the connections between legal and ethical principles and the research process, consider the following modified version of the clinical case from Chapters 1 and 2, "Complex physical and mental health needs of rural incarcerated women" (Kane & DiBartolo, 2002) (Appendix A-2). The RN in the prison clinic recognizes that A.K.—the 20-year-old woman who is incarcerated in a minimum security prison to serve a 10-month sentence for possession of cocaine—needs both education and support in preparation for her maternal role. Remember that the patient in our clinical case is 5 months pregnant, she has tested positive for HIV, and the nurse realizes that A.K. fits the criteria for a research study that is being implemented in her prison clinic. The study describes maternal bonding in women diagnosed as HIV positive, replicating an earlier study but using a sample of patients who have a history of substance abuse. The researcher for the study has met with all the staff in the prison unit and has oriented them to the study protocol, including the informed consent process that must be completed before any patient is enrolled in the study. The RN certainly wants to help with any research that will eventually serve patients, but she also wants to be sure that she does not cause A.K. any harm or introduce additional stress by asking her to decide whether to participate if the study is not worthwhile. This chapter first discusses how the RN can determine that more good than harm should come from the study of maternal bonding and that the study has a likelihood of contributing to our knowledge. The chapter then describes some of the problems that can arise when recruiting a sample for a study and how that can affect the usefulness of the study for clinical practice.

WHICH NURSING ACTIONS ARE RESEARCH AND REQUIRE SPECIAL ETHICAL CONSIDERATION?

One important notion regarding research ethics is being able to understand when a particular nursing action is research and when it is a care practice. Research actions require full patient consent and institutional review board (IRB) authorization (concepts we will discuss shortly). However, practice actions are held to a different standard. Sometimes nurses may be asked to collect new data or to perform their care actions in a different manner. It is important for the nurse to be able to determine if the new action is research or if it is new care practice in order to safeguard the patient.

While both research and practice can often look alike and can actually occur together, they are different primarily in the purpose and expected outcome. The Belmont Commission Report (1979) defined ethical principles for the protection of human subjects of research and in doing so provided guidelines for deciding if an action is research or if it is practice. **Practice** is comprised of actions that are planned and implemented exclusively for the enhancement of health and the improvement of the well-being of an individual. Research, on the other hand, is comprised of systematic actions that are planned and implemented exclusively to test a hypothesis, to examine a phenomenon, to allow for conclusions to be drawn, or to generate new knowledge or confirm past knowledge. Research does not have any outcome that specifically improves the patients' health or well-being.

Two professional documents exist to help an RN make decisions regarding the ethics of research. These documents are from the American Nurses Association

(ANA) and from the International Council of Nurses (ICN). The ANA's Code of Ethics for Nurses was approved by the ANA House of Delegates in 2001 and provides details on the ethical standards of RNs (ANA, 2001). The ICN Code of Ethics for Nurses (ICN, 2000) is an international code of ethics for nurses and was first adopted by the International Council of Nurses in 1953, revised and reaffirmed at various times since, and most recently revised in 2000. Both of these documents assert that nurses have fundamental responsibilities to promote health, prevent illness, restore health, and alleviate suffering. Inherent in these ethical statements is the belief that nursing is integrally involved with respecting human rights, including the right to life, to dignity, and to be treated with respect. Nursing research, as an action in which nurses are involved, carries the need to safeguard these rights of patients.

The two mentioned documents are predicated on three ethical principles important to research. They focus on autonomy, beneficence, and justice. Autonomy, as it pertains to research, is a fundamental ethical principle that underpins both self-determination and the right of every person to give clear and knowledgeable informed consent. If autonomy is not safeguarded, a nurse has failed to uphold the ethical standards of the profession. Remember that a patient may, appropriately, be asked to participate in research that carries great risk. The research is not inherently unethical as long as the person's autonomy rights have been addressed and the person's decision to be involved in research is a fully informed decision. There is no requirement that researchers only propose studies that involve no risk. Researchers and the nurses involved must, however, fully reveal any potential risk and assist patients to be fully informed so that patients can make unencumbered decisions about whether or not to enter the study.

The second ethical principle, beneficence, is the basis of the ability of nurses to act in the best interest of the research subject and to always function in an advocacy role as patients consider becoming research subjects. The third principle, justice, is fundamental in research and identifies how subjects should be recruited and treated during the research study. Justice assumes that nurses will ensure that research subjects are always selected from a wide array of the population and are not recruited in coercive ways.

INFORMED CONSENT

The RN in our clinical case has been oriented to the study being carried out on her unit, and realizes that a patient's consent to participate is important; she also knows that, as a professional, she is ethically obligated to follow the three ethical principles of autonomy, beneficence, and justice. She decides to review the consent form so that she can plan how she will respond to any questions that A.K. might have. As she reads through the consent form in preparation for her discussion with A.K., she realizes that there are three distinct components to the consent form: (1) a description of the study, including specifically what the subject will be asked to do as a research participant; (2) a description of any potential risks and any potential benefits to participating in the study; and (3) a description of the subject's rights if he or she chooses to participate. Each of these sections of an informed consent relates to at least one of the **five human rights in research** that have been identified by the ANA guidelines for nurses working with patient information that may require interpretation. They are:

1. Right to self-determination
2. Right to privacy and dignity
3. Right to anonymity and confidentiality
4. Right to fair treatment
5. Right to protection from discomfort and harm (ANA, 1985)

Table 7-1 defines these rights, and we discuss them as they relate to the process of research.

Informed consent is the legal principle that an individual or his or her authorized representative can make a decision about participation in a research study only after being given all the relevant information pertaining to the study as well as being given a reasonable amount of time to consider the decision to participate. The written consent form is a legal document indicating that the principle of informed consent has been adhered to. This document, along with a relatively detailed description of the study, is generated by a researcher before beginning a study and is

TABLE 7-1

Definitions of the Five Rights of Human Subjects in Research (ANA, 1985)

Right	Definition/Description
Right to self-determination	Individuals are autonomous and have the right to make a knowledgeable, voluntary decision that is free from coercion as to whether or not to participate in research or to withdraw from a study.
Right to privacy and dignity	Individuals have the right to the respect of choosing what they do and what is done to them and to control when and how information about them is shared with others.
Right to anonymity and confidentiality	Individuals should be afforded the respect of having information they share or that is gathered about them kept in a manner that does not connect them to the individual information and the respect of choosing for themselves who knows that they are participating in a research study.
Right to fair treatment	Individuals have the right to nondiscriminatory selection of participants in a study, to nonjudgmental treatment that honors all agreements established in the consent, and to resources to address any concerns or problems that should arise during participation in the research.
Right to protection from discomfort and harm	Individuals have the right to be protected from exploitation and to be assured that every effort is made to minimize any potential harm from a study, while maximizing the potential benefits of the study.

reviewed and approved by an entity called an **institutional review board**. An IRB is a board created for the explicit purpose of reviewing any proposed research study to be implemented within an institution or by employees of an institution. Most hospitals have an internal IRB, whereas small clinics may share one or use one associated with a local hospital or university. The individuals who sit on the IRB always represent a variety of backgrounds and interests and usually include members who are researchers, one or two lay members from the community, and individuals, such as ministers, who have a special knowledge and interest in ethics. The diversity of the members' backgrounds helps to ensure that a proposed research study is evaluated from numerous perspectives. The IRB does not examine the scientific merit of the proposed study, only the ethics of what is being proposed and what is being asked of the study subject.

The establishment of IRBs occurred in response to incidences of unethical and dishonest research practices in the past. Best-known examples include the Nazi medical experiments brought to light during the Nuremberg War Crimes Trial following World War II and the Tuskegee Syphilis "Study" that withheld treatment for syphilis from men from a poor black community in the South without their knowledge in order to study the progression of the disease. To address the concern of ethics in research, the National Research Act, Public Law 93-348, was signed on July 12, 1974. This law created the National Commission for the Protection of Human Subjects of Biomedical and Behavioral Research. This federal commission was empowered to identify the ethical principles that should be included in the planning and conduction of all research involving human subjects. They further were empowered to develop guidelines to ensure that research is conducted in accordance with those principles. The results of this commission still impact research today and include (1) identifying the differences between research and activities that are routine care practices; (2) establishing the importance of reviewing the risk:benefit ratio in order to determine the ethical nature of planned research; (3) establishing guidelines for the selection of human subjects for participation in research; and (4) identifying what is required in the informed consent process for various types of research. The findings of this commission were released in the previously mentioned *Belmont Report* (1979).

The Belmont Report's name was derived from the Smithsonian Institution's Belmont Conference Center, where the commission met to finalize the report. It remains the most important modern document that identifies basic ethical principles and guidelines that should be applied to all research involving human subjects. The report was published in the *Federal Register* and is still the guiding document whose principles are used by IRBs as they consider research proposals. Although the majority of researchers are honest and ethical, there have been continued occasions when researchers have falsified data, failed to disclose risks, or failed to report adverse events that have occurred during their research. IRBs exist to guard against these types of unethical and dishonest practices.

The function of an IRB is to ensure that the research project includes procedures to protect the rights of its subjects. It is also charged with deciding whether the research is basically sound to ensure that the time and potential risk to the participant is outweighed by the potential scientific gain that could come from the study.

A research study that asks anything of individuals is, at a minimum, using their time. A study that is not well planned or has a major flaw will make the results meaningless and wastes its participants' time and effort. It is the IRB's responsibility to make sure, as best can be determined, that this is unlikely to happen.

Beyond ensuring the soundness of a research study, an IRB also looks at the balance between the risks and benefits of the study. This evaluation of the risk:benefit ratio is integral to protecting a study subject from discomfort and harm. A **risk:benefit ratio** is a comparison of the level of risk present for subjects compared with the level of benefit. A study that proposes to ask healthy college-age students to take an experimental acne drug that has a high potential of causing kidney failure has a very poor risk:benefit ratio and would not be approved. But a study that asks terminal cancer patients to take an experimental cancer drug that may cause kidney failure has a much better risk:benefit ratio and would likely be approved.

Researchers are obligated to identify any potential risks to participation in their study and describe how they will try to prevent these risks, how they will monitor for their occurrence, and what they will do if they occur. If the researcher's plan is considered inadequate, the proposed research will not be approved. Some studies entail risks to life or health that simply are too great, regardless of their potential benefit and despite efforts made to minimize those risks.

CORE CONCEPT 7-1

It is unethical and illegal to implement a research study that uses animal or human subjects without institutional review board approval.

One potential risk to research participants is considered so important that it is viewed as a separate right. This is the risk of a breach in anonymity, confidentiality, or both. A participant in research is considered **anonymous** when no one, including the researcher, can link the study data from a particular individual to that individual. **Confidentiality** is related to anonymity because although the researcher knows the identity of the participant, it ensures that neither the identities of participants nor any information that participants provide individually will be revealed to anyone. Because many nursing studies examine sensitive areas such as abusive relationships, HIV status, sexual function, anxiety, and substance use, merely being identified as a participant in a study can reveal personal and private information about an individual. A study that follows subjects over time cannot ensure anonymity until the study is complete because the researcher must know who the participants are to stay in touch with them throughout the study. However, researchers can guarantee that participation in and responses of individuals in the study are kept confidential and that only the researcher(s) has access to the data. Once a study is completed, all links between individuals and specific data can be destroyed; this ensures that future work with the research data will be anonymous. As with any potential risks in a study, a researcher must tell the IRB in writing how the confidentiality and anonymity of subjects in the study will be achieved and how the security of any collected data will be maintained.

The IRB members address the subject's right to fair treatment by reviewing the researcher's plan for recruiting subjects. A subject recruitment plan must give all the members of the population of interest an opportunity to participate and may not target vulnerable groups simply because it is "easier" to get their participation. Vulnerable populations include groups such as (1) prisoners, as they are available and may feel compelled to participate as a show of good behavior; (2) the homeless, who may be unduly influenced to participate because of such incentives as payment rather than from a true desire to participate; or (3) the mentally ill, who may be less able to fully consent to treatment or who may feel coerced to participate. Additionally, researchers cannot avoid inclusion of individuals who are more difficult to recruit or who have more risk considerations. An example of this would be women. Women, especially during reproductive years, always carry an increased need to consider risks, as they may become pregnant and may be unaware of this during their early participation in a study. Because women have been actively avoided in past research, new studies must now include women and children as well as men, if at all appropriate to the research question, and must include individuals with diverse economic and racial characteristics. Additionally, the researcher must make the IRB aware of the location for data collection, the strategies used to recruit subjects, and any criteria for participation.

In Chapter 6, we discussed that the criteria for participation define the population and are used to either purposely seek diversity or to limit and control for factors that may confound the study findings. In the "Motherhood in the context of maternal HIV infection" study used in Chapters 1 and 2 (Sandelowski & Barroso, 2003) (Appendix A-1), only adults over the age of 18 were recruited. It is likely that the researcher presented an argument that the perception of motherhood and HIV status of those under age 18 is different from those of adults over the age of 18 and that including both those groups in one study may provide confusing data. Similarly, the article used in Chapter 3, "Correlates of recovery among older adults after major abdominal surgery" (Zalon, 2004) (Appendix A-3), indicated that individuals with a diagnosis of cancer or who were exhibiting psychotic symptoms were excluded from the study. The researchers did not do this because of a lack of concern for those with cancer or psychosis, but probably because the presence of these health states could confuse understanding of "recovery," making it difficult to separate that factor from the variables under study. Whatever the criteria for inclusion in a study, the IRB will review them carefully to be sure that they are fair.

CORE CONCEPT 7-2

The goal of research with human subjects is always to minimize the risks and maximize the benefits.

Ensuring the right to self-determination as well as the right to privacy and dignity are also the IRB's responsibility. These rights are reflected in the informed consent document by providing a clear explanation of the study, what will be required of individuals who participate, and the actual or potential risks and benefits of participation. The intent is that a potential research subject can make a knowledgeable decision based on the information provided in the consent form. In addition, respect for the potential subject is indicated through allowing them the freedom to decide what they will or will not do or share. Self-determination is also included as a direct right within any study consent form in a statement that says that the subject has the right of **withdrawal** from the study at any time, without penalty, until the study is completed. Once a study is complete, all data become anonymous, and it is no longer possible to withdraw information received from any specific individual. All research consent forms are expected to clarify with subjects that if they start in a study and later change their mind about participating, for any reason, that they retain the right to self-determination and are free to withdraw.

Another aspect of self-determination is the right to decline participation in a study without consequences. A researcher must assure the IRB that individuals who either decline to participate in research or later withdraw after initial consent will not be punished. This is particularly relevant if the study is being conducted in a health care setting where it is possible that a patient might feel direct or indirect coercion to participate. **Coercion** involves some element of controlling or forcing someone to do something. In the case of research, coercion would occur if a patient felt forced to participate in order to receive a particular test, service, or treatment; to "please" a provider of care; or to receive the best quality of care. Even if not forced to agree to participate in a study, a potential subject still experiences coercion if he or she feels that the best possible care will not be given if the choice is made not to participate. Therefore, any consent form for research where withholding or modifying treatment would be possible will include a clear statement that treatment and care will not be influenced by whether the individual participates in the study.

The right to privacy and dignity also is related to the right to anonymity and confidentiality. A researcher must inform a potential subject if participation in a study will involve invasive questions or procedures, again ensuring the respect of being in charge of deciding what will or will not be shared or exposed without the subject's approval. This reflects the participant's right to privacy. Clearly, once data become anonymous, there is no longer a risk of breaching privacy, but until that point, it is the responsibility of the researcher to ensure the right to privacy.

The last aspect of informed consent is a statement about the rights of the participant to care if some untoward effect should occur from participating in the research and the provision of the specific names and telephone numbers of the researcher(s) and an IRB representative. These sections of the form give the potential participant access to both the researcher and an independent resource, usually the IRB representative, if he or she has questions or problems. Individuals who agree to participate must be given a copy of the consent form so that they can contact the researcher or IRB representative as needed throughout the research and after it is completed.

Throughout this section, we have discussed the responsibilities of IRBs, which are in place to guarantee an organization that any research carried out within that organization or by its employees conforms with, protects, and respects the rights of their subjects. Although IRBs have the responsibility for review, it is always the primary responsibility of the researcher to plan for and guarantee the protection of subjects. If a nurse researcher were to plan a study in which no IRB review was provided, it would still be the ethical and legal responsibility of that researcher to ensure the guarantee of this protection.

Let us return to the RN in our clinical case. Box 7-1 shows an informed consent form that might have been developed had a researcher chosen to perform a replication of a maternal bonding study. As discussed in Chapter 2, a replication study essentially repeats an earlier study with a different sample to see if the same results are found. Having reviewed the informed consent form that she will be presenting to A.K., the RN recalls that for this study to have been approved by her institution's IRB, the board must have reviewed the basic soundness of the study in addition to its risk:benefit ratio. This provides her with some assurance that A.K.'s participation would not be a waste of her time or effort. It also provides some assurance that the risks to A.K. are probably reasonable, given the potential benefits from the study.

When reviewing the first section of the informed consent, the RN sees a description of the purpose of the study, duration of the study, and procedures. The first thing she notes is that the consent clearly states under the purpose that participation in the study is voluntary and will not be connected to A.K.'s care in any way. She knows that this is an important point to convey so that A. K. does not feel coerced to participate in the study. She also notices that maternal bonding has been defined as the processes that result in a feeling of connectedness between mother and child, and that the language of the consent form is generally not technical. Despite this, the RN realizes that she may need to explain to A.K. what is meant by talking about her perceptions and what is meant by periodic questionnaires, so she will need to be prepared to use more common language if necessary. The RN also knows that the idea of discussing HIV and drug use may be unpleasant to most patients. She must find an approach to explaining the use of procedures that gives a fair and impartial explanation but also allays any unreasonable fears that A.K. may have.

By considering these aspects of explaining the consent form, the RN is honoring the rights to self-determination, dignity, and protection from discomfort. Only by fully and correctly understanding the purpose and procedures of the study can A.K. make a knowledgeable decision with regard to her participation, ensuring self-determination. By being sure that A.K. fully understands the nature of the procedure that may be performed and the reasons for that procedure, her rights to dignity and protection from discomfort will be ensured as well.

CORE CONCEPT 7-3

The five human rights in research are first and foremost the responsibility of the researcher(s) and are linked to the three ethical principles of autonomy, beneficence, and justice.

<table>
<tr><td>**Box 7-1**</td><td>Fictional Informed Consent Form for Participation in a Study of Maternal Bonding in HIV-Positive Women With Histories of Substance Abuse</td></tr>
</table>

Prison Hospital XYZ
INFORMED CONSENT

PRINCIPAL INVESTIGATOR: Jane J. Doe, RN, PhD

TITLE OF PROJECT: Replication study of factors predictive of maternal bonding in HIV-positive women with histories of substance abuse.

PURPOSE: The purpose of this study is to understand how the maternal bonding process occurs, what factors influence that process, and to examine the relationships among maternal bonding and the experience of substance abuse. Maternal bonding is defined as the processes that result in a feeling of connectedness between mother and child.

DURATION: Volunteering for this study will involve being monitored throughout the last trimester of your pregnancy and into the first month of activity with your infant. Participation in this study is entirely voluntary, and deciding not to participate will not affect your care now or in the future in any way.

PROCEDURES: Participation in the study means allowing the nursing staff to meet with you weekly during the end months of your pregnancy and to discuss with them how you are feeling about motherhood. Additionally, you will be asked to fill out questions at intervals that will ask your perceptions of your past history of substance abuse and your HIV health status. Finally, a nurse will observe your interaction with your new baby and ask you to discuss how you are feeling in the maternal role. These observations and interactions with the nurse will be provided to you at no cost. In addition, participation in this study means that the researcher will collect some information from your chart about your diagnoses, medications, general health, and lab test results.

POSSIBLE RISKS/DISCOMFORTS: Becoming a new mother, having HIV, and having a history of drug abuse are all private aspects of each person's life, and therefore, discussion of these issues may be embarrassing or upsetting to you. There may be some discomfort in discussing these issues. There are no other known risks to participation in this study.

POSSIBLE BENEFITS: The possible benefit to participation in this study is having access to a health professional to whom you can ask questions and who is interested in how you are doing. The other possible benefit is the knowledge that you are contributing to a study that may help people like yourself in the future.

CONTACT FOR QUESTIONS: If you have any questions or problems, you may call Jane J. Doe at 423-965-0811 or Bob L. Smith at 423-965-0912. You may call the Chairman of the Institutional Review Board at 423-965-7777 for any questions you may have about your rights as a research subject.

CONFIDENTIALITY: Every attempt will be made to see that your study results are kept confidential. A copy of the records from this study will be stored in the Department of Acute Nursing, Room 100, at ABC University for at least 10 years after the end of this research. Your conversations with the nurse may be tape recorded, but all reasonable efforts will be made to protect the confidentially of your information. The results of this study may be published and/or presented at meetings without naming you as a subject.

(continued)

Box 7-1   Fictional Informed Consent Form for Participation in a Study of Maternal Bonding in HIV-Positive Women With Histories of Substance Abuse (*continued*)

Although your rights and privacy will be maintained, the Secretary of the Department of Health and Human Subjects, the ABC University Institutional Review Board, the Food and Drug Administration, and the Department of Acute Nursing have access to the study records. Your records will be kept completely confidential according to current legal requirements.

COMPENSATION FOR MEDICAL TREATMENT: ABC University will pay the cost of emergency first aid for any injury that may happen as a result of your being in this study. It will not pay for other medical treatment.

VOLUNTARY PARTICIPATION: The nature, risks, and benefits of the project have been explained to me as are known and available. I understand what my participation involves. Furthermore, I understand that I am free to ask questions and withdraw from the project at any time, without penalty. I have read and fully understand the consent form. I sign it freely and voluntarily. A signed copy has been given to me.

Your study record will be maintained in strictest confidence according to current legal requirements and will not be revealed unless required by law or as noted.

_____

SIGNATURE OF VOLUNTEER OR LEGAL REPRESENTATIVE & DATE

_____

SIGNATURE OF INVESTIGATOR & DATE

When the RN reviews the sections describing the possible risks/discomforts and benefits, she finds that these are clearly stated and include an explicit acknowledgment that personal disclosure is difficult. The consent form seems neither to exaggerate nor to minimize the risks and benefits of this study for A.K. The next two sections of the consent form directly address A.K.'s rights by providing her with the names and telephone numbers of the researchers and of an independent source of information, the chairman of the IRB. The consent form also tells A.K. that her records will be kept confidential, the location of those records, and for how long they will be kept.

Finally, the consent form tells A.K. that she has a right to compensation for any emergency care that might be needed because of her participation in the study. This statement may cause alarm in A.K. because nothing in the form has suggested that there could be a need for emergency care. The RN knows that she must explain that this is a legally required statement that probably has limited applicability for this particular study.

The last paragraph of the consent form confirms that A.K. has read and understands the study and that she will always have the right to withdraw from the study, if she chooses to do so. The right to withdrawal without any consequences is as important as the right to decline to participate and assures the patient the right to

TABLE 7-2

The Five Basic Rights and Relevant Components of the Informed Consent Form

Basic Right	Components of Informed Consent
Right to self-determination	Description of purpose of study Description of procedures in study Description of possible risks/discomforts Description of possible benefits Statement of right to withdraw from study Statement of voluntary nature of participation without consequences if person chooses to not participate Information about contacts for questions
Right to privacy and dignity	Description of possible risk/discomfort Description of confidentiality
Right to anonymity and confidentiality	Description of confidentiality
Right to fair treatment	Description of purpose of study Description of procedures in study Description of any compensation for medical treatment
Right to protection from discomfort and harm	Description of procedures Description of potential risks/discomforts Description of potential benefits

self-determination and fair treatment throughout participation. Table 7-2 summarizes the links between the five human rights in research and the specific sections of the consent form that we have discussed. After a careful and thoughtful review of the consent form, the RN is prepared to approach A.K. professionally for her consent to participate in the study.

One last point must be understood about informed consent. So far, we have been discussing informed consent to participate in a study, meaning agreement based on a full understanding that assumes the ability to understand and make rational decisions. Occasionally, in research, the potential subject is not able to understand fully and make rational decisions regarding participation, as is often the case for children and persons with cognitive disorders or severe mental or physical illness. Under those circumstances, a researcher is obligated to seek consent from a designated legal representative of the potential subject, such as a parent, guardian, or other relative.

However, the subject may have a level of function that allows the researcher to seek his or her assent. To **assent** means to agree or concur and, in the case of research, reflects a lower level of understanding about the meaning of participation in a study than consent. Assent is often sought in studies that involve older children or individuals who have a level of impairment that limits their ability but does not preclude their understanding of some aspects of the study. Suppose that A.K. was so ill that she could neither read the consent form nor discuss it in any detail with the RN. Because A.K.'s sister is legally designated as her representative if she becomes unable to participate in decisions about her own care, the RN would explain the study and review the consent form with the sister. Her signature would be needed to include A.K. in the study. However, the RN and A.K.'s sister could seek A.K.'s assent to be in the study by asking her briefly if she would mind helping in a study that looks at maternal bonding and involves the nurses in closely monitoring her process of bonding. If A.K. agrees, we would consider that she has assented to participate in the study: She has agreed without completely understanding all the aspects of the study, and it will be her sister who will make the knowledgeable decision, assuring A.K.'s full rights.

CRITICALLY READING REPORTS OF SAMPLING AND RECOGNIZING COMMON ERRORS

Informed consent, as well as the problems that can arise in samples described in Chapter 6, can affect the answer to the question "To what types of patients do these research conclusions apply—who was in the study?" The most common error found in a sampling report related to the ethics of a study is the failure to tell us enough to let us judge the occurrence of potential problems. Almost every study report will include some descriptive information about the sample, and most will indicate the source of the subjects or the location of the study subjects. However, this information may not be adequate for evaluating the sampling process for ethical principles.

An example of a study in which additional information about the process of sampling in terms of ethical concerns would have been useful is the "Needs of family members of patients with severe traumatic brain injury" used in Chapter 6 (Bond, Draeger, Mandleco, & Donnelly, 2003) (Appendix A-5). The authors tell us that consent forms were signed and that seven family members participated. The authors also include some important information that assures us that the rights of these research subjects were guaranteed by discussing consent form procedures. However, we do not know if a lot more than seven family members were available, if they were the only ones approached about the study, or why they were the participants. These are issues because they may give us a sense of whether the level of burden involved in the study in some way precluded inclusion of participants and/or led to participants dropping from the study.

As you critically read reports of research, there are two questions to ask that directly address ethical considerations in sampling. These are the fourth and fifth questions listed in Box 6-2 in Chapter 6. The fourth question asks, "Was enough information given for me to understand how rights of human subjects were protected?", and the fifth question asks, "Would my patient population have been placed at risk if they had participated in this study?" In "Needs of family members of patients with severe traumatic brain injury" (Appendix A-5), the authors do give us enough information to understand how the rights of their subjects were protected; however, they might have given a bit more information about subjects refusing to participate or dropping so that we could better answer whether participation in this type of study would be a risk for one's own patient population.

PUBLISHED REPORTS—WHAT DO THEY SAY ABOUT CONSENT AND THE SAMPLING PROCESS?

As we look at the research studies found by the RNs in our four clinical cases, it is important to realize that when considering sampling as a factor in the utilization of research findings, the clinical nurse often is the expert. We have discussed the meaning of several terms used in research to describe sampling strategies and actual samples, and these are important for understanding the conclusions of a research study. What we have not discussed is that often it is the practicing nurse who most readily recognizes the limits to IRB protection and sampling process because those in practice understand their patients' needs, functionality, and characteristics. If the nurse researcher is not directly involved in patient care with the population of interest, he or she may not realize that a certain segment of the population is not represented in the sample or has special ethical needs. Therefore, once the RNs in our clinical cases understand the sampling language and the IRB process, they are likely to be the best judges of whether a study sample reflects real patient populations and is appropriate to a particular research question.

The RNs in the clinical cases now have a much greater understanding with regard to which types of patients these studies can be applied. Legal and ethical principles have been considered and applied appropriately in all of the studies, and all of the samples have strengths as well as some limitations. The next challenge for the RNs is to reach a better understanding of why and how data were collected from the individuals in these samples. Just as the sample affects the meaningfulness of a study for practice, the measures used and approach taken to procuring data can affect the knowledge gained.

OUT-OF-CLASS EXERCISE

What Goes Into a Questionnaire?

Before proceeding to Chapter 8, look at the in-class questionnaire that you completed at the beginning of your course. If you did not have an in-class study, look at the questionnaire included in Appendix C.

As you read the questionnaire, write down your impressions regarding the following questions.

1. As you look at each question, what do you think is the variable of interest?
2. Do some of the questions fit together to measure just one variable? Which variable? Do you think the questions are all logically connected?
3. What makes the questionnaire easy to read and answer?
4. What makes the questionnaire confusing? Are any particular questions more confusing than others? Why?
5. Do any aspects of the organization of the questionnaire or the wording of questions make it difficult for some people to answer the questionnaire?

After you have responded to these questions, to which there are no correct or incorrect answers, you are ready to read Chapter 8.

References

American Nurses Association (ANA). (1985). *Code for nurses with interpretive statement*. Kansas City, MO: Author.

American Nurses Association (ANA). (2001). *Code of ethics for nurses with interpretive statements*. Silver Spring, MD: Author.

Belmont Report: *Ethical principles and guidelines for the protection of human subjects of research*. (1979). The National Commission for the Protection of Human Subjects of Biomedical and Behavioral Research.

Bond, A. E., Draeger, C. R. L., Mandleco, B., & Donnelly, M. (2003). Needs of family members of patients with severe traumatic brain injury: Implications for evidence-based practice. *Critical Care Nurse, 23*(4), 63–72.

International Council of Nurses (ICN). (2000). *The ICN code of ethics for nurses*. Geneva, Switzerland: Author.

Kane, M., & DiBartolo, M. (2002). Complex physical and mental health needs of rural incarcerated women. *Issues in Mental Health Nursing, 23,* 209–229.

Sandelowski, M., & Barroso, J. (2003). Motherhood in the context of maternal HIV infection. *Research in Nursing & Health, 26,* 470–482.

Zalon, M. L. (2004). Correlates of recovery among older adults after major abdominal surgery. *Nursing Research, 53*(2), 99–106.

Resources

LoBiondo-Wood, G., Haber, J., & Krainovich-Miller, B. (2002). Overview of the research process. In G. LoBiondo-Wood & J. Haber (Eds.), *Nursing research: Methods, critical appraisal, and utilization* (5th ed.). St. Louis: Mosby.

Locke, L. F., Silverman, S. J., & Spirduso, W. W. (1998). *Reading and understanding research*. Thousand Oaks, CA: Sage Publications.

Polit, D. F., & Beck, C.T. (2003). *Nursing research: Principles and methods* (7th ed.). Philadelphia: Lippincott Williams & Wilkins.

DATA COLLECTION METHODS

How Were Those People Studied—Why Was the Study Performed That Way?

LEARNING OBJECTIVE:

The student will relate the data collection methods of a study to the meaning of its results and conclusions.

Revisiting Study Variables

Methods for Constructing the Meaning of Variables in Qualitative Research

Errors in Data Collection in Qualitative Research
  Trustworthiness
  Confirmability
  Transferability
  Credibility

Methods to Measure Variables in Quantitative Research

Errors in Data Collection in Quantitative Research
  The Quality of Measures—Reliability and Validity
  Errors in Implementation of Quantitative Data Collection

Common Errors in Written Reports of Data Collection Methods

Critically Reading Methods Sections of Research Reports

Connecting Data Collection Methods to Sampling, Results, and Discussion/Conclusion

Published Reports—Would You Use These Studies in Clinical Practice?

KEY TERMS

Audit trail	Inter-rater reliability	Structured questions
Confirmability	Items	Test-retest reliability
Construct validity	Likert-type response scale	Theoretical definition
Content validity	Member checks	Transferability
Credibility	Operational definition	Triangulation
Criterion-related validity	Participant observation	Trustworthiness
Error	Questionnaire	Unstructured interviews
Field notes	Reliability	Validity
Group interviews	Rigor	Visual analog
Instrument	Scale	
Internal consistency reliability	Semistructured questions	

CLINICAL CASE

M.J. is a 34-year-old woman who was discharged from the hospital one day after a right mastectomy surgery for stage II cancer. An RN has been assigned to provide home care to M.J., and when the nurse makes her first home visit, she finds M.J. crying and expressing feelings of discouragement. While checking M.J.'s incision and her vital signs, the RN listens supportively as M.J. talks about her feelings. The RN has had several cases of postoperative care for women following breast surgery, and she wonders how she might improve the home care she provides to these patients, particularly in the areas of psychosocial needs and self-care. She looks for research evidence that might guide her practice by doing a literature search and finds one report of research that seems particularly relevant titled "Efficacy of an in-home nursing intervention following short-stay breast cancer surgery" (Wyatt, Donze, & Beckrow, 2004). This article is presented in Appendix A-6. We will be using the information in the methods section of this report as examples throughout this chapter. Table 8-1 summarizes the RN's clinical question for this clinical case.

REVISITING STUDY VARIABLES

The unique language of research associated with data collection is extensive, as a quick glance at the Key Terms listed at the beginning of this chapter shows. The abstract of the article found by the RN indicates the study tested an intervention for breast cancer that may relate to the needs of M.J. and other patients like her. After reading the article, however, the RN realizes that understanding how complex aspects of health such as "quality of life" (QOL), "anxiety," and "functional status" were measured is essential to her understanding of the results and conclusions of the study. She begins to read the methods section to help her achieve this understanding.

To examine the measurement approaches taken, the RN first has to identify the variables in the study. We discussed variables in Chapters 4 and 5, defining them as some aspect of interest that differs in a variety of groups or situations. Both qualitative and quantitative studies have variables, but only quantitative studies use the categories of independent and dependent variables. Independent variables are those factors in the study that are used to explain or predict the outcome of interest and

TABLE 8-1

Statement of Clinical Question From the Clinical Case

What interventions are effective in supporting breast cancer patients with their psychosocial and self-care needs postoperatively?

The *Who*	Breast cancer patients
The *What*	Psychosocial and self-care functioning
The *When*	After breast surgery
The *Where*	In home
Key search terms to find research-based evidence for practice	Breast cancer
	Home health
	Self-care
	Psychosocial well-being

are sometimes called *predictor variables* because they are used to predict the dependent variable. In the article, the RN read about the efficacy of an in-home intervention, and the authors determined efficacy by testing the effects of an intervention as their predictor or independent variable. Dependent variables are the variables that depend on other variables in a study or are the outcome variables of interest. The efficacy of an in-home intervention article refers to the dependent variables as outcome variables.

As a review, remember that it is not the variable itself but how it is used that makes it either independent or dependent. For example, in one study, the purpose might be to describe the effects of chemotherapy on patients' levels of stress. In such a study, the outcome or dependent variable is stress. Another study might seek to understand how factors such as education, stress, and perceived benefits lead to nonadherence of diet restrictions. In such a study, we also see the variable "stress," but now it is an independent variable because it is being used to predict the outcome of adherence.

The variables studied in the article about the in-home intervention are listed in Table 8-2. This article is a quantitative study that uses both the intervention itself and demographic characteristics as independent or predictor variables. The outcomes examined include functional status, activities of daily living (ADL), QOL, anxiety, self-care education, and health service utilization. In other words, the study examined whether or not the intervention and demographic characteristics would predict those variables.

Before we continue, let us look at how we determine the variables in a study. Although it is logical that variables differ across groups or situations, many research reports will not explicitly identify or list the study variables. For example, the efficacy of in-home intervention report never really lists or clearly states the independent and dependent variables used in the study, but careful reading lets us do this, as shown in Table 8-2. Obviously, variables should reflect the topic of interest, which, in turn, should be described in the purpose, background, and research questions, sections of a research report discussed in depth in Chapter 10. Because a qualitative study usually begins with one or more broad questions and uses open-ended approaches to collecting data, the variables of interest often are clearly identified within the research questions. In contrast, reports of quantitative studies should clearly describe the variables even if they are not explicitly labeled as such because the data collection methods in quantitative research are specifically aimed at measuring study variables as objectively as possible.

The data collection section of a report of a quantitative study should describe how each variable was measured and identify each variable. The RN in our clinical case found the outcome variables identified under a section titled "Measures," and the intervention that was the predictor variable was described under the section titled "Procedures." Both the Measures and the Procedures sections are actually subsections under the general heading of "Methods." By reading carefully the methods section then, the RN should be able to find the description of the measures used and, thus, identify the study's variables.

Variables also can be identified and discussed in terms of their definitions rather than whether they are independent or dependent. Variables can be defined at two

TABLE 8-2

Types and Definitions of Variables From the Study of Efficacy of In-Home Care for Short-Stay Breast Cancer Surgery

Variable	Type	Theoretical Definition	Operational Definition
Self-care intervention	Predictor or independent variable	Focused nursing intervention that targets the needs of women following short-stay breast cancer surgery	Protocol consisted of a minimum of two home visits and two phone calls by an RN during the 2 weeks immediately following surgery and 24-hour access to a nurse by pager
Surgical recovery and self-care knowledge	Dependent or outcome	None	"Yes/no" questions in four areas: (1) infection status and antibiotic use; (2) surgical arm range of motion; (3) breast self-exam technique, and (4) lymphedema prevention knowledge
Use of health services	Dependent or outcome	None	Health Service Utilization Instrument
Functional status	Dependent or outcome	None	Rand Health Insurance Experiment and Medical Outcomes Research instrument: 10 items that measured functional status
Anxiety	Dependent or outcome	None	State-Trait Anxiety Inventory: Self-report on 20 items
Quality of life	Dependent or outcome	Well-being in four life domains—biological, social, psychological, and spiritual/existential	Functional Assessment of Cancer Therapy–Breast (FACT-B) scale: Six subscales addressing physical well-being, social/family well-being, relationship with physician, emotional well-being, functional well-being, and additional concerns

levels: the theoretical level and the operational level. A **theoretical definition** is one that is described and understood conceptually, not concretely. Because it is stated conceptually, this definition is not always clearly measurable. Therefore, a second type of definition called the *operational definition* is needed. An **operational definition** is one that is defined in specific, concrete terms that allows us to see how we might actually measure the variable. If researchers do not have a clear understanding of the theoretical meaning of a concept, then they may be inconsistent in their measurement of that concept, leading to disagreement about what was actually measured and questions about the overall meaning of the study.

CORE CONCEPT 8-1

The measures in a quantitative study should reflect the specific variables under study.

For example, the variable "stress" can be operationally defined as an individual's perceptions that an event is threatening and that he or she has no way to manage the threat. This definition is conceptual, giving the reader a clearer idea of what is meant by the word *stress,* but it does not tell us how that variable might actually be measured. An operational definition of stress might be an individual's summed score regarding his or her ratings on a four-point scale of the perceived level of threat from 40 life events. Or, still using the same theoretical definition, stress could be operationally defined as the number of beats per minute that the heart rate increases when a person looks at pictures of negative events. These two definitions are concrete and tell the reader exactly how the variable "stress" will be measured.

Although some variables such as temperature or heart rate are concrete and may only be defined operationally, many variables of interest to nursing are relatively abstract and may need both a theoretical and an operational definition if they are going to be used in a quantitative study. Examples of these types of variables include QOL, pain, anxiety, mobility, and patient knowledge. If a researcher believed that we had a theoretical understanding of the QOL variable, he or she might break it down into one or more concrete components that would then comprise an operational definition. For example, he or she might operationally define, or operationalize, QOL as was done in the article found by the RN in the clinical case. In that study, the researchers operationalized QOL as scores on the Functional Assessment of Cancer Therapy–Breast (FACT-B) scale (Wyatt et al., 2004). Alternatively, a researcher might operationalize QOL as a single item rated on a 10-point scale, as was done in the article about caregiving experience used in Chapters 4 and 5 (White, Mayo, Hanley, & Wood-Dauphinee, 2003) (Appendix A-4). Almost any variable can be operationalized, but the correctness and accuracy of that operationalization must be evaluated. You can think of an operational definition, or the operationalization, of a variable as a form of translation: The researcher is translating an abstract theoretical idea into a concrete set of measures.

CORE CONCEPT 8-2

Operationalizing variables is like translating a phrase from one language to another. The researcher is translating an abstract, theoretical variable into a concrete measure or set of measures.

When a variable is not measured with 100% accuracy, we say that there is error in the measurement. In research, **error** refers to the difference between what is true and the answer we obtained from our data collection. If we operationalized gender as the data collectors' assessment of gender based on observation, that observation might be wrong probably only 1 in 1000 times. Think about that: If we had a data collector sit in a hospital waiting room and record the gender of a person walking in the room, occasionally he or she might misperceive or be confused by odd dress or appearance. In almost all measurement, there could still be some error because an observational assessment would be wrong occasionally. The difference between the gender of 1000 people and the measurement of gender through observation would be the error in the measurement of that variable. In Chapter 2, we compared qualitative research with creating an artist's rendition of a new home as well as compared quantitative research with developing the blueprints for that home. An artist can misunderstand the specifications for a new home and create distortions or illusions in a painting, just as an architect can make errors in measurement that can lead to plans that are inaccurate, incomplete, or wrong. In both cases, error in measurement will occur.

Remember that we said measurement is about translation. If you have experienced having someone translate your words into another language, you know that translation is open to interpretation and even error. Qualitative research does not operationalize variables because it does not presume to know enough about the variables of interest to be able to select appropriate and accurate concrete measures. Yet, qualitative research does translate specific experiences or observations into theoretical concepts or descriptions of variables during the process of data collection and analysis. Therefore, qualitative research is open to errors in interpretation during the data collection process. For example, a researcher may get focused on an idea that one or two participants who are trying to quit smoking discuss, such as "fear of failure," and start looking for that theme in other interviews. The researcher may then hear statements about discouragement as well as about disappointing significant others as variations of the fear of failing when, in fact, discouragement or disappointment are important and different themes that warrant exploration.

Because quantitative research often examines abstract variables that require both a theoretical and an operational definition, the opportunities for error in measurement can be even greater. Error can occur in the translation from theoretical to operational, and it can occur in the operationalized measurement process. Therefore, both qualitative research and quantitative research are open to problems in the translation of variables. We will discuss how those potential problems with translation can affect the meaning of the results of a study for practice later in this chapter.

Before looking at specific approaches used to collect data for studies, let us apply the ideas of theoretical variables and operational definitions to the fictional article in Appendix B about nursing students' choices of field of practice. The author of the article tells us in the first paragraph, under the heading of "Measures," that the questionnaire used in this study had three sections: One that asked about demographic characteristics; one asked about education, well-being, and career choice; and one asked about automobile preferences. Demographic variables are usually fairly concrete and commonly understood, so the author does not offer theoretical definitions of them. However, the author does tell us indirectly that these variables were measured by self-report because they were measured through a questionnaire that was completed by the students. Therefore, the operational definition of age in this study is the actual reported age. The variable age then might be translated to be "the subject's report of his or her age in years." Age also could have been operationally defined by asking for the subject's birth date, which the researcher could then have used to compute age to the day using a computer calculation that subtracts date of birth from the current date. The fictional article does not tell us whether the questionnaire asked for age in years or for birth date, so we do not know exactly how the age variable was operationalized.

The second section of the questionnaire was used to operationalize several variables in the study, including educational background, well-being, and student preference for clinical practice after graduation. Educational background was operationalized by the answers to two questions: (1) if the student was currently licensed to practice as an RN or a licensed practical nurse (LPN) and (2) the total number of years of the student's postsecondary education. Well-being was operationally defined as the student's rating of his or her health on a four-point scale. Anticipated field of choice was operationally defined as choice from a list of career options. In each case, a variable has been translated into a specific measure or measures, and alternate translations could have been used. Equally important, there is room for error both in the translation of a variable to a measure and in the measuring process itself. The remainder of this chapter discusses the measurement process and how error may occur.

Finally, the researcher in the fictional article included in the questionnaire an open-ended question regarding life experiences that led to choice of field of practice. In this last question, the researcher does not concretely translate a variable but asks the subjects to share experiences that may help her to develop a definition of the variable "life experiences affecting choice of field." Because this variable is not concrete, the researcher will have to start by developing a theoretical translation or definition before considering an operational definition. The fictional article provides several examples of operationally defined variables but includes no theoretical definitions. As we discuss some specific methods for collecting information about variables, we see examples of theoretical definitions that were in the article found by the RN in the clinical case (see Table 8-2 for the theoretical and operational definitions of those variables).

Qualitative

METHODS FOR CONSTRUCTING THE MEANING OF VARIABLES IN QUALITATIVE RESEARCH

For this section, we will refer back to the article from Chapter 6 that reports on a study of the needs of family members of patients with traumatic brain injury (Bond, Draeger, Mandleco, & Donnelly, 2003) (Appendix A-5). [Note that the RN in the clinical case from this chapter found a quantitative article, which we will use as an example as we later talk about quantitative measurement.] As you recall, the Bond et al. (2003) study examined the needs of family members, and the report contains only the one major variable of family needs, which the authors have indicated is a factor not well understood and, therefore, needs a theoretical definition. A study that is using a qualitative approach should examine variables and increase understanding of something that is abstract and unknown by asking for, or looking for, specific examples, experiences, or perceptions. However, because a qualitative study does not attempt to measure variables concretely, we do not expect to find operational definitions included in a report of the study methods.

The primary purpose of many qualitative studies is to develop a clear theoretical definition of a variable so that it might eventually be operationally defined and concretely measured. For example, the theoretical variable of family needs is the focus of the qualitative study we are using as an example. Because the purpose of that study was to increase our understanding of family needs, neither a theoretical nor an operational definition was offered. A concrete definition would presume that we already had a relatively clear understanding of family needs and could concretely measure it. Whereas, in fact, the researchers were trying to construct a theoretical definition of family needs that then could be translated into an operational definition.

In qualitative research, the study methods used to collect data are intended to allow the researcher to construct a description of the meaning of the variable(s) under study. Remember that a qualitative approach assumes that truth is a moving target. The more we can know, feel, or understand about a variable of interest, the closer we will come to a full and complete meaning, but that meaning will always be context laden and, therefore, changing and evolving. A qualitative method for data collection, then, does not aim to measure specifically or make concrete a variable of interest. Rather, these data collection methods aim to expand our understanding about a variable or variables on as many levels as possible.

Qualitative methods of data collection depend on the participants' open sharing of their thoughts, feelings, and experiences verbally, visually, in writing, with music, and within life activities. Although it may not be surprising that participants can share through speaking and writing, other means of expression, such as music or cooking a meal, are probably less frequently considered but can be meaningful avenues for understanding a participant's experiences or feelings. Therefore, the data methods include interviews, journaling, participant observation, and art analysis. Interviews are probably the most frequently used methods for collecting data in qualitative research, with two broad categories of interviews used: those that are unstructured and those that use groups.

Unstructured interviews involve asking questions in an informal and open fashion, without a previously established set of categories or assumed answers, to gain understanding about a phenomenon or variable of interest. Unstructured interviews in qualitative research assume that the product of the interview reflects the interactions among the interviewer, participant, and interview environment or setting. Depending on the type of qualitative study, the researcher may identify and purposely set aside or bracket his or her knowledge, beliefs, or expectations about the variable, or he or she may not bracket and instead may carefully document and incorporate his or her knowledge, beliefs, and perspectives into the data collection process. In any case, data collection using an unstructured interview includes not only the actual words of the participant but also notes the participant's tone, expressions, and associated actions, and what is occurring in the setting. These notes are often called **field notes** because they are a record of the researcher's observations about the overall setting and experience of the data collection process while in that setting or field itself. Field notes are used to enrich and build a data set that is thick and dense.

Not all interviewing techniques are unstructured. However, qualitative research does not generally use either semistructured or structured interviews because these types of interviews assume and control options for answers to questions. As such, semistructured and structured interviews do not fit with the perspective of a qualitative researcher that it is the participant's own ideas and language that extend our knowledge and understanding of a phenomenon.

Unstructured interviews may take several forms, including in-depth interviews, oral histories, storytelling, and life reviews. In all forms, the intent is to openly explore the understanding and experiences of the study participants. As was done in the family needs study, unstructured interviews usually are tape-recorded or videotaped, then transcribed verbatim into a written form that will include notes on pauses; vocalizations that are not actual words, such as sighs; and even voice tone at times.

A related method of data collection is **participant observation**. In this type of observation, the researcher intentionally imbeds himself or herself into the environment from which data will be collected and becomes a participant. From the perspective of active participation in the experiences and lives of those studied, the researcher/participant records observations, feelings, conversations, and experiences regarding the phenomenon of interest. The family needs study report does not indicate whether or not observations of participants in the study were included in the data collected, so we must assume that the major sources of data in that study were the participants' own words. However, we can imagine that observations of family experiences and reactions while they were in the ICU with their patient would have added to the depth and richness of the data used to develop a theoretical understanding of family needs.

Group interviews also are used to collect data in qualitative research and involve collection of data by interviewing more than one participant at a time. The data collected, then, are not just the participant's responses, but are also the responses that occur due to the interaction of the participants as they hear and respond to each other. Group interviews may take the form of focus groups, in which a preset topic is addressed in an open-ended fashion and the researcher keeps the focus of the group on that topic. Another form of group interview is brainstorming, in which no particular focus or direction is established, and group dialogues about a broad topic in an unstructured discussion. Group interviews may occur spontaneously in a setting where a researcher finds or facilitates two or more participants in naturally dialoging about a phenomenon of interest. For example, a researcher studying the experience of receiving government assistance and observing a group of women waiting for their food stamps might see several women talking about what it is like to shop with the stamps. The researcher might introduce himself or herself, obtain consent, and join the discussion, asking a few questions and listening to what the women have to say. In general, group interviews are rich in data and can be a relatively inexpensive method of data collection. However, use of group interviews may limit hearing and knowing unique individual perspectives or ideas because groups limit some individual expression.

Use of journals is another approach that can be used to collect data in qualitative studies. In journaling, a researcher can ask participants to describe, in writing, their ongoing experiences with a phenomenon of interest. This type of data collection can provide continuous and evolving information from an individual perspective that cannot be collected in face-to-face interviews. However, it clearly depends on the participant's ability and willingness to write on a regular and detailed basis. The researcher also depends on the participant's own description of the setting and interactions related to an experience under study because he or she is not present during the journaling. A more limited form of written data can be collected by directly asking participants to write a response or description about a phenomenon on the occasion of data collection. This approach is often called a *free write*. The fictional article in Appendix B about students' choices of fields of nursing used a limited version of written data collection by asking an open-ended question about students' experiences that had affected their choices of field in nursing. This can be considered to be a form of qualitative data collection because it does not constrain or limit the responses that students can give and lends itself to providing data about the meaning of life experiences for future life choices.

A similar form of data collection involves the use of expressional media or art forms such as art, music, or poetry. Here, data such as drawings or photography are collected, as it is assumed that they reflect the participant's perception and interpretation of certain experiences. When art is used, an interview often is included so that the participant can share or interpret his or her art to the researcher. For example, homeless individuals might be given disposable cameras and asked to take photographs that reflect their experiences of being homeless. The researcher might then analyze the photographs for common subjects or common reflected moods.

Another form of data collected in qualitative research is documents and records. These types of data are used in historical research and may include personal and business letters, logs, contracts, accounts, and other written records. These data are compiled and examined to create a clear picture of some past aspect and are particularly useful when the phenomenon of interest has evolved over time, such as the elimination of wearing nursing caps in the clinical setting.

In all of these methods, the researcher is not collecting discrete, clearly defined, and limited information. Qualitative data are used to develop theoretical meaning by creating a verbal, a visual, or an auditory picture of a variable of interest. Although data collection in qualitative research is not structured and objectified, it is carefully planned and thought through, and it involves clearly identified methods for the overlapping processes of collecting, handling, and analysis.

ERRORS IN DATA COLLECTION IN QUALITATIVE RESEARCH

In qualitative research, error can be introduced into a study in two major ways. Problems can occur with the processes of data collection and analysis, or both. When considering the aspects that can create error, qualitative researchers aim to ensure the rigor of both processes. **Rigor** is a strict process of data collection and analysis as well as a term that reflects the overall quality of that process in qualitative research. It is reflected in the consistency of data analysis and interpretation, the trustworthiness of the data collected, the transferability of the themes, and the credibility of the data. Qualitative researchers use several tools and processes to guarantee that each of these aspects of rigor is ensured.

Trustworthiness

Trustworthiness refers to the honesty of the data collected from or about the participants (Lincoln & Guba, 1985). To collect trustworthy data, the researcher must have a meaningful relationship with the participants, which may require time to develop. Participants also must want to share information so that they can communicate their feelings, insights, and experiences without feeling pressured or wanting to censor what they share (Lincoln & Guba, 1985). For example, the family members who participated in the family needs study (Appendix A-5) were not likely to share their experiences and perceptions honestly and openly unless they believed that the researcher had a real interest in their perceptions and an acceptance of them and their life experiences. Participants do not develop such openness without first getting to know the researcher, at least to some extent. For example, the researcher in the family needs article used a private hospital waiting room to provide privacy for initial interviews (Bond et al., 2003). In this manner, the trust and a relationship of respect was established early in the study process. The same researcher then visited the family member each day until the patient either died or left the ICU, thus maintaining and building the trusting relationship. The strategies used throughout the data collection process were carefully thought through and were implemented to ensure trustworthiness.

Trustworthiness of data collection may also be supported by using a consistent protocol in data collection. Use of a protocol may seem contradictory to the open-ended nature of most qualitative data collection methods. However, a protocol can provide a broad framework for data collection and ensure a similar setting and interaction, without structuring the data collected. The family needs article describes a protocol when the authors state that they first interviewed each family member in the waiting area and then daily in the ICU, and the subsequent interviews were carried out by telephone if needed (Bond et al., 2003).

Confirmability

A second aspect of ensuring rigor in qualitative data collection is **confirmability**—that is, the consistency and repeatability of the decision making about the process of data collection and data analysis (Lincoln & Guba, 1985). One approach taken to ensure confirmability of data in qualitative research is developing and maintaining an audit trail. An **audit trail** is an ongoing documentation regarding the researcher's decisions about the data analysis and collection processes. Documentation from the audit trail may include field notes about the process of data collection, theoretical notes about the working hypotheses or developing ideas during the analysis, or methods notes regarding approaches to categorizing or organizing the data. The audit trail can be used to assist the researcher in being consistent as well as to demonstrate the presence of consistency when sharing the data.

Qualitative researchers often use computer software programs, such as NU.DIST and N.VIVO, to help them to organize and analyze data. These programs do not perform the thinking and conceptualizing that is at the heart of qualitative data analysis, but they can be used to examine the data efficiently, to organize it around themes and dimensions as they are identified in the data, and to synthesize large volumes of data. As the researcher begins to identify a data theme, different units of language or observations can be categorized under this theme. As new themes arise, the data can be reorganized consistently by the software. In addition, a record of the evolving decisions about themes and the classification of data are maintained, ensuring that the researcher is consistent in the analysis of all the data and assisting the qualitative researcher in maintaining an audit trail.

Taking a simple example, suppose that the researcher for the choice of field study reported in the fictional article (Appendix B) had broken down the students' written answers describing experiences that contributed to their choices of field into units that were the individual sentences and then stored them within a computer program. The researcher might decide that whenever students described some kind of experience with fiction about health care, such as a novel or television series, that this reflected a theme. The researcher now must explore the data to decide what are and are not examples of experiences with fiction about health care. For example, novels, plays, movies, and television series may all clearly fit into the theme of fiction, but are advertisements that depict health care also part of this category? As she decides and tells the program that references to television, radio, literature, film, and theater all reflect exposure to media, the computer will find and place into a category and sentences with those references. When the researcher later adds some additional data from another class of students, she might decide that identification with selected actors or actresses is a separate theme from the broader media exposure. The computer can be told to reorganize the data, looking for references to particular actors or actresses, but it will also retain the information about how the original category was formed. This provides the researcher with a powerful ongoing record of decisions, enhances the ability to work with large data sets, and decreases the possibility of the researcher defining or describing a category inconsistently from one time to another.

Transferability

A third aspect of rigor in a qualitative study is the transferability of the concepts, themes, or dimensions identified. **Transferability** refers to the extent to which the findings of a study are confirmed by or are applicable to a different group or in a different setting from where the data were collected (Lincoln & Guba, 1985). Transferability is different from generalizability because the focus is not on predicting specific outcomes in a general population. Rather, the focus is on confirming that what was meaningful in one specific setting or with one specific group is also meaningful and accurate in a different setting or group. One of the methods used to ensure transferability is to describe themes that have been identified in one sample to a group of similar participants who did not contribute to the initial data collection to determine if the second group agrees with the themes. This procedure is sometimes called *external checks*. Transferability also can be ensured if the researcher actively seeks sources of data that contradict the ideas that are emerging from the data. If disconfirming data are found, they can be used to modify or reinterpret the total body of data to develop more comprehensive and credible findings. Findings that reflect the breadth of experiences or ideas will then be more easily transferred or related to different groups.

Credibility

Credibility, the fourth aspect of rigor of concern to qualitative researchers, overlaps with transferability and trustworthiness. **Credibility** refers to the confidence that the researcher and user of the research can have in the truth of the findings of the study. Lincoln and Guba (1985) suggest that the credibility of qualitative data can be supported by a researcher performing several actions, including seeking feedback from participants regarding evolving findings and interpretations and seeking participants whose perceptions differ from those already included in the study. The former activity is often referred to as *member checks*. **Member checks** means just what it sounds like—that the data and findings from data analysis are brought back to the original participants to seek their input concerning the accuracy, completeness, and interpretation of the data. In the family needs study, Bond et al. (2003, p. 66) indicate that "Appropriate follow-up and probing questions were included as required" (Appendix A-5), thus suggesting that they may have confirmed their interpretation of the data with the study participants.

Credibility also is ensured through processes that guarantee trustworthiness and transferability, such as spending time with the participants and maintaining thorough, phenomenon-focused observations. It can be further ensured through the use of triangulation. **Triangulation** is the process of using more than one approach or source to include different views or to look at the phenomenon from different angles (Lincoln & Guba, 1985). This process focuses on the data, seeking different types of sources of information regarding a phenomenon, or it can focus on the use of more than one investigator, the use of several theories, or the use of numerous methods in the study (Denzin, 1989). When multiple sources of data all lead to the same conclusions, the credibility of those findings is increased.

Table 8-3 summarizes the aspects of rigor that we have discussed. As we read and consider using results from qualitative research in practice, we must consider the rigor of the data collection methods and analysis. The greater the rigor in the

TABLE 8 - 3

Aspects of Rigor

Aspect	Definition	Methods
Trustworthiness	The honesty of the data collected from and about participants	Establishment of ongoing or meaningful interactions Use of a protocol
Confirmability	The consistent repeatable nature of the data collection and analysis	Use of computer software to organize and analyze data Audit trails
Transferability	The extent to which findings relate to other settings or groups	External checks Seeking disconfirming cases or outliers
Credibility	The confidence in the truth of the findings	Triangulation Member checks

study, the more we can be confident that the findings are meaningful truths that we can use to understand our patients. What helps us to be confident includes the use of processes to ensure the trustworthiness of the data, such as the researcher's establishment of meaningful interactions and maintenance of ongoing contact with participants. That the data are confirmable can be indicated by the researcher stating that an audit trail was maintained or that selected software was used to assist in data analysis. Use of approaches such as external checks and searching for participants who differ or have dissenting views can help to ensure us of the transferability of the data. The credibility of the data can be supported by member checks and triangulation.

METHODS TO MEASURE VARIABLES IN QUANTITATIVE RESEARCH

Quantitative

In quantitative research, the methods used for data collection aim to measure the variables of interest clearly, specifically, and accurately. Earlier, we said that an operational definition of a variable is a description of how it will be measured and that a researcher doing a quantitative study almost always must decide how to measure the variable of interest, even when it is as concrete as a subject's gender. Remember also that the goal in quantitative research is to measure variables numerically so that they can be statistically described and analyzed. Therefore, the methods used for data collection in quantitative research include physiologic measurements, chemical laboratory tests, systematic observations, and written measures containing carefully defined questions, questionnaires, and/or scales.

In quantitative studies, variables often are discussed and defined at theoretical and operational levels because the goal in a quantitative study is to examine discrete factors as concretely as possible. The efficacy of in-home intervention study includes a variable called *quality of life*. Because this variable can have many conceptual meanings, the authors provide a theoretical definition by stating that "this study was based on the holistic framework for QOL developed by Wyatt & Friedman (1996). This model includes four life domains: biological, social, psychological and spiritual/existential" (Wyatt et al., 2004, p. 324) (Appendix A-6). That definition is included in the background section of the research report immediately before the authors list their research questions. The authors then provide a concrete operational definition of QOL that describes how it was measured in their section describing measures.

Although all variables in a quantitative study should have an operational definition, not all variables in quantitative research will have a theoretical definition. Concrete variables, such as gender, weight, platelet count, or oxygen saturation, do not have or need a theoretical definition. There is a common understanding of the conceptual meaning of "gender," so it does not need a theoretical definition. But even concrete variables need an operational definition when they are being examined in research because several approaches can be taken to measure them. For example, we can operationally define gender in at least three different ways: (1) the presence or absence of a Y chromosome, (2) a self-reported characteristic, or (3) an observed characteristic. In most cases, we will get the same result no matter which way we define and measure gender. However, in rare cases, some people perceive themselves to be the opposite gender from that indicated in their chromosomal composition, and some people are androgynous enough that a superficial observation might lead to incorrect categorization. Therefore, even a variable as concrete as gender must be operationally defined so that we can understand exactly what was measured.

CORE CONCEPT 8-3

In a quantitative study, every variable should have an operational definition that specifies how the variable was measured.

Physiologic measurement is probably the most concrete type of data collection in quantitative research and may include anything from a simple measurement of blood pressure to the calculation of pulmonary function values. As was pointed out with the gender variable, physiologic measures still must be defined operationally because most of them can be measured in several different fashions and with different levels of accuracy. A research study that examines a physiologic variable should report specifically how the physiologic parameter was measured so that the accuracy and appropriateness of that measure can be evaluated. Similarly, a study that includes a variable measured by a laboratory test should specify the actual test or procedure used to arrive at the study values. For example, if blood sugar were measured in a study, the report should indicate whether it used a capillary sample or a venous sample and what type of control and calibration measures were used to ensure consistency and accuracy.

A second method of measuring variables in quantitative research involves systematic observation of the variable of interest. Measurement by systematic observation differs from the observation data collection methods used in qualitative research because it is structured and defined to ensure that each measurement is accurate and comparable to earlier or later measures. As a result, systematic observation does not try to collect as much detail and variation as possible but has a narrow focus on specific components of the variable under study.

For example, in a study that was trying to describe factors affecting fecal incontinence, the researchers would need to operationalize the variable fecal incontinence, perhaps by stating that the specific observation required to indicate the presence of fecal incontinence is the presence of uncontrolled release of stool and/or soiled clothing. Thus, the variable is clearly defined, and the data collection focuses on the specific components of the definition. Therefore, data collectors would not be interested in factors such as urinary incontinence, skin condition, type of bedpan, staffing ratio, or the subject's ability to use the call button. Data collectors will look for and record reports by the staff or the client of involuntary release of stool, and they will count the presence or absence of the defined components to give each subject a value of "yes" or "no" for the variable fecal incontinence.

A third method for measurement in quantitative research is use of an instrument. The word **instrument** is used in research to refer to a device that specifies and objectifies the data collecting process. Instruments are usually written and may be given directly to the subject to collect data or may provide objective description of the collection of certain types of data. The FACT-B is an example of a written instrument used in the efficacy of in-home intervention study to measure quality of life (Wyatt et al., 2004) (Appendix A-6). Some instruments provide directions for observations, and the measure depends on observers noting certain specified and defined types of behaviors, counting the presence or absence of those behaviors, and converting them into a final numeric score. For example, the authors might have used an observational measure of anxiety that required visiting the breast surgery patients in their homes and observing for specific factors, such as rapid speech, fine tremors, restlessness, and disjointed ideas. When a researcher uses this type of observational measurement, the components that define the variable have been specified before data collection begins, and the study does not seek to expand the understanding of the components of that variable, as would a qualitative approach, but seeks to count the extent to which they are present.

We have said that instruments are devices that define and objectify the data collection. Some quantitative studies collect data using **semistructured questions** in order to collect data that specifically target objective factors of interest. For example, telephone surveys often consist of semistructured questions, such as "tell me how you use television to relax in the evening." Or a quantitative study might use a **structured question** that establishes what data is wanted ahead of the collection and does not allow the respondent any flexibility in how to answer. For example, the question "how many members of the household eat breakfast daily?" is a structured question. In contrast, unstructured questions are like unstructured interviews and seek to determine what data, experiences, or ideas are relevant and meaningful without previous narrowing of the definition or specification.

Many instruments used in nursing research collect data in a written form, provided directly by the subjects in the study. These instruments are also called *questionnaires* or *scales,* and the terms are sometimes used interchangeably. *Instrument* is the broadest term and, as we have said, can include interview questions, directed observations, or written collection of data. A **questionnaire** is an instrument used to collect specific written data, and a **scale** is a set of written questions or statements that, in combination, are intended to measure a specified variable. The questions or statements included on a scale are often called **items**. The language of research when discussing measurement of variables can become confusing, but grasping the basic meanings of some of these terms will allow you to better understand the meaning of a study for your clinical practice. Box 8-1 summarizes and gives an example of each of the frequently used terms in quantitative measurement. The FACT-B described in the efficacy of in-home intervention study (Appendix A-6) is an instrument that defines and objectifies the quality of life experiences of women who have had breast surgery using six subscales.

Many of the abstract concepts that we want to measure in nursing research are operationalized by using written scales of one type or another. Because the concepts are abstract, it is not logical or reasonable that we could measure them with a single question. For example, suppose we want to measure the concept of "stress." One could simply ask subjects "Are you stressed—yes or no?" However, answers to this question alone will not capture levels of stress, negative versus positive stress, sense of managing or not managing stress, or the nature of the stresses. To collect a fuller

---

Box 8-1 | Definitions and Relationships Among an Instrument, Questionnaire, Scale, and Item

Instrument—a device that specifies and objectifies the process of data collection
Example: Written instructions for a focused observation of behaviors indicating pain
↓

Questionnaire—An instrument that is completed by the study subjects
Example: Three-page written form that asks subjects about their personal characteristics, medications, past medical history, and pain
↓

Scale—a set of written questions or statements that measures a specified variable
Example: Three questions that ask the subjects to rate how often they experience pain in different situations
↓

Item—the individual question or statement that comprises a scale
Example: How often do you wake up in the night because of your pain?

0	1	2	3
Never	Rarely	Occasionally	Frequently

and more complex measure of stress, one needs more than one simple question, hence the use of scales that consist of several statements or items related to the concept being measured.

The first step in developing a scale to measure an abstract concept is to identify items or questions that are relevant to the concept. Identification of items may be based on previous research about the concept, theory related to the concept, experts' knowledge regarding the concept, or individuals' experiences with the concept. Often, items for a scale are created based on several of the sources described. For example, a list of items to measure stress might first be developed based on a theory of stress and coping, then reviewed by experts in the field of stress and coping for suggestions, and finally, reviewed or tested with small groups of individuals who are experiencing stress to see what they think about the items. The result might be five items such as those listed in Box 8-2. (*Note:* This is not an existing and established stress scale; it is simply intended to be an example.)

In addition to developing items that all are intended to address the same abstract concept or variable, scale development requires deciding how subjects will be asked to respond to the items. One type of response asks subjects to respond whether an item is true or false. A second approach to responding is called a **Likert-type response scale**. This type of response asks for a rating of the item on a continuum that is anchored at either end by opposite responses. For example, a Likert-type response scale that asks subjects to rate the frequency with which they experience what is described in each item that reflects stress from Box 8-2 might range from "always" at one end to "never" on the other end, as illustrated in Figure 8-1. Another example that could be used with the same items intended to measure stress could ask about frequency of experiencing what is described in the item with four options: 0 = never, 1 = once a week, 2 = two to three times a week, and 3 = daily. Likert-type scales may include from three to as many as eight or more choices, although the usual number of responses ranges from four to six. Notice that the answers to these questions are structured so that the subject cannot answer anything that he or she wishes such as "once every other week" or "sometimes." Use of this scale to measure stress would result in a number between 0 and 15, which is a sum of the number for each item. The score on the scale could be considered to reflect the stress of the individual subject with subjects who answered "never" for all items, getting a score of 0, and subjects who answered "daily" for all items, getting a score of 15.

Visual analog is another response format that can be used in scales that differs from true/false, yes/no, and Likert-type scale responses. A visual analog consists of a straight

---

Box 8-2 Sample Stress Measurement Items

1. How often do you feel anxious?
2. How often do you have difficulty sleeping at night?
3. How often do you feel overwhelmed?
4. How often do you feel tired, even after a good night's sleep?
5. How often do you feel angry for no identifiable reason?

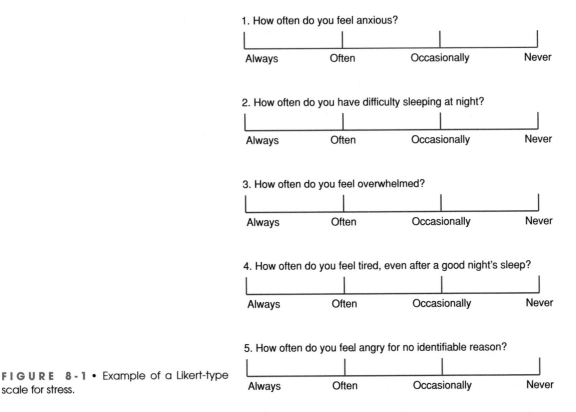

1. How often do you feel anxious?

Always   Often   Occasionally   Never

2. How often do you have difficulty sleeping at night?

Always   Often   Occasionally   Never

3. How often do you feel overwhelmed?

Always   Often   Occasionally   Never

4. How often do you feel tired, even after a good night's sleep?

Always   Often   Occasionally   Never

5. How often do you feel angry for no identifiable reason?

FIGURE 8-1 • Example of a Likert-type scale for stress.

Always   Often   Occasionally   Never

line of a specific length that has extremes of responses at either end but does not have any other responses noted at points along the line. Subjects are asked to mark the line to indicate where they fall between the two extreme points. Often, the line is 100 mm because a line that size fits easily on a standard piece of paper, and the subject's response is scored from 1 to 100, depending on the placement of his or her mark. For example, a subject might be asked to rate the level of stress that different situations cause for him or her, ranging from no stress to extreme stress, as illustrated in Figure 8-2.

The efficacy of an in-home intervention study uses a number of instruments to operationalize the variables in the study, including the State-Trait Anxiety Inventory, the Health Service Utilization instrument, the functional status instrument from the Rand Health Insurance Experiment and Medial Outcomes Research study, and the FACT-B that measures quality of life (Wyatt et al., 2004). In each case, the authors tell us about the scale itself. Information about the scales usually includes the number of items, the general nature of the items, how subjects are asked to respond to the items, and how to interpret the numbers from the scale. For example, the FACT-B includes six subscales that measure well-being. The FACT-B instrument defines and objectifies the QOL experiences of women who have had breast surgery using six subscales, including well-being in the physical, social/family, emotional, and functional areas as well as relationship with doctor and additional concerns. The authors tell us that items on the scales are rated on a 5-point scale ranging from 0 = not at all to 4 = very much. They go on to write about reliability of this scale and do

Rate your level of stress in each of the following situations by placing an "X" on the line below each situation. The left side of the line represents NO STRESS, and the far right side of the line represents EXTREME STRESS.

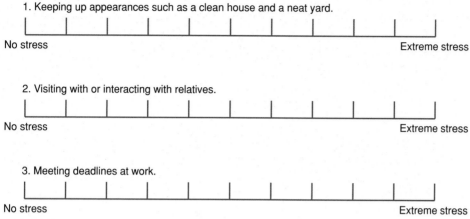

1. Keeping up appearances such as a clean house and a neat yard.

No stress   Extreme stress

2. Visiting with or interacting with relatives.

No stress   Extreme stress

3. Meeting deadlines at work.

No stress   Extreme stress

FIGURE 8-2 • Example of a visual analog scale.

not tell us how many items there are in each subscale or about the range of possible scores. After reading this description of the measure of QOL used in the efficacy of in-home intervention study, the RN in our clinical case has a clearer idea about what was meant by QOL and how it was measured. Although she might want a bit more information, what has been provided allows her to consider whether the measure is relevant to what she has observed in clinical practice.

We have now discussed methods to collect data and specific measurement approaches. We also have mentioned that at times error can occur in the methods or in the process of measurement and in the earlier section talked about potential errors in qualitative measurement. The potential for error occurs in both qualitative and quantitative methods of data collection. Understanding how this error can occur is important so that you can consider what that potential error means for understanding and using research in clinical practice.

ERRORS IN DATA COLLECTION IN QUANTITATIVE RESEARCH

In quantitative research, the data analysis process usually is separated from the data collection process. There are two general areas in which error can occur in quantitative data collection: (1) in the quality of the measures used to collect data and (2) in the implementation of those measures or the data collection process itself. These two areas are not entirely discrete and do overlap. We start by talking about the quality of the measures used to collect quantitative data.

The Quality of Measures—Reliability and Validity

Accuracy and consistency in measurement are at the heart of successful quantitative research. As an intelligent reader and user of research, you must ask yourself two questions about any measure used in a quantitative study: (1) How consistently does the instrument, questionnaire, or procedure measure what it measures? and (2) Does the instrument, questionnaire, or procedure measure what it is supposed to measure? The first question addresses the reliability of a measure, and the second question addresses its validity.

CORE CONCEPT 8-4

Consistent measurement is reliable measurement. Accurate or correct measurement is valid measurement.

Reliability means that a measure can be relied on consistently to give the same result if the aspect being measured has not changed. Consider, for example, measuring the gender of a sample: If three independent observers each record the gender of 1000 adults as they individually walk into a room, there will be a quite high level of consistency in the final count of the numbers of men and women in the sample. However, if even five or six of the sample are androgynous in their appearance, there may be some small differences in the final counts provided by the three observers. We have already said that this leads to some small error in the measure. If we changed our sample to 1000 diapered infants all dressed in white, we would expect much more inconsistency in the final totals because gender identification of infants by observation is much more difficult to do consistently. If, instead, three laboratories conducted genetic testings of each of the 1000 infants, there should be no differences in the final totals for boy and girls (assuming no laboratory error). Thus, the data collection on gender (particularly for infants) using the method of observation is less reliable than the data collection on gender using the method of genetic testing.

The reliability of a measure becomes more difficult to ensure as the measurement process becomes more complicated because complexity allows for more opportunities for error through inconsistency. Several approaches are taken to ensure or examine the reliability of measurement in quantitative research, depending on the type of measurement being used. When data are being collected by observation, a researcher often trains the observers and then tests them with different cases until all the observers agree on their observations the majority of the time. Earlier, we used a hypothetical example of observations to create a score for anxiety. If there were such a measure, the observers might be asked to practice making the observations needed with different "practice patients" to obtain a score on the anxiety scale until they each reached the same score at least 95% of the time.

In addition, when data are being collected by observation, researchers often report a inter-rater reliability score. **Inter-rater reliability** is present when two or more independent data collectors agree in the results of their data collection process. So, perhaps, in our hypothetical case of a rating of anxiety, a researcher might report that actual inter-rater reliability was 97%. This means that in 97% of the occasions, two independent raters got the same score. By providing this information, a researcher would help the RN in our clinical case to know that this complicated procedure to get a measurement of anxiety was used consistently across the different subjects. That consistency in use decreases the chances that any differences between subjects were due to inconsistent measurement rather than real differences. Assurances of reliability of a measure allow us to be comfortable that little error occurred in the measurement because of inconsistent use of the scale or instrument.

When a measure of a variable in a study is a written questionnaire or scale, two other types of approaches can be taken to ensure that the measure is reliable. The first is to test the measure before it is used in the study by having individuals complete the questionnaire or scale at two or more time points that are close enough together that we would not expect the "real" answers to have changed. This kind of reliability is called **test-retest reliability**; what we hope for is consistency in the answers in the different time points. If a scale or questionnaire is confusing or does not have a lot of meaning for a subject, his or her responses from one time to another are likely to differ. This means that the scores from the measure will not be consistent, and differences found may occur because of a lack of reliability of the measure rather than because of actual differences. For example, in the efficacy of an in-home intervention study, the authors report that the FACT-B had "Test-retest reliability correlations ranged from .82 to .92 in a sample of 70 outpatients with various cancer diagnoses" (Wyatt et al., 2004, p. 326) (Appendix A-6). This means that the measure was given to the 70 outpatients at two different time points, and their answers to the items were the same in between 82% and 92% of the items. This tells us that the FACT-B scale is completed with relatively good consistency.

Similarly, one would expect that nursing students' choices of field of practice would not change much during a week. If the author of the fictional article (Appendix B) had administered her questionnaire to the students twice, a week apart, and found big differences in choice, we would believe that the questionnaire was not measuring this variable consistently. That inconsistency would then shed significant doubt on the findings of the study because we could not be sure that the study truly measured choice of field.

A second way that reliability is often measured for quantitative measures is by calculating a statistic called an *alpha coefficient*. This statistic reflects a computation of how closely the answers to different questions or items within a scale are related and is, therefore, often called the *internal consistency reliability coefficient*. **Internal consistency reliability** is the extent to which responses to a scale are similar and related. Remember that we said that many abstract concepts in nursing and other fields are measured using scales consisting of several items or questions that all relate to the same aspect being studied. If, in fact, all the items or questions address the same aspect or variable, we would expect a consistent pattern in how subjects respond to or answer the items.

Let us go back to the five items that we are pretending were developed to measure stress (Box 8-2). We would expect that a highly stressed person would indicate that most of the experiences listed were happening regularly. If, instead, we found that subjects indicated that one or two of the items were occurring regularly but that others were not occurring at all, there would be a low internal consistency among the items. Alpha coefficients, often called the *Cronbach alpha* after the statistician who developed the test, can range from 0 to 1.0, with a value of 0 indicating that there are absolutely no relationships among the responses to the different items in a scale, and a value of 1.0 meaning that the answers to the items were all completely connected or related to each other. In general, researchers hope for an alpha coefficient of greater than 0.7, indicating a relatively strong relationship or connection among the responses to the different items on any particular scale.

Many quantitative studies that use scales to measure variables report internal consistency reliability coefficients or alpha coefficients to let the reader know how internally consistent that measure was. For example, the RN in our clinical case reads that for the FACT-B instrument, the "pre- and post-test alphas of the whole instrument for the current sample were .89 and .91 respectively" (Wyatt et al., 2004, p. 326) (Appendix A-6). This tells her that the FACT-B, which we previously learned consisted of six subscales, was answered relatively consistently throughout the study.

To summarize, the reliability of a measure reflects how definite we can be that the measure will yield the same data consistently if the actual or "real" variable stays the same. When quantitative data are collected using observation, the rate of agreement, or inter-rater agreement, tells us the consistency of the observational measure. Test-retest reliability can tell us if a measure stays consistent over time when the aspect measured has not changed. Internal consistency reliability or a Cronbach alpha coefficient is a statistic that tells us how consistently subjects responded to a set of items or questions. In all three cases, the goal in quantitative research is to use measures that will most consistently measure the variables of interest.

Validity is the second aspect of measurement that must be considered when deciding on use of research in clinical practice. **Validity** reflects how accurately the measure yields information about the true or real variable being studied. A measure is valid if it measures correctly and accurately what it is intended to measure. Validity becomes more of an issue the more abstract the variable to be measured is; with a concrete variable such as gender, validity is not a great concern. We are generally confident that gender self-report will yield a true measure of gender. However, let us look at another demographic variable that may seem as concrete: the variable of race. To measure this variable, researchers might ask subjects to indicate their race by checking one category from a list that looks like the one in Box 8-3. On initial inspection, we might assume that this list is clear and should yield valid results. However, although the use of the term *Native American* to represent those

---

Box 8-3   Potentially Invalid Forced Choice Race Item

Please check the item below that best describes you.

_____ Black   _____ Latino/Latina
_____ White–non-Hispanic   _____ Asian–not Pacific Islander
_____ Native American   _____ Pacific Islander

individuals who represent the indigenous peoples of the Americas is considered politically correct, it also can be interpreted to mean "born in America." If many subjects interpret an item asking about race in this way, then the measure will yield inaccurate information about race.

A second example of an invalid measure might come from Box 8-2, where we listed five fictional items that a researcher might use to measure stress. Looking at those items more closely, one might wonder if they are really measuring stress, or if they more accurately measure depression. Certainly, feelings of anxiety and anger, trouble sleeping, and feeling overwhelmed are classic symptoms of depression. Thus, this measure may be an inaccurate measure of stress because it may actually be measuring depression, which is an entirely different concept. The issue of validity of a measure becomes much more complex in scales used to measure variables such as depression, stress, efficacy, motivation, or coping. Scales or written instruments that are developed to measure abstract concepts such as these must find a way to describe or ask about factors that are specific to the concept and are clear enough to avoid confusion with other concepts. Three types of validity are sometimes described within reports of research: content validity, criterion-related validity, and construct validity.

The simplest of the three, and the one that is most easy for a reader of research to assess, is content validity. **Content validity** asks whether the items or questions on a scale are comprehensive and appropriately reflect the concept that they are supposed to measure. Put simply, the question becomes "Is the *content* of the scale complete and appropriate?" Researchers who have to develop their own measure of a concept will try to establish the content validity of the measure by asking a group of experts to review the items on the scale for completeness and appropriateness. If researchers are using a measure that has only been used a few times in other research, they may describe what type of assessment was made of the measure when it was developed to ensure content validity. As a user of research, you can assess what is called the *face validity of a measure,* which is simply one person's (perhaps not an expert's) interpretation of content validity. Face validity is a judgment of how clearly the items on a scale reflect the concept they are intended to measure.

As we have said, if we consider the face validity of the items listed in Box 8-2 that were proposed to measure stress, we might begin to question them. In fact, the items listed in that box generally reflect the symptoms that we expect to see when someone is experiencing depression rather than stress. Although depression and stress may be related, we do not necessarily expect everyone who is experiencing significant negative stress to also be depressed. Therefore, the face validity of these items must be questioned. In all likelihood, if a panel of stress experts reviewed these items, they would decide that the items were not valid items for a stress scale.

The RN in our clinical case can make some of her own judgments about the face validity of most of the scales used in the efficacy of an in-home intervention study because the authors give the reader information about the content of the items on several of the scales. In the example of the State-Trait Anxiety Inventory the authors make this comment:

The State Anxiety scale consists of 20 statements that assess how respondents feel "right now, at this moment." The essential qualities evaluated include feelings of apprehension, tension, nervousness and worry (Wyatt et al., 2004, p. 326) (Appendix A-6).

The RN can think about her experience with anxious patients and decide whether these areas of feelings are inclusive of the major signs and symptoms of anxiety. In thinking about this, the RN is making her own judgment about the face validity of the scale; if she decides that it is not valid, she may then decide that the results of the study connected with this variable are questionable for use in practice.

The second type of validity that may be described in a research report is criterion-related validity. **Criterion-related validity** is the extent to which the results of one measure match those of another measure that is also supposed to reflect the variable under study. The question asked with this type of validity is "Do the results from the scale relate to a known criterion relevant to the variable?" If a researcher were trying to test the criterion-related validity of the five-item "stress" scale in Box 8-2, subjects might be asked to answer those five items and then to rate their stress level on a scale from 1 to 100. If scores from responses on the five items closely matched ratings of stress on the 100-point scale, they might be considered to provide some evidence for the criterion-related validity of the five-item scale. The criterion used in this example is a direct self-rating of stress level, and the example is one of a test for concurrent criterion-related validity. That is, the test looked for a relationship between two measures concurrently, or at the same time.

A second type of criterion-related validity looks for a relationship between the scale being tested and some measure that should be closely related that occurs in the future. This type of validity is called *predictive validity*. An example of predictive validity for the State-Trait Anxiety Inventory might be found in the fact that anxiety scores decreased over the 6 weeks of the study, and subjects' additional concerns on the QOL scale also decreased over that time (Wyatt et al., 2004). One would expect that anxiety and concerns would be related, therefore suggesting that the measure of anxiety was accurately measuring what it was supposed to measure. The authors of the efficacy of an in-home intervention study do not report the finding of parallel decreases in anxiety and decreases in concerns as predictive validity, but it could be described that way.

The last type of validity that is sometimes discussed in a report of research is construct validity. **Construct validity** is the broadest type of validity and can encompass both content and criterion-related validity because it is the extent to which a scale or an instrument measures what it is supposed to measure. The construct validity of a scale or an instrument is supported with time if results using the measure support theory about how the construct (variable) being measured is supposed to behave. This may include predictive validity and concurrent validity but also will include other less direct predictions that arise from theory. Several approaches can be taken to measure the construct validity of a scale or an instrument, including use of statistical procedures such as factor analysis or structural equation modeling, comparison of results from the measure to closely related and vastly differing constructs, and the development of hypotheses that are then tested to provide support for the scale. In all cases, the goal is to build evidence that the construct, or abstract variable, is being measured by the scale.

There is a relationship between the validity and reliability of measures: A scale can be reliable but not valid. However, a scale cannot be valid and also not be reliable. A scale may consistently measure something (reliability) but not the something it is supposed to measure (validity). However, if a scale measures what it is supposed to measure (validity), then it will inherently also be consistent (reliable). So a scale must have reliability in order to have the possibility of being valid. For example, we have suggested that the five items in Box 8-2 have questionable validity as a measure of stress, but it is possible that subjects might answer those five questions consistently, giving us reliable data about something—just not about stress.

One last note about reliability and validity is related to data collection from sources such as medical records. In nursing research, using medical records to collect certain types of data is quite common. However, some unique issues surrounding this data must be considered. As all nurses know, we can be confident that whatever is documented on a record has a high likelihood of having occurred. Therefore, if we are collecting data about pain level and we find notations regarding the patient's pain complaints, we can be sure they are accurate. However, we cannot be as confident that the absence of a notation about pain means that the patient did not have pain. If a great deal happened during a particular shift and a patient's pain was not exceptional in some way, it is possible that the pain was not charted. Thus, the reliability of certain types of data from medical records—that is, the consistency with which the kinds of data are documented—must be considered when choosing to use medical records to measure study variables. This is not to say that records are unreliable, only that there is inconsistency in the documentation of certain care aspects in records.

In summary, the different types of reliability and validity that must be considered when understanding quantitative studies are detailed in Table 8-4. Although reliability focuses on the consistency of a measure, validity focuses on the accuracy or correctness of a measure. Three types of validity are considered by researchers. Content validity refers to the extent to which the scale or instrument is comprehensive and addresses the concept or variable of interest. Criterion-related validity can be either concurrent or predictive and refers to how closely the results on the measure in question relate to results on other measures of the same concept in the present or future. Construct validity refers to the overall ability of the scale to measure what it is supposed to measure and is established only after the repeated use of a measure yields results that reflect the theoretical expectations for the concept being measured. An instrument of measurement can be reliable but not valid. However, if a measure has been shown to be valid, then it will be reliable.

Errors in Implementation of Quantitative Data Collection

We said that error can be introduced into the measurement of variables in quantitative research because of problems with either the quality of the measure or the

TABLE 8-4

Aspects of Reliability and Validity

Aspect	Definition	Methods
Reliability—how consistent is the measure?		
Inter-rater reliability	Agreement between two or more independent data collectors about the results of their data collection process	Carefully structured instruments Practice until a high level of agreement is reached
Test–retest reliability	Consistency in answers on tests when we would not expect the real answers to have changed	Repeated administration of measures or tests to calculate consistency in responses
Internal consistency reliability	The extent to which responses to a scale are similar and related	Calculation of a Cronbach alpha coefficient
Validity—how accurate is the measure?		
Content validity	The comprehensiveness and appropriateness of the measure to the concept it is intended to measure	Expert panel review Face validity
Criterion-related validity	The extent to which results of one measure match those of another measure that examines the same concept	Concurrent validity Predictive validity
Construct validity	The extent to which a scale or instrument measures what it is supposed to measure	Content and criterion-related validity Hypothesis testing Statistical procedures such as factor analysis

process of implementing the measure. Although reliability and validity speak to the quality of a measure, even a reliable and valid measure can be implemented incorrectly and lead to error. Implementation of data collection requires careful and detailed planning to ensure that the process is consistent and does not invalidate the measures. For example, a researcher could be using a reliable and valid measure of blood sugars, but subjects may fail to understand the dietary restrictions of fasting before samples are collected, thus introducing errors into the data. A procedure that confirms true fasting status would ensure that the measure yielded meaningful data. Another example of an implementation error occurs when a written scale that may have been shown previously to be reliable and valid is administered with incorrect directions, or the subjects are prompted in a way that sways their responses to a measure. Pointing out that the financial support for an agency depends on positive reviews before asking subjects to complete a satisfaction survey is an obvious example.

The order in which subjects are asked to complete questionnaires also can affect their responses. For example, if subjects are asked to complete a scale that asks several questions about symptoms of depression and then are asked to rate their level of overall depression, the scale likely will have increased their awareness of how depressed they really are, thus affecting their total depression ratings. In addition, different timing and environments affect data collection. For example, asking nursing students about their choices of field when they have just completed an exciting clinical rotation in the emergency room could lead to more of them selecting the emergency room than would have selected it if they had been asked at some time after that rotation.

Other types of error that can occur in the measurement process include sloppy handling of data, resulting in a loss of some of it. Failure to keep careful records can lead to missed opportunities for repeat measures because subjects' addresses or telephone numbers are misplaced or not accurately recorded. This is a problem, particularly in longitudinal studies such as the efficacy of an in-home intervention study, in which subjects are asked to complete measures at two different time points.

Finally, the implementation of data collection can introduce error by arbitrarily changing a measure through translating it to another language or administering it in a format other than that which was intended. Measures that are reliable and valid have been successfully translated into other languages, but this requires a careful translation process and then translating the measure back into the original language by independent translators to ensure that the meanings of items on a scale remain intact when the language changes. An issue similar to translation to another language exists when a measure that was developed to be read by a subject is instead read to a subject. The subject is then hearing the words rather then seeing them, and this can definitely affect his or her understanding and potential response to the items.

In summary, measurement in quantitative research must be carefully planned and controlled. The variables to be measured must be clearly defined. If the variables are abstract, we should expect to see both a theoretical definition and an operational definition so that we can judge both the meaning of the variable and how well that meaning was translated into data through measurement. Errors in measurement can be present because of problems with the measure itself or incorrect implementation of the measure.

The measurement language in both qualitative and quantitative research can be complex and confusing. Overall, the important points are that data collection must be trustworthy, confirmable, and consistent as well as transferable, credible, and accurate. Both the process and actual measures in data collection must be considered as we decide how to use the results of research in practice. To decide how measurement in a study has affected results and conclusions, we must receive complete and clear information about the measures. This leads us to consider what might be some common problems with written reports of data collection.

COMMON ERRORS IN WRITTEN REPORTS OF DATA COLLECTION METHODS

Probably the most common error that occurs in written reports of research studies is provision of incomplete information. This was somewhat of a problem with the article read by the RN in our clinical case (Appendix A-6) because the report does not provide as much detail about the different instruments used in the study as we might like. For example, we know neither how many items were in each of the six subscales for the FACT-B, nor what the possible range of scores would be. We also do not know as much as we might like about the 20 items on the State-Trait Anxiety Inventory; we only know examples of the kinds of feelings addressed.

Similarly, the fictional article (Appendix B) leaves several gaps in the information provided about the collection of the data. For example, the author does not give us a clear theoretical or operational definition of the dependent variable in this study—choice of field. Theoretically, "choice" could be defined as what students would really like to do if all options were open to them, or it could be defined as what students expect to do given current openings and other aspects of their personal situations. The results section of this report does give us some idea about how "field of choice" was operationally defined because those categories that were elected by the students are listed. We know that the students were not permitted to write in their choice but were given a list of nursing career options from which to select. However, the author does not tell us what was included in the original list of options, so we do not know if the final categories reported in Table 1 from the fictional article included all the possible options or if there were options that were not selected or were collapsed into one of the reported categories. In other words, we are not clear about the operational definition for the dependent variable either. This lack of clear information jeopardizes the usefulness of the research for practice because it becomes difficult to be comfortable with conclusions based on measurement that we do not understand or believe was consistent or accurate.

A second common error with written reports of data collection is a failure to organize clearly the information in a manner that makes it understandable. Although the efficacy of an in-home intervention article provides a wealth of information about the measures used in the study, the information is not easily understood in the winding narrative format in which it is presented. A table summarizing the variables and measures used in the study would have been helpful to the reader for understanding the measurement used in this study.

A third error that occasionally occurs is a failure to reference the source of measures used in a study. Although the practicing nurse may not choose to do so often, the option of reading other studies that previously used a measure that was used in the new study should be available. Referencing reports of previous studies that indicated the reliability and validity of a measure is particularly important because it gives the reader the option to learn more about that specific measure and increases one's confidence in the quality of the measure.

CRITICALLY READING METHODS SECTIONS
OF RESEARCH REPORTS

There are seven questions you can ask yourself as you read the methods section of a research report, and these are listed in Box 8-4. The first and probably simplest question to ask yourself is "Did the report include a clearly identified section describing methods used in this study?" The efficacy of an in-home intervention included a methods section with several pertinent subsections. The next question to ask is "Do the methods make this a quantitative or a qualitative study?" In this chapter, more than any up until now, we have been able to clearly separate qualitative and quantitative methods because these two approaches to collecting data differ so markedly. Thus, if you read that a researcher is planning a qualitative study using a written questionnaire with 25 items that will measure well-being, you will have to immediately wonder about the match between stated approach and actual methods used. You also will be surprised to find a quantitative study report that does not provide information to operationally define the variables in the study. The article may not call the description of measurement *operational definitions,* but if no explanation of measurement is present or the measurement is open-ended and unstructured, you may question the fit between approach and methods.

In critically reading the methods section of a research report, you should ask a third question, "Do I understand what my patient population would be doing if they were in this study or a study using a similar method?" If you are not sure what they would be asked to do, or how often they would be asked to do something, then the methods section is probably not as detailed as needed. Without enough detail about study measurement and procedures, it is impossible to evaluate the usefulness of study results. In particular, if one does not know how a variable was measured, it is

---

Box 8-4 | How to Critically Read the Methods Section of a Research Report

Does the report answer the question "How were those people studied—why was the study performed that way?"

1. Did the report include a clearly identified section describing methods used in the study?
2. Do the methods make this a quantitative or a qualitative study?
3. Do I understand what my patient population would be doing if they were in this study or a study using similar methods?
4. Do the measures and procedures in this study address my clinical problem?
5. Do I think that the measures used in this study would provide helpful and useful information when used with my patient population?
6. Do I think what the researcher collected and how it was collected was the best way to address the clinical question?
7. Do I think that the researcher(s) should have planned the study differently in order to answer my clinical question?

not possible to decide whether the measurement was appropriate. A related question is "Do the measures and procedures in this study address my clinical problem?" Again, without enough detail, one cannot answer that question; however, if adequate detail is provided, you will want to ask critically if you think that the methods used address your clinical concern. For example, the RN in our clinical case is interested in short-term psychosocial needs of patients after breast surgery. The study that she found measured their outcomes before surgery and again four weeks later. This measurement period may be too long to capture the more immediate psychosocial needs of patients in the first couple weeks after discharge. Thus, the methods used may not match the RN's clinical question.

The next two questions to consider address "Do I think that the measures used in this study would provide helpful and useful information when used with my patient population?" and "Do I think what the researcher collected and how it was collected was the best way to address the clinical question?" In a qualitative study, one needs to consider trustworthiness, confirmability, credibility, and transferability of the data based on what is told about the data collection process and the measure used. Similarly, in a quantitative study, reliability and validity of measures used in the study and whether potential error was introduced through the data collection process need to be considered. If the report does not provide enough information for you to answer these questions, then you may not be able to use the findings in your clinical practice.

Finally, it is important to consider "Do I think that the researcher(s) should have planned the study differently in order to answer my clinical question?" Again, the RN in our clinical case might believe that a shorter time interval or more measurement points would have improved her ability to use the study in clinical practice. Similarly, you might decide that a quantitative study that had trouble operationalizing an abstract variable perhaps should have started with a qualitative approach in order to collect data about that concept. This last question directly leads you to consider the overall study design, and that will be the topic of Chapter 9.

CONNECTING DATA COLLECTION METHODS TO SAMPLING, RESULTS, AND DISCUSSION/CONCLUSION

At the beginning of this chapter, we said that the RN needed to understand how the study variables were measured to comprehend the meaning of the results of the studies about efficacy of an in-home intervention for breast surgery patients. One thing that may have become clear to the RN as she learned more about research methods is that sampling and data collection methods are linked in both quantitative and qualitative research. Particularly in qualitative studies, data collection and analysis drive the sampling because additional participants often are sought purposely to focus on aspects of the phenomenon that are emerging from the data. We also discussed trustworthiness and the use of both member and group checks. These aspects of rigor in data collection require sampling strategies that ensure a trusting and open relationship with the data collector. Further, a researcher may ask the right questions about a phenomenon but may fail to gain access to the right groups to answer those questions; so, as we read about data collection, we must consider the sampling process as well.

In quantitative research, sampling is most connected to data collection in follow-up for repeated measures over time. However, the data collection process also can be affected by the nature of the sample or vice versa. For example, a study of homeless patients that uses measures written in English that have no established Spanish version may exclude a group of Spanish-speaking subjects. Another problem in data collection that is closely related to sampling is the educational level assumed in the measures. A complex written scale that uses language aimed at a high school reading level may become unreliable when used with subjects who have a lower education level. Thus, sampling and data collection can be closely linked in quantitative research as well as in qualitative research.

Throughout this chapter, we have stressed that if variables are not clearly defined or are not consistently and accurately measured, the results of the study must be questioned. Similarly, if rigor is not maintained through both data collection and analysis, the results of qualitative research are jeopardized; the results of a study are only as good as the data that went into those results. Therefore, understanding how data were collected and recognizing how potential sources of error in the data collection were addressed is closely linked to our ability to accept the results of a study. This, in turn, clearly affects our willingness to accept and adopt the conclusions of a study.

A last link between data collection and the rest of the research process is the link between data collection and the section of a research report that speaks to limitations of a study. Despite the best plans and efforts, problems do arise with data collection. These may be mentioned in the write-up of the data collection itself, but the implications of those problems for the conclusions of a study are often addressed when the author discusses limitations. For example, in the efficacy of an in-home intervention study report, the authors identify the lack of validity and reliability data for their interview measures used in the study as a limitation that may have affected the results of their study (Wyatt et al., 2004). Thus, the conclusions of a study are directly linked back to the measurement process.

PUBLISHED REPORTS—WOULD YOU USE THESE STUDIES IN CLINICAL PRACTICE?

Our RN was concerned about how to help M.J. and other breast surgery patients with their needs after coming home from the hospital. After considering the data collection methods in the efficacy of an in-home intervention article, the RN is comfortable that a self-care for physical and psychosocial needs intervention has some potential to empower her patients in their own self-care. The researchers in the study followed a clearly described procedure and mainly used measures that have reports of validity and reliability. The RN believes that the outcomes examined—anxiety, use of health care, QOL, and function—are clinically relevant in her experience with patients. However, the study found only limited differences between the groups who did and did not receive the self-care intervention, and the study only collected data

4 weeks after the patient's surgery, leaving the RN uncertain as to whether she should actively try to develop a self-care education intervention for her patients. The RN is not sure why the researchers chose to have three groups in their study, or why the researchers did not repeat their measurement more frequently. In order to answer this question, she will have to read the section that describes the research design for this study.

OUT-OF-CLASS EXERCISE

Free Write

The next chapter continues to address the question of why a study included the people it did and it was done the way it was by talking about research designs. Before reading that chapter, consider the question of whether being in nursing school affects the students' well-being. If you were going to conduct a study to address this question, how would you go about it? What do you think would be the best way to conduct a study to answer this question, and what do you think would be the most realistic approach? Are they the same or different, and why? Think about this, then write in as much detail as possible your ideas about how to conduct a study to determine if and how being a nursing student affects well-being. Wherever you can, write your rationale for conducting the study in the manner on which you have decided. After you have completed this assignment, you will be ready to move on to read about research designs in Chapter 9.

References

Bond, A. E., Draeger, C. R. L., Mandleco, B., & Donnelly, M. (2003). Needs of family members of patients with severe traumatic brain injury. *Critical Care Nurse, 23*(4), 63–72.

Denzin, N. K. (1989). *Interpretive interactionism.* Newbury Park, CA: Sage Publications.

Lincoln, Y. S., & Guba, E. G. (1985). *Naturalistic inquiry.* Beverly Hills, CA: Sage Publications.

White, C. L., Mayo, M., Hanley, J. A., & Wood-Dauphinee, S. (2003). Evolution of the caregiving experience in the initial 2 years following stroke. *Research in Nursing & Health, 26,* 177–189.

Wyatt, F. K., Donze, L. F., & Beckrow, K. C. (2004). Efficacy of an in-home nursing intervention following short-stay breast cancer surgery. *Research in Nursing & Health, 27,* 322–331.

Resources

Campbell, D. T., & Russo, M. J. (2001). *Social measurement.* Thousand Oaks, CA: Sage Publications.

Denzin, N. K., & Lincoln, Y. S. (Eds.). (1998). *Collecting and interpreting qualitative materials.* Thousand Oaks, CA: Sage Publications.

LoBiondo-Wood, G., Haber, J., & Krainovich-Miller, B. (2002). Overview of the research process. In G. LoBiondo-Wood & J. Haber (Eds.), *Nursing research: Methods, critical appraisal, and utilization* (5th ed.). St. Louis: Mosby.

Locke, L. F., Silverman, S. J., & Spirduso, W. W. (1998). *Reading and understanding research.* Thousand Oaks, CA: Sage Publications.

Polit, D. F., & Beck, C. T. (2003). *Nursing research: Principles and methods* (7th ed.). Philadelphia: Lippincott Williams & Wilkins.

RESEARCH DESIGNS: PLANNING THE STUDY

How Were Those People Studied—Why Was the Study Performed That Way?

LEARNING OBJECTIVE:

The student will interpret the strengths and weaknesses of research designs in relation to sampling, data collection methods, and the meaning of the results and conclusions.

Continued

Phenomenology	Reactivity effects	Selection bias
Pretest–post-test	Repeated measures	Testing
Prospective designs	Research design	
Quasi-experimental designs	Retrospective designs	

CLINICAL CASE

A nurse is working in the ICU unit of a small rural hospital. He is on duty the night that D.M., a truck driver, is admitted to the unit following an accident, where he ran off the road and into a ditch. D.M. overturned his truck, sustaining a crushing injury to his chest. He was in the ditch for 30 minutes before help arrived, and it took another 30 minutes to extricate him from the vehicle. D.M. specializes in long-distance hauling, and he lives almost 3,000 miles from the site of the accident. He is married, has two small children, and has a sideline business of race-dog breeding, an endeavor that he calls "Loves—I Love Those Mutts to Death." D.M. is still in critical condition and will be in the ICU for some time, as he is currently too unstable to transfer.

The RN assigned to care for D.M. is a recent graduate who has just completed his orientation period to the ICU. He wonders how D.M.'s recovery will be impacted by the great distance that separates D.M. from his home and family. The RN is concerned about what nursing interventions will assist with D.M.'s adjustment and how that can be matched to his lack of close psychosocial support. The charge nurse tells the RN that she recently read a nursing study about assisting the psychosocial needs of ICU patients and wonders if the nurse would find it helpful. According to the charge nurse, the study findings indicate that feeling safe is the most important need of critically ill ICU patients. The RN decides to find and read this article and to search for additional information about the psychosocial needs of his ICU patients. He finds the article, entitled "Feeling safe: The psychosocial needs of ICU patients" (Hupcey, 2000). This article is available in Appendix A-7. Read it before you continue with this chapter so that the examples discussed will be more meaningful. Table 9-1 identifies the clinical question of the RN and the key search terms that he might use in his search.

We also will return to many of the articles used in the earlier chapters as further examples, so it would be a great idea to review them as well. Remember, all the articles used as examples are available in full text throughout Appendix A.

RESEARCH DESIGNS: WHY ARE THEY IMPORTANT?

As we have considered how to interpret and use research findings in nursing practice, we have been moving from the end of research reports toward their beginning. We have learned that the conclusions of a report usually do not provide enough information

TABLE 9-1	
Statement of Clinical Question From the Clinical Case	
What interventions will assist the adjustment of patients in the ICU who do not have psychosocial support?	
The *Who*	ICU patients
The *What*	Adjustment
The *When*	Family not available
The *Where*	In ICU
Key search terms to find research-based evidence for practice	ICU, support, adjustment, family

to allow us to fully understand or apply the findings. The usefulness of the study results depends on the sample and the methods used to collect data. We have learned also that various approaches to sampling and data collection have differing strengths and weaknesses. Thus, we need to better understand the overall purpose and nature of research designs because they direct the sampling and data collection processes. This chapter discusses research designs to help explain why a study is planned and implemented using any particular design and how different designs affect approaches to sampling and data collection, which, in turn, influence the study results and conclusions.

The RN in the clinical case reads in the feeling safe study that a qualitative research design was used, but he is not sure why this methodology was selected. He also notes that one critique of the current knowledge about psychosocial needs of ICU patients is that while we have studies that identify some needs, there is little evidence on how to best meet these needs. The RN knows that much of nursing research is not qualitative and wonders how a qualitative design will produce information that is useful for his practice. He remembers from school that quantitative research designs, such as randomized or experimental studies, are considered "strong" and he wonders if qualitative will be the "best" type of design to use in assisting him to care better for D.M.

A **research design** is the overall plan for acquiring new knowledge or confirming existing knowledge. In Chapter 1, we said that research is characterized by a systematic approach to gathering information to answer questions, which is in contrast to those approaches that use intuition, seek expert advice, or follow tradition. The research design is the plan for that systematic approach, conducted in a way that ensures the answer(s) found will be as meaningful and accurate as possible. The design identifies how subjects will be recruited and incorporated into a study; what will happen during the study, including timing of any treatments and measures; and when the study will end. A research design is selected with two broad purposes: (1) to plan an approach that will best answer the research question and (2) to ensure the rigor and validity of the results. We will discuss each of these purposes in general terms, and then we will look at specific approaches to research design.

Answering the Research Question

The first purpose in selecting a research design is to plan a systematic collection of information that will answer the question of interest. Two considerations are important: (1) the fit of the design to the research question and (2) the functionality of the design for the purpose of the study. Fit refers to how well the design matches the question of interest. It is in considering fit that we begin to address the question the RN in our clinical case has asked about meeting the psychosocial needs of a long-distance trucker. In the simplest terms, not all research questions can be answered through experiments because **experimental designs** answer questions requiring that we already know a great deal about the topic in order to set up a meaningful experiment. For example, simply setting up an experiment would not answer a research question regarding the characteristics of student nurses who select nonacute settings for their first practice after graduation. Why? Because an experiment assumes that we know some factors that we want to manipulate in order to see if and how they affect an

---

Box 9-1   General Types of Research Questions

- Questions that describe
- Questions that connect or link factors or concepts
- Questions that predict or examine effects of manipulation

---

outcome. If we do not know what factors are influencing the outcome of interest—in this example, the choice of practice after graduation—we have nothing to manipulate!

Research questions can be broadly categorized as questions that seek to describe or understand, questions that seek to connect or relate, and questions that seek to predict or study the effects of manipulation (Box 9-1). Generally, if we do not have adequate knowledge about a phenomenon of interest to nursing, we have to start by describing and understanding it, and the researcher will select a design that best allows for meeting that need. Once such studies are done and we have some idea of the meaning of the selected aspects of the phenomenon, we can ask questions about connections or relationships among those aspects. To answer those questions, the researcher will need a different form of design. Only after we know something about the connections and relationships can we begin to ask questions that seek to predict or manipulate aspects of the phenomenon, and there are designs specifically matched to this as well.

Now we are more aware that a research design must fit the type of question asked in order to provide appropriate and effective answers. A research design intended to answer questions about prediction will not be useful or appropriate for questions that seek to describe a phenomenon. Similarly, a design meant to allow meaningful description will not answer questions that seek to predict. The fit of a design to a research question depends on the function of the design and on how much is known about the topic of the study. In other words, different research designs serve different functions and, therefore, are particularly well suited to one type of research question, but not to another.

The functions of specific research designs can be broadly categorized, just as types of questions can be categorized. The functions include

1. Designs for describing or understanding
2. Designs for connecting or relating
3. Designs for manipulation and prediction

CORE CONCEPT 9-1

The type of research question being asked affects the type of research design that will and can be used.

Two other important considerations are designs that include timing or time as a factor in the study and designs that seek to control or not to control. Although several other factors differentiate types of research designs, the framework we will use for understanding how research designs influence the meaningfulness of research for practice focuses on three factors: (1) the overall function of the design, (2) how time or timing is incorporated into the design, and (3) whether the design seeks to control or not control study factors. Figure 9-1 depicts these broad factors and how they relate. We will discuss specific designs that fit into each category later in the chapter.

In summary, when deciding on a design, a researcher must consider several factors, including the functions of a design and the fit of those functions to the purpose of the research. Research designs differ in terms of the type of questions they can answer, whether they include time as a factor, and whether they focus on control within the study. The fit and functionality of a research design significantly influence whether the study can answer the research question of interest.

Ensuring Rigor and Validity

In addition to examining function and fit to answer the research question, the research design has as a purpose to ensure the rigor and validity of a study. In Chapter 8, we discussed these concepts in the context of specific strategies for data collection and

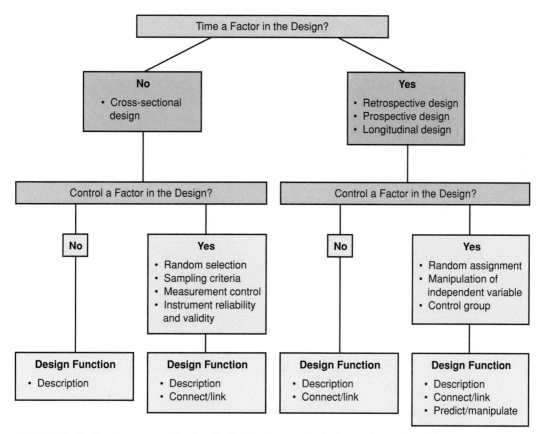

FIGURE 9-1 • Three broad factors that affect research design and associated terms.

measurement. The terms *rigor* and *validity* also are used in a broader sense to refer to the overall study. In Chapter 8, we said that rigor is a strict process of data collection and analysis as well as a term that reflects the overall quality of that process in qualitative research. It is in the broader sense of this quality that we consider rigor when discussing study design. Designs in qualitative research usually are more flexible and often are described as "emerging" to indicate that the design may be altered as the study progresses. Nevertheless, the design must still have a function that fits the research question and provides the foundation ensuring the accuracy of the study.

Like the term *rigor, validity* is used in research to refer both to specific ways that measures can correctly and accurately reflect their intended variable and to the accuracy of the overall results. Although use of the word *validity* in reference to measurement and design may be confusing, remember that the validity always has the same general meaning: accuracy or correctness. Content validity, criterion-related validity, and construct validity all refer to aspects of the accuracy of a measure. Validity of a study refers to its accuracy.

Study designs in quantitative research provide the foundation that ensures overall validity. Two types of validity are mentioned frequently when discussing research design. The first type, called **internal validity**, is the extent to which we can be sure of the accuracy or correctness of the findings of the study. Thus, it refers to how accurate the results are within the study itself, or internally. The second type, called **external validity**, is the extent to which the results of a study can be applied to other groups or situations. In other words, external validity refers to how accurately the study provides knowledge that can be applied outside of, or external to, the study. Figure 9-2 summarizes and illustrates the relationships among measurement validity, internal validity, and external validity.

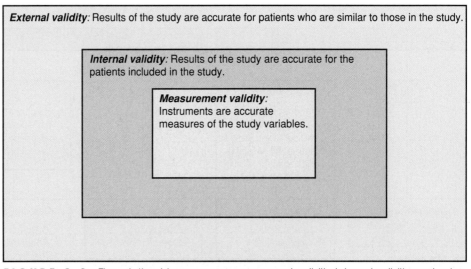

External validity: Results of the study are accurate for patients who are similar to those in the study.

Internal validity: Results of the study are accurate for the patients included in the study.

Measurement validity: Instruments are accurate measures of the study variables.

F I G U R E   9 - 2 • The relationships among measurement validity, internal validity, and external validity.

Research designs can affect both internal and external validity, and these two types are related in many research designs. Generalizability, discussed in Chapter 6, is a big aspect of external validity because it refers to the ability to infer that findings for a particular sample can be applied to the entire population. External validity also includes the extent to which the findings from a study in one setting can be applied to other similar settings. Logically, if a study lacks internal validity, it automatically lacks external validity: If the results are not accurate within the study, they clearly will not be accurate in other samples or settings. Similarly, if a study lacks measurement validity, it will lack internal validity. However, a study can have measurement validity and not have internal validity, or it can have correct findings and thus be internally valid but not externally valid. That is, the findings of a study may be real and correct to the specific sample and setting of the study but not applicable to the general population or to other settings. This relationship is illustrated in Figure 9-2 by the nesting of the three boxes representing the three types of validity.

Several aspects of study design can potentially lead to problems with rigor and internal and external validity. These problems are referred to as *threats to validity* because they threaten the accuracy of internal findings or the ability to apply the findings to other samples or settings. The threats to rigor and internal and external validity often discussed in research literature are listed in Table 9-2.

Threats to the Rigor of a Qualitative Study

Qualitative

As was indicated in Chapter 8, the rigor of a qualitative study is reflected in the consistency, trustworthiness, transferability, and credibility of the study. Qualitative designs or methods are based on distinct philosophical perspectives and have clearly defined systematic methods associated with each design. When we talked about these concepts in Chapter 8, we focused on the process of data collection, but in this chapter, we will focus on the process of implementing the entire study. For example, when considering these concepts in reference to the overall rigor of a study, we must consider *consistency* in the application of the study design throughout the study, or

TABLE 9-2

Threats to Rigor and Internal and External Validity

Rigor—Accuracy of Findings of a Qualitative Study	Internal Validity—Accuracy of Findings Within a Quantitative Study	External Validity—Accuracy of Findings of a Quantitative Study to the Settings and Samples Outside of the Study
Trustworthiness	History	Reactivity effects (Hawthorne effect)
Confirmability	Maturation	Measurement effects
Credibility	Testing	Novelty effects
Consistency	Instrumentation	Experimenter effects
	Mortality	
	Selection bias	

consider *credibility* given the researchers' accurate use of the study method. Thus, the language used to speak about overall study rigor in qualitative research is essentially the same as that used to discuss the data collection process, but the focus is broadened to the implementation of the study as a whole, and method and standards will differ a little.

Quantitative

Threats to Internal Validity

Threats to internal validity are potential problems that can affect the accuracy or correctness of findings within a study. They include problems of history, maturation, testing, instrumentation, mortality, and selection bias. These threats are summarized in Box 9-2.

The threat referred to as **history** is some factor outside those examined in a study affecting the outcome or dependent variable. The term *history* is used because some past event has influenced the dependent variable. For example, in the "Evolution of the caregiving experience in the initial 2 years following stroke" study (White, Mayo, Hanley, & Wood-Dauphinee, 2003) (Appendix A-4), if partway through that study Medicare benefits had changed to increase available coverage for home health aid care, caregiver outcomes may have improved, making the findings of the study invalid.

Maturation refers to a change in the dependent variable simply because of the passage of time. In the caregiver article (White et al., 2003), some caregivers might have ended up with changes in their outcomes that simply occurred due to aging. Thus, the natural aging process, a type of maturation with time, might lead to decreased daily functioning, regardless of whether the subjects were providing care to a family member. Those studies with a design that did not include a control group would be vulnerable to maturation. We talk more about the role of control groups shortly.

The threat called **testing** refers to changes in a dependent variable that result because it is being measured or because of the measure itself. For example, the mere presence of a nurse asking patients about the amount and quality of their psychosocial supports might increase a patient's anxiety, changing his or her self-report. Another possible example is a study in which a pretest of depression might make a subject more aware of how bad he or she feels, thus increasing the depression. A related threat to internal validity, called **instrumentation**, refers to changing the measures used in a study from one time to another. For example, suppose that the number of injections of pain medication for a postoperative cardiac patient's pain was being examined in a research study. Suppose that the timing of when the researcher collected data on the injections and the way in which the researcher documented the injections changed midway through the study. The change in the measurement might lead to different results; thus, values using the first method would not be directly comparable to values from the revised method.

The last types of threats to internal validity frequently considered when selecting a research design are *mortality* and *selection bias*. We examined both of these threats in Chapter 6 during the discussion of potential problems with sampling, although we did not use that exact terminology. **Mortality** refers to the loss of subjects

> ## Box 9-2 Summary of Threats to Internal Validity
>
> Internal validity is threatened because some *outside factor* **(history)** or *time* **(maturation)** affects the dependent variable, because the *measurement process* itself **(testing)** or *changes in a manner* **(instrumentation)** affect results for the dependent variable, or because the sampling process is biased *by loss of subjects* **(mortality)** or *selection of subjects* **(selection bias)**.

from a study because of a consistent factor related to the dependent variable. Occasionally, the loss of subjects is from death. At other times, mortality refers to subjects withdrawing from a study. The author of the feeling safe article found by the RN in the clinical case for this chapter does not indicate if any subjects in the study were excluded or lost. Given that the subjects were ICU patients, this loss might be expected. Nevertheless, if even two or three of the critical subjects for this study had died or been dropped from the study, we would have to wonder whether some factor directly related to psychosocial needs may have been associated with their death or being dropped and how that factor then affected the accuracy of the findings.

Selection bias refers to subjects having unique characteristics that in some manner relate to the dependent variable, raising a question whether the findings from the study resulted from the independent variable or the characteristics of the sample. Remember, we examined random assignment in Chapter 6 and learned that the times when we randomly assign subjects, any possible systematic bias in a sample has an equal chance of being present in the subjects of either group. This negates the potential threat of selection bias when comparing two groups.

Suppose that in the article used in Chapter 3, "Correlates of recovery among older adults after major abdominal surgery" (Zalon, 2004) (Appendix A-3), some of the patients required an additional piece of equipment by the bedside, such as a suction machine, that made it more difficult to get out of bed or to easily change position from supine to lateral. As a result, the researchers might have inadvertently introduced bias into their study by selecting patients who needed the suction machine at the bedside. The bias would occur because the health problem requiring the use of suction might also affect the recovery rates, thus confounding any differences that might occur solely because of the other variables of pain or depression.

Threats to External Validity

Threats to external validity are potential problems in a study that affect the accuracy of the results for samples and settings other than those of the study itself. As we said earlier, threats to internal and external validity are related, and in fact, overlap exists in the language used to describe the different threats. Because we are discussing the ability to apply the results of a study to other samples and settings, research literature often refers to threats to external validity as the effects of a threat to validity. Several effects are considered when selecting a research study design to ensure external validity. They include the effects of reactivity, measurement, experimenter, and/or novelty.

CORE CONCEPT 9-2

Studies with problems in internal validity automatically will have problems in external validity. Having internal validity, however, does not guarantee that the study will have external validity.

Reactivity effects refer to the responses of subjects to being studied. Threats to internal validity, such as testing, may cause reactivity. However, reactivity also can occur in a broader sense simply because subjects know that they are being studied. For example, the correlates of recovery after the major abdominal surgery article (Zalon, 2004), presented in Chapter 3 (Appendix A-3), depended on data collected from multiple surveys. Clearly, the subjects were aware that their answers would be scrutinized closely, and although they may not have known what specific aspects of their answers were expected by the researchers, the mere fact of their thinking about how their answers would be perceived might change how the subjects might respond.

In another example, let us say that the data being collected were based on observations of doctor–nurse interactions. Just because the subjects knew that they were being observed, they may have altered somewhat how they usually would interact. If being observed, in fact, greatly affected the behavior, the results of that study would differ in settings where behavior was not being observed. This then would be considered a threat to external validity. Another term sometimes used to describe reactivity is the **Hawthorne effect**. This name was derived from a study at the Hawthorne Electric Plant in which productivity of workers improved simply because they were being studied, no matter what intervention was applied. Reactivity and the Hawthorne effect are the same concept.

Measurement effects are changes in the results of a study resulting from various data collection procedures. This effect sounds similar to instrumentation and testing (threats to internal validity). Remember that any threat to internal validity automatically affects external validity negatively, and overlaps between internal and external validity can become confusing. Just as there are other forms of reactivity effects besides those inherent in threats to internal validity, there are other forms of measurement effects that are not threats.

For example, suppose that being asked about one's quality of life and anxiety before having breast cancer surgery (as was done in the "Efficacy of an in-home nursing intervention following short-stay breast cancer surgery" study) (Wyatt, Donze, & Beckrow, 2004) (Appendix A-6) led to increased awareness and expectations about how the surgery would affect quality of life. Then, the lack of an effect from the intervention found in the study may be valid for patients who have been questioned about these factors—that is, those who received these measures before the surgery—but would not be valid for patients who did not receive the questionnaire. The measurement of QOL in the study did not jeopardize the validity of the findings since all three groups of subjects received the same measure. However, the intervention might have had more effect if the measures had not been used; thus, there might have been a measurement effect on the external validity of the study.

The last two effects for us to consider are novelty effects and experimenter effects. Both involve uncontrolled or unmeasured effects from being in a study. **Novelty effects** occur when the knowledge that what is being done is new and under study somehow affects the outcome, either favorably or unfavorably. Once the independent variable is used outside the context of a study, the enthusiasm or doubts that affected the results are no longer present, so the results are no longer accurate in a setting that is not known to be a study. For example, using a self-help intervention for smoking cessation might be associated with success in quitting smoking, leading the researchers to conclude that the self-help intervention was effective. However, in fact, it was the novelty of the intervention and the subjects' knowledge that it was a new approach that actually led to their success in quitting, and when the intervention was later used in a clinical setting without a study being implemented, the success rate decreased.

Experimenter effects occur when some characteristic of the researcher or data collector influences the study results. For example, subjects may answer the questions the way they believe a researcher wants them to answer so that results change when subjects are not responding to cues from the researcher.

No matter which threat affects external validity, it reflects some problem with the environment or the research process that may make the study results less valid or accurate for other samples or settings. The names of the different effects and threats are intended to reflect the threat or effect, but they can be confusing. What is most important for the RN in our clinical case is not only to know that research designs are selected for their function and fit to the research question, but also to do the best possible job of ensuring the rigor and validity of the study. To review, rigor refers to the overall quality of a qualitative study; internal validity refers to the accuracy of the overall results within a quantitative study; and external validity refers to the accuracy of the overall results of a quantitative study in relation to settings and samples that are different or external to that study. Different research designs have varying strengths and weaknesses in relation to rigor and validity. The next two sections of this chapter describe some of these specific designs considering their functions, timing, and efforts at control.

QUALITATIVE RESEARCH DESIGNS

Qualitative

Figure 9-3 places qualitative designs within the framework of the broad factors of function, time, and control. As has been said throughout this book, the goal of qualitative research is to gain knowledge that informs our practice broadly and holistically, understanding that all knowing is evolving and contextual. That means that a design or method for a qualitative study will never focus on controlling factors to isolate specific aspects of a phenomenon. Rather, the methods focus on acquiring the richest possible data—that is, data with the greatest complexity and variety. Therefore, the designs intentionally seek to avoid external control over setting and factors.

Earlier, we said that there are three broad types of research questions: those that seek to describe and understand, those that seek to connect or relate, and those that

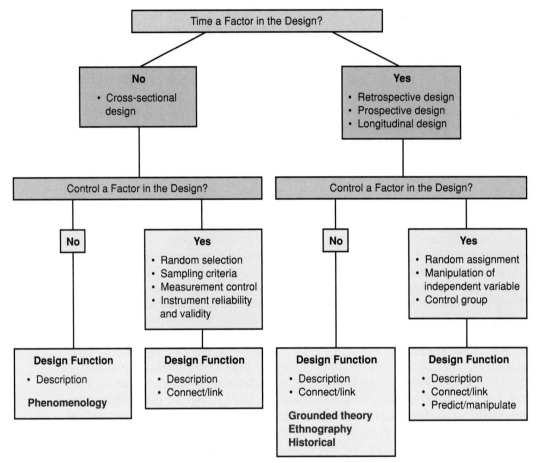

FIGURE 9-3 • Three broad factors that affect research design, with associated terms and associated qualitative designs.

seek to predict or manipulate. Qualitative research questions seek to describe, understand, and connect or relate, but they do not seek to predict or manipulate. Qualitative studies are most often done when we know the least about the topic of interest. As we gain understanding, the researcher will shift to methods other than qualitative.

There are three broad functions of qualitative research designs, including increasing understanding, promoting participation or immersion, and linking ideas and concepts. Designs that function to facilitate understanding answer **descriptive design** questions. Designs that seek to promote participation or immersion answer questions of both description and connection. Designs that seek to link ideas and concepts answer questions of connection or relationship. We will discuss four general types of designs or methods for qualitative research. Within each method are variations that are often associated with the names of the methodologists who developed

TABLE 9-3	
Methodologists Commonly Associated With the Major Qualitative Methods	
Major Method	**Specific Methodologists**
Phenomenology	Parse
	van Kaam
	Colaizzi
	Giorgi
	Paterson and Zderad
	Munhall and Boyd
	van Manen
Grounded theory	Glasser and Strauss
	Strauss and Corbin
	Stern
Ethnography	Goodenough (ethnoscience)
	Geertz (ethnographic algorithms)
	Sanday (ethnobehavior)
	Leininger (ethnonursing)
History	Bullough
	Hamilton

them. Some reports of qualitative studies use these specific names rather than the more general method name. It is beyond the scope of this book to describe these variations, but Table 9-3 lists some of the names frequently associated with each of the four methods.

Phenomenology

Phenomenology, or the phenomenologic method, is a qualitative method used to discover and develop understanding of experiences as perceived by those living the experience. As with all qualitative studies, the method seeks to avoid external control by going as directly as possible to those who have lived or are living the experience being studied. The method assumes that lived experiences can be interpreted or understood by distilling their essence. The "Needs of family members of patients with traumatic brain injury" study (Bond, Draeger, Mandleco, & Donnelly, 2003) (Appendix A-5) from Chapter 6 used phenomenologic methods to identify the essence of what families need when their family member has suffered a devastating critical injury. It may be helpful to go back and read the methods section of that research report for an example of a study using phenomenology.

There are several variations on the phenomenologic method (Spiegelberg, 1976; van Kaam, 1966; Giorgi, 1971; Colaizzi, 1973), but in general, the method includes identifying the people who are living or have lived the experience of interest and seeking, usually through unstructured interviewing, their perceptions. As data are collected, the researcher uses the processes of intuiting, analyzing, and describing to discover essential themes in the experience of the phenomenon (Parse, 2001). Skilled interviewing is needed to promote the most open and rich sharing of experiences as participants lived and perceived them.

As presented in Chapter 4, phenomenology uses a spiraling process of data collection and analysis, and detailed field notes of observations during data collection augment the richness and fullness of data. Time is not necessarily a major factor in phenomenologic methods, except as the participants in the study experience it. In fact, the method supports seeking participants who are both currently experiencing the phenomenon of interest and have already experienced it to get a breadth of perceptions of experiences.

In phenomenologic methods, neither length of time for collecting data nor number of participants is defined before the study starts. Rather, data are collected until all information is redundant of previously collected data—until saturation occurs. Sampling in phenomenology is always a convenience sample because only those who have had the experience of interest are sought, and neither limits nor criteria are placed on who can be a participant, other than the ability to communicate about and having lived the experience. Depending on the specific phenomenologic method used, the researcher often starts by identifying his or her own perceptions or expectations about the phenomenon to be studied and then attempts to consciously bracket them—hold them separate—so that they will not color either the data collection or the analysis process (Spiegelberg, 1976).

In the family needs in traumatic brain injury (TBI) article (Bond et al., 2003) (Appendix A-5), the authors describe going to a waiting room of a hospital to collect data. The authors worked with TBI patients, giving them insight into the experience of dealing with this health state. The interviews consisted of unstructured questions regarding, for that day, the families' needs and concerns. The duration of each interview and the overall study were not established ahead of time. The number of participants reflected the point of data saturation. The sample is described as purposive because families who were in the hospital setting with their family member were sought for the study. No effort was made, however, to control factors such as gender, race, age, or length of time the family member had been hospitalized. This study highlights the major characteristics of the phenomenologic method.

Ethnography

The second method commonly used in qualitative research is the ethnographic method, or **ethnography** (Spradley, 1979). A closely related method that was developed by Leininger (1991) within nursing is called *ethnonursing*. This method originated in the discipline of anthropology, and its purpose is for the researcher to participate or to immerse himself or herself in a culture to describe a phenomenon or phenomena within the context of that culture. Ethnography and ethnonursing assume that culture exists, even though it is not visible, and that the only way to know a culture is to get both an insider's view and an outsider's perspective. The insider's view is sometimes called an *emic perspective*.

Let us say in our clinical case that the RN discovers that the trucker was actually drunk at the time of the crash. The RN further finds out that the trucker's family is coming for a visit, and the wife has stated that she plans to bring their 15-year-old son, who is struggling with his emotions regarding his father's drinking while driving. The RN wonders what he might suggest to the mother that would help the adolescent cope. He finds another article reporting a study called "Qualitative evaluation of a school-based support group for adolescents with an addicted parent" (Gance-Cleveland, 2004). This article is available in Appendix A-8. The study used an ethnographic method to understand the features, critical attributes, processes, and benefits of school-based support groups for adolescents with an addicted parent. Reviewing that study report will give you an example of this method.

Again, controlling the environment or aspects of the study is not part of this qualitative method. The researcher tries to become part of the culture studied to acquire an insider's understanding so that he or she can then translate it into a common language understood by those outside the culture (Spradley, 1979). Because cultures are by nature complex, ethnographic methods take time, and the concept of time may be studied within the culture, but there is no set use of time within the method itself. This means that there is no structured plan concerning when data are collected or when the study ends. In general, data are collected as they happen and as opportunities present themselves, although the researcher may seek specific opportunities to interact within the culture. The researcher collects and analyzes data simultaneously so that he or she immediately uses knowledge gained to guide additional data collection. Therefore, there is no structured format for the collection of data.

In the qualitative evaluation of school-based support group article, the author tells us that she was the cofacilitator of the groups from which data were derived. She gives this information to indicate her immersion within the culture that she was studying. The general purpose of this research was to examine support groups for adolescents with an addicted parent, and the author realizes that these students are a unique cultural community. Some other aspects of ethnographic methods are less obvious in this particular article because the author does not directly talk about cultural aspects of adolescents in school settings. The entire study, however, reflects the unique culture of schools. In addition to studies with recognized cultural groups, ethnographic methods frequently are used in nursing to describe unique subcultures, such as adolescent drug users, people living in homeless shelters, and people residing in halfway houses.

Grounded Theory

Grounded theory is the third qualitative method commonly used in nursing research (Glaser & Strauss, 1967). The function of **grounded theory** is to study interactions to understand and recognize links between ideas and concepts or, in other words, to develop theory. The term *grounded* refers to the idea that the theory developed is based on or grounded in participants' reality rather than on theoretical speculation. Grounded theory is best used to study social processes and structures, hence the focus on links and interactions among ideas or categories. The article found first by the RN in our clinical case, "Feeling safe: The psychosocial needs of ICU patients" (Hupcey, 2000) (Appendix A-7), used a grounded theory method and provides you with a good example of this method.

Grounded theory methods often incorporate time into the study because the focus usually is on processes or change. The method itself, however, does not specify any particular timing to the data collection and analysis process. Sampling in grounded theory usually will be purposive—that is, purposely seeking participants experiencing the process or changes under study (Strauss & Corbin, 1994). Data collection in grounded theory can include interviews and careful observation of interactions and processes. As with all qualitative methods, grounded theory has a goal of avoiding placing limits or external controls on the processes being studied because the function of the method is to ground theory in natural reality. In the feeling safe article, the grounded theory method was particularly appropriate to her research question because she was interested in studying psychosocial needs, and grounded theory focuses on social processes, such as those within families. The results described for this study identified social processes that changed over time as the person was in the hospital, demonstrating that the function of the method is to describe processes and linkages.

Historical

The last general qualitative method sometimes used in nursing research is called the **historical** research method. Its function is to answer questions about links in the past to understand the present or to plan the future. Historical research methods require the researcher to define a phenomenon in a manner that can be clearly delineated so that data sources can be identified. For example, a phenomenon that might lend itself to historical research is to understand the process of nurse practitioners' legitimization as health care providers. Nurse practitioner legitimization, however, is too undefined to be approached using the historical method because it is not clear what time period or data sources would be relevant. The phenomenon of credentialing of nurse practitioners as a vehicle to legitimization of the role, on the other hand, defines a focus for data sources as well as a time period because the development of credentialing occurred throughout a definable number of years. Data sources in this example would target the development and implementation of the process of credentialing nurse practitioners and how that process related to perceptions of the legitimacy of the role of nurse practitioners.

Data sources in historical research may include records, videotapes, photographs, and interviews with people involved in the phenomenon or review of published reports. As with the other qualitative methods discussed, the researcher tries to acquire as broad a sample of data sources as possible. Unlike the other methods, in the historical method, a focus of data collection includes evaluation of data sources for their reliability. For example, an editorial in the *Journal of the American Medical Association* regarding the process of nurse practitioner credentialing might reflect a bias that makes the description of the process questionable. That same editorial, however, might be a reliable data source about the professional climate in which credentialing developed. A researcher using the historical method would evaluate the data source and consider this potential bias when deciding how to use it.

We have not had a research study that has used the historical method as an example in this text. However, an article that does use this method, "Historical analysis of siderail use in American hospitals" (Brush & Capezuti, 2001), can be found in Appendix E.

We have now discussed four different methods used in qualitative research, the functions of which vary. Phenomenologic methods provide in-depth data about a particular life experience and, therefore, are particularly useful in answering descriptive questions, especially when very little is known about the topic of interest. Ethnographic methods provide immersion and active participation in a particular culture or subculture and assist in answering descriptive and linkage and connection questions. Grounded theory methods provide data about social interactions, which can be built into a theory based on reality. These methods are particularly useful in answering questions about interactions or links among social processes. Historical methods provide data about past processes to gain insight about the present and future. They answer questions about links and connections.

All the qualitative methods we have examined specifically attempt to avoid introducing external control into the study design because all are interested in gathering data that are as complex and rich as the real world. Nevertheless, all four methods entail a systematic process for sampling, data acquisition, and data analysis. Strict criteria for timing are not part of any of the methods, but time is an inherent component of the historical method, is often a part of the culture studied using ethnography, and is usually an aspect of interactional processes reported in grounded theory studies.

Throughout this section discussing qualitative design, the word *methods* has been used more frequently then the word *design*. This is because design suggests a more formalized and standardized plan than is often present within qualitative methods. Qualitative research designs are consciously and intently unstructured and flexible to reflect the unpredictable and complex nature of phenomena as they occur in life. As we will see in the next section that discusses quantitative designs, the word *design* is more appropriate in quantitative research because quantitative methods seek to standardize as well as formalize the process of sampling, data collection, and data analysis.

QUANTITATIVE RESEARCH DESIGNS

Quantitative

We will once again use the three broad factors of function, time, and control to categorize quantitative designs (Figure 9-4). The language used to describe quantitative designs can be confusing initially because terms are used in different combinations to define different methods. Rather than start with the functions of differing designs, we start by discussing the language used to address time and control when referring to quantitative research design.

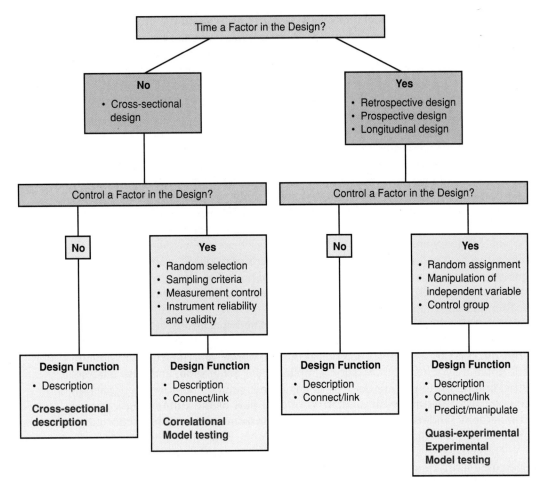

F I G U R E 9 - 4 • Three broad factors that affect research design, with associated terms and quantitative designs.

Time

Whereas time is a factor to study or incorporate into the fabric of a method in qualitative research, time is a specific factor that defines different research designs in quantitative research. Quantitative designs are described as either retrospective or prospective. **Retrospective designs** are those in which data are collected about past events or factors. **Prospective designs** are those in which data are collected about events or variables as they occur, moving forward in time. In addition to considering whether data are collected moving backward or forward in time, designs are described in terms of point of time of measurement. Research designs are **cross sectional** if they collect all data at one point in time. Research designs are called **longitudinal** if they collect data at different time points. Therefore, a prospective study automatically is longitudinal as well. A cross-sectional study, however, does not have to be retrospective.

Consider for example a study of patient satisfaction with care. A retrospective and cross-sectional study would collect data from patients at some point after they visit a clinic, perhaps 1 or 2 weeks later, and ask them to recall their level of satisfaction during their visit. Data are collected at one time point looking at past experience. A study of patient satisfaction that surveys patients as they leave a clinic also would be cross sectional because data are collected at only one time point for each subject. However, it would not be retrospective because it is not going back in time; data are being collected about variables in the present. A prospective longitudinal patient satisfaction study might collect data before a visit to a clinic, immediately after the visit, and 1 week later, looking for changes in selected variables over time. At each measurement point, the question might be "How satisfied are you right now with the clinic care?" Thus, data are not being collected about past experiences or perceptions, even when they are collected 1 week after the visit. From this example, it should be clear that it is a combination of factors that define research designs in quantitative research. This idea is important to grasp.

Terms used to describe the use of time in quantitative research designs include those we have discussed and another important term: *repeated measures*. **Repeated measures** mean just what the words say—a design using repeated measures repeats the same measurements at several points in time. When you see this term, it suggests that a variable or variables were measured more than just two or three times, and you can expect that the analysis of the study examines the pattern of change in the variable over time.

CORE CONCEPT 9-3

The labels for quantitative research designs usually are combinations of words or terms that define the design's function, use of time, and use of approaches to provide control.

A longitudinal prospective study may or may not have repeated measures. We have reviewed several longitudinal studies throughout this book, but only some of them included repeated measures. For example, the evolution of caregiving experience article (White et al., 2003) (Appendix A-4), used in Chapters 4 and 5, was longitudinal and used repeated measures because the same data about the same variables were collected in the same way regularly over time. In contrast, if we look at the efficacy of an in- home intervention study (Wyatt et al., 2004) (Appendix A-6), that study was longitudinal but only measured the variables at three time points—before the intervention and 1 and 6 months following the intervention. Although the measures were used more than once, this study would not be considered a design using repeated measures; rather it is using a pre- and post-test design.

Control

In addition to differences in how they consider the factor of time, quantitative research designs differ in the amount of control of extraneous factors that they attempt to impose on a study. Remember that quantitative research seeks to clearly define and measure specific variables. To do so, research designs seek to ensure that outside factors not specifically defined and measured in the study are not allowed to affect what is included in the study. Outside or extraneous factors not considered and measured within a quantitative study are sources of error. In Chapter 8, we discussed error in measurement in relation to measurement reliability and validity. We are now considering error in a broader manner, just as we examined validity of an entire study previously in the chapter. Designs in quantitative research seek to ensure the internal and external validity of the study by minimizing error. They do so by imposing different controls on the sampling, data collection, and analysis.

The areas within which research designs seek to create or to impose control include the sampling and measurement processes. Control in the sampling process can be imposed by establishing criteria for inclusion or exclusion that attempt to prevent some outside difference among subjects from confusing the findings of a study. Another method of control is the use of random sampling, by which the entire population is enumerated, and everyone has an equal chance of being asked to be in the study. A third method is random assignment because all subjects have an equal chance of being included in any particular group in the study. Thus, any differences in the subjects will likely be distributed equally within different groups that will be compared. We reviewed each of these approaches to control in Chapter 6. Quantitative research designs partly reflect and define the sampling approach that a study will take.

Control within the data collection process can be imposed by ensuring the validity and reliability of the measures or by ensuring that the measurement process itself is consistent, avoiding instrumentation threats. Control in measurement also can be imposed by creating **comparison group(s)** so that either exposure to the factors studied is manipulated in a controlled fashion or the timing of the measurement process is manipulated around a factor of interest. Study designs that include a comparison group create control by comparing subjects in two groups who differ in an independent variable of interest. Inclusion of a comparison group eliminates such threats to internal validity as history and maturation because both groups experience the same history or process of maturation. A design using a comparison group attempts to ensure that two groups are as similar as possible on most factors that could affect the dependent variable of interest and assume that they differ clearly in an independent variable. Therefore, such designs hope to isolate the influence of that independent variable on the dependent variable of interest. Study designs that include a **control group** create a greater level of control by manipulating the independent variable of interest so that the control group is not exposed to it, whereas the experimental group is. Again, a dependent variable is examined for differences to see if the factor manipulated affects that dependent variable.

Functions of Quantitative Research Designs

Having considered the factors of time and control, we will now discuss specific quantitative designs considering these two factors as well as overall function. Quantitative research designs vary in the level of control that they impose from limited in descriptive and correlational studies to more control in quasi-experimental studies to the most control in true experimental designs.

Descriptive Designs and Correlational Studies

Descriptive designs function to portray some phenomenon of interest as accurately as possible. Correlational studies use a descriptive design to describe interrelationships among variables as accurately as possible. Researchers generally consider studies that look at correlations to be a subtype of descriptive designs and refer to them as *studies* rather than the broader term *design*. Clearly, descriptive designs are used to answer research questions that seek to describe. **Correlational studies** are used to answer research questions that seek to link or connect. Both types focus on exerting control through the quality of the measurement—that is, by using reliable and valid measures as discussed in Chapter 8 and through sampling criteria or procedures. Descriptive and correlational studies may impose control by establishing certain criteria for inclusion or exclusion from the study. Remember, this also can be called *purposive sampling* or *use of a convenience sample*. Both types of design can impose even greater control over extraneous factors by using randomly selected samples.

Descriptive and correlational designs can be longitudinal or cross sectional, and they can be retrospective or prospective. Decisions about how time is a factor are based on the nature of the question, the potential sample, and the measures. Some phenomena, such as growth or productivity, clearly entail a time element that would make it logical for a researcher to use a longitudinal design. However, as we discussed in Chapter 6, finding, following, and maintaining subjects over time can be difficult and costly, so some studies may use a single cross-sectional design to avoid problems of following subjects over time. Certainly, some measures can be repeated easily, whereas others cannot, because they measure stable concepts unlikely to change or because the measurement process is too intrusive to repeat often. For example, the concept of an individual's sense of coherence is a stable sense of the world and oneself within the world and, although a researcher may be interested in measuring this as a variable in a study, it would not be helpful to measure it more than once because it will remain stable. An example of an intrusive measure might be a bone marrow analysis. It could be that data from weekly bone marrow tests would be ideal in evaluating a new cancer drug. However, this test is too intrusive and painful to repeat at that kind of interval.

A special type of correlational study is a design for **model**. A model is the symbolic framework for a theory or part of a theory. In Chapter 2, we discussed Lazarus's theory of stress, also shown as a model in Figure 9-5. A design testing such a model identifies measures for each concept and examines how the concepts relate. A study testing Lazarus's theory would identify ways to measure the variables of

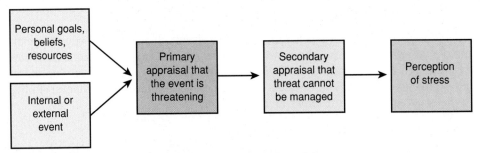

FIGURE 9-5 • Schematic model of Lazarus's theory of stress.

personal beliefs and resources, the event, primary appraisal, secondary appraisal, and stress. Then, the study would statistically analyze relationships among the results on these measurements of the variables to see if the relationships found were of the type and direction predicted by the model.

Often, designs for model testing are longitudinal, so some parts of the model are measured at one time point and other aspects are measured at a later time point. This allows researchers to propose causal relationships between concepts in the model. Therefore, model testing designs often attempt to answer questions that predict as well as relate.

In summary, descriptive designs function to portray a phenomenon of interest and may be retrospective, prospective, cross sectional, or longitudinal. They also may impose varying levels of control through sampling strategies, such as purposive samples or random sampling. Correlational designs function to describe or identify inter-relationships among factors of interest; they also may be retrospective, prospective, cross sectional, or longitudinal. Because correlational designs describe relationships, you will occasionally see them called *descriptive correlational designs*. Correlational designs may use the same range of sampling strategies used in descriptive designs. Model testing designs are a special type of correlational design that usually incorporate time in some manner, either through longitudinal data collection or through use of measures that combine retrospective and concurrent data collection.

Quasi-Experimental and Experimental Research Designs

Quasi-experimental and experimental research designs function to answer questions involving prediction and the effects of manipulation. Quasi-experimental differs from experimental primarily in the amount of control imposed. Both types include control of an independent variable, but a true experimental design always includes a control group and random assignment to groups. Remember, a control group is a group of subjects who do not receive an intervention so that the control group can be compared with those who do receive the intervention (Box 9-3).

When researchers discuss quasi-experimental and experimental designs, they often use a set of symbols to diagram the particular form of design used. When they do this, they use the symbol "O" to indicate occasion of observation or measurement,

---

Box 9-3 Components of Experimental Designs

- Manipulation of the independent variable
- Random assignment of subjects to groups
- A control group

---

with a subscript number designating the time point of the observation. They use the letter "X" to denote the intervention, meaning the independent variable, and they use "R" to denote that subjects were randomly assigned to groups. Figure 9-6 is an example of this type of diagram. It translates to mean that two groups were formed using random assignment (R). Each group had measurements taken (O_1), one group received the intervention (X), and both groups had a second measurement taken (O_2). This design includes manipulation of the independent variable, random assignment, and a control group; therefore, it is experimental. Because it includes an observation both before and after the intervention, the type of design in Figure 9-6 is called a **pretest–post-test** experimental design.

Although most quasi-experimental and experimental designs are longitudinal, it is possible for an experiment to be implemented at only one time point. Figure 9-7 shows how a single time point experimental design would look. Because experimental designs always involve manipulation of an independent variable, they are never retrospective. Finally, **multifactorial** is a term sometimes associated with experimental design that refers to several independent variables being manipulated in a study. The examples we have considered have all had a single independent variable; however, some studies control and manipulate two or more independent variables.

A **quasi-experimental design** lacks either a control group or random assignment. It may not include two groups at all. Instead, it may involve a series of observations, followed by an intervention and then another series of observations (Figure 9-8). In this case, there is manipulation of the independent variable but no control group. The threats to internal validity in this type of design include instrumentation and testing as well as selection bias and mortality. There also are quasi-experimental designs that have two groups of subjects, but the groups are nonequivalent because subjects are not randomly assigned to each group. Such a design is referred to as a *nonequivalent control group pretest–post-test quasi-experimental design,* and

$$R \quad O_1 \quad X \quad O_2$$

$$R \quad O_1 \quad \quad O_2$$

FIGURE 9-6 • Schematic of pretest–post-test experimental design.

$$R \quad X \quad O_1$$

$$R \qquad O_1$$

FIGURE 9-7 • Schematic of an experimental design with only one point of measurement.

it entails observations of two groups, followed by one group receiving the intervention and then a second set of observations. Because both groups receive the same measurement, this quasi-experimental design is less threatened by instrumentation and testing but still is threatened by selection bias and mortality. Thus, a rather long name for a design tells us a great deal about how the research study was implemented. What if we were interested, for example, in studying the effect of positioning changes on the pain levels of hospitalized patients? If we were to find a study that randomly assigned patients to two groups and then manipulated a variable for one group but not the other, we would say that the study was most likely experimental in design. A design must include manipulation of an independent variable, a control group, and random assignment in order to be classified as experimental.

Another phrase applied to methods that we need to discuss further is repeated measures. We have already said that this phrase means that multiple measures of the same variable were taken over time. In our hypothetical study of the effect of positioning, let us assume that the researcher chose to measure a variable such as heart rate before turning the person, immediately after turning, and 5 minutes after turning, then 10, 15, and 25 minutes after turning, for a total of six measures. This is a good example of the frequency of measures you would expect if a design is said to use repeated measures. If a study lacked true random assignment to the intervention groups, and/or lacked a control group, the study would be labeled as quasi-experimental.

In summary, the language used to describe quantitative research designs reflects their function, such as descriptive, correlational, or experimental. Other language used to describe designs reflects how time is a component, such as retrospective, cross sectional, or longitudinal. Finally, the language of designs reflects the level of control imposed in the study, with experimental designs imposing the greatest control over extraneous variables. We have reviewed several of the studies used throughout this book as examples of various designs. To provide familiar examples of several research designs, Table 9-4 categorizes each of the eight studies in this text thus far according to type of research design used.

$$O_1 \quad O_2 \quad O_3 \quad O_4 \quad X \quad O_5 \quad O_6 \quad O_7 \quad O_8$$

FIGURE 9-8 • Schematic of repeated measures quasi-experimental design.

TABLE 9-4

Categorization of Research Designs of the Eight Articles Used in This Text

Chapter and Reference	Research Design
Chapters 1 & 2: Sandelowski, M., & Barroso, J. (2003). Motherhood in the context of maternal HIV infection. *Research in Nursing & Health, 26,* 470–482.	Metasynthesis of qualitative studies
Kane, M., & DiBartolo, M. (2002). Complex physical and mental health needs of rural incarcerated women. *Issues in Mental Health Nursing, 23,* 209–229.	Descriptive cross sectional
Chapter 3: Zalon, M. L. (2004). Correlates of recovery among older adults after major abdominal surgery. *Nursing Research, 53*(2), 99–106.	Descriptive correlational
Chapters 4 & 5: White, C. L., Mayo, N., Hanley, J. A., & Wood-Dauphinee, S. (2003). Evolution of the caregiving experience in the initial 2 years following stroke. *Research in Nursing & Health, 26,* 177–189.	Longitudinal descriptive
Chapter 6: Bond, A. E., Draeger, C. R. L., Mandleco, B., & Donnelly, M. (2003). Needs of family members of patients with severe traumatic brain injury. *Critical Care Nurse, 23*(4), 63–72.	Phenomenology
Chapter 8: Wyatt, G. K., Donze, L. F., & Beckrow, K. C. (2004). Efficacy of an in-home nursing intervention following short-stay breast cancer surgery. *Research in Nursing & Health, 27*(5), 322–331.	Randomized clinical trial
Chapter 9: Hupcey, J. E. (2000). Feeling safe: The psychosocial needs of ICU patients. *Journal of Nursing Scholarship, 32*(4), 361–367.	Grounded theory
Gance-Cleveland, B. (2004). Qualitative evaluation of a school-based support group for adolescents with an addicted parent. *Nursing Research, 53*(6), 379–386.	Ethnography

HOW CAN ONE GET THE WRONG DESIGN FOR THE RIGHT QUESTION?

Let us return to the question that our RN in the clinical case was considering about why all studies are not experimental. We have already addressed one part of the answer to that question: The research question must ask about prediction or the effects of manipulation before an experimental design will fit. For a question seeking to examine the effects of manipulation or to predict, we must have certain baseline knowledge already in place. The other reason that experimental designs are not the right design for every question involves the strengths and weaknesses of the design itself. Experimental designs are strong on control; therefore, they have the fewest threats to internal validity. That same control, however, makes experiments dissimilar from the "real" world of patient care, where variety and complexity are the rule. Therefore, the results of a study using an experimental design are generally accurate, and we can trust highly that the findings are correct. However, the findings may not be easily applied or generalized to clinical practice, where many of the factors controlled in the experiment will not be controlled.

For example, if subjects in a study on the effects of a new multiposition bed had to receive a two-dimensional CAT scan or an echocardiograph to confirm physiological changes when the bed moved, the availability of technology would automatically reflect a certain level of hospital and, in most cases, a certain level of insurance coverage. Thus, uninsured patients and those from rural settings without access to tertiary care centers would more than likely be underrepresented or not represented in such a study. Yet, being uninsured or living in a rural setting are factors that may affect physiologic functioning and resilience. The very controls that ensured that the patients did have physiological changes related to the multiposition bed also may limit the generalizability of the study. In reality, the controls exerted in this example probably do not greatly influence the utility of the results for more general practice; however, this example gives you an idea of why the aspects that provide control in a design also may limit the clinical usefulness of the results.

Quasi-experimental studies lose some of the internal validity of an experimental design but often gain some applicability to real life. Often, a quasi-experimental design is selected to answer a research question when the implementation of a true experimental design is not feasible. For example, researchers who want to study HIV-prevention programs with homeless women would face great difficulty in randomly assigning homeless women to different programs because homeless people generally do not follow schedules or have circumstances that would enable them to attend programs that are not conveniently located. If the researchers tried to implement several different programs in one shelter (randomly assigning the women in the shelter to a program), it is likely that the women would share activities from the different programs, causing the programs to blur and making it impossible to isolate the effects of one compared with the other. Therefore, a researcher testing an HIV program with homeless women would likely use a quasi-experimental design, selecting homeless shelters to either receive or not receive the intervention to be tested. In contrast, if the researchers want to test HIV-prevention programs with high school students, they might more easily randomly assign subjects and create a true experiment. Nevertheless, results with high school students would not be easy to apply to the different lives and experiences of homeless women. Therefore, the very control possible with high school students would preclude the study being as useful for homeless women.

As we move to descriptive and correlational designs, control decreases even further because the researcher no longer controls the independent variable. Selection criteria or random selection, however, can still provide some control. In addition, measurement reliability and validity increase our confidence about the accuracy of the factors being studied. Because descriptive and correlational designs still impose control through sampling and measurement, the richness and diversity of real-life clinical situations is limited. Phenomenologic, ethnographic, and grounded theory designs impose the least control over the process of research and, therefore, capture the greatest detail and depth of real experiences. Yet, they can become so subjective or conceptual that the results also may be difficult to apply to real practice. Qualitative designs are not intended to develop knowledge about predictions; but, we often seek knowledge that will allow us to predict in nursing.

Therefore, the answer to the question "How can one get the wrong design for the right question?" involves feasibility in terms of who or what is being studied, what measures are available, and what is already known about the problem or phenomenon. A study of the process of tobacco addiction cannot ethically manipulate the variable of exposure to tobacco, so it will, by necessity, be nonexperimental. A study of drug efficacy requires careful control of as many extraneous factors as possible, lending itself to experimental design. However, withholding drug treatment in some cases may be unethical, leading to the use of quasi-experimental design. Studies of subjective experiences, such as pain, grief, or satisfaction, require understanding best acquired through seeking the insights of those who have experienced or are experiencing the phenomenon, lending themselves to qualitative designs. Yet, a researcher may not be skilled in qualitative methods and so may choose a cross-sectional descriptive design instead.

What should be evident at this point is that study design shapes the approach taken to sampling, measurement, and data analysis. Understanding the basic language of design will allow you to understand many of the decisions made by the researcher(s) regarding the study, clarifying the approaches taken to acquiring subjects or participants and to the data collection itself. Recognizing that the terms used in quantitative design are combined differently to specify the function, control, and time factor in a design will help you to better understand the types of designs described in published research.

In addition to terms that reflect the function of and the use of control and time in a design, some designs are described as mixed methods. **Mixed methods** refers to some combination of methods in relation to function, time, or control. A study that collects retrospective data by asking parents to complete a questionnaire about family history of heart disease, their children's level of physical activity, and the parents' smoking behavior is an example of collecting data about how things were, thinking back in time. In addition, if this study then collects data of cholesterol level, blood pressure, and HgA_1, this could be classified as a longitudinal study because it links data from the past about activity, history, and smoking with data from the present about blood pressure, cholesterol, and HgA_1.

Another use of the term *mixed methods* is to refer to a combination of qualitative and quantitative methods. The fictional article from Appendix B about nursing students' choices of clinical practice uses a somewhat mixed method because it includes data collection by use of a pen-and-paper quantifiable questionnaire and a written open-ended question that was analyzed using methods associated with qualitative research. As nursing research develops, more and more researchers are recognizing the value of both qualitative and quantitative methods to more fully answer questions of interest to nursing. This has led to increased use of a combination of qualitative and quantitative designs in single studies.

Before beginning this chapter, you were asked to consider how you might best conduct a study of the effects of nursing school attendance on well-being. Now that we have examined various research designs and some of the advantages and disadvantages of each, let us consider some choices you would need to make if you were going to conduct such a study.

First, you could approach a study of the effects of nursing school attendance on well-being from a qualitative perspective or a quantitative perspective. The decision would depend partly on what is already known, such as what is known about influences on well-being in college students, how nursing programs differ from other undergraduate programs, and whether nursing students differ from other undergraduate students in some important ways that might affect well-being. If little is known about any of these factors, a qualitative study of the lived experiences of nursing students in terms of sense of well-being while in school might be the research design to use. If little is known about well-being and nursing students, a researcher might implement a grounded theory design to examine interactions that affect well-being.

A researcher also might decide to do a descriptive correlational study measuring well-being and other factors that would logically be relevant, such as general health, age, family commitments, work schedule, and grade-point average, to see how they relate. If implementing a quantitative study, the researcher could decide to do measurements only at one time point and perhaps include students just entering school, those halfway through school, and those preparing to graduate. Such a study would be cross sectional. To address problems with internal validity, the researcher would need to consider how comparable students in the three different classes were in factors that affect well-being other than nursing school attendance.

Alternatively, a researcher might decide to do a longitudinal study, following a group of nursing students from the time they enter school to graduation. This type of study would take much time and many resources; it also would be open to such threats to internal validity as mortality, testing, and instrumentation. The question of effects of nursing school attendance and well-being probably does not lend itself to or fit with either quasi-experimental or experimental designs, unless something already has been shown to be a factor that could be manipulated to try to change well-being.

This example demonstrates why studies addressing approximately the same question may use different research designs. As an intelligent user of nursing research, you do not have to decide what type of design to use, but it is helpful for you to understand some considerations that go into selecting a design as well as the meaning and strengths and weaknesses of different research designs.

COMMON ERRORS IN PUBLISHED REPORTS OF RESEARCH DESIGNS

As you read published studies, such as those the RN found in our clinical case, there may be problems with the amount of information provided about the study design. One common problem is a lack of detail about the design, leaving the reader uncertain concerning the methods used. In some cases, the only thing we are told is that a particular method or design was used. This happens more in published reports of qualitative studies than in reports of quantitative studies and may occur partly because qualitative methods were less well known or used in nursing in past years. A written report of a study design should not simply tell the reader the label for the design; it also should describe enough of the actual process of the research study to assure the reader that the design was implemented appropriately.

For example, a study that states it uses phenomenologic methods also should tell you enough about the subjects to assure you that they were rich and appropriate sources of data and, generally, how data were collected and analyzed. A study that tells you it used an experimental design also should provide specific information about the random assignment process, creation of the control group, and manipulation of the intervention.

As with measurement in research, a study design can be complex. Nevertheless, it is the responsibility of the author(s) to communicate in writing all the essential aspects of the design so that the reader can intelligently read and understand the study. The use of a time line often helps readers to understand a study design, particularly if it is longitudinal. The other aspect that occasionally is lacking in published reports is a rationale for the choice of research design. We have discussed that a researcher has to make several decisions when selecting a design. Occasionally, the rationales for decisions, such as not including a control group, can help the reader to better understand the problems of the study and how they may affect usefulness for clinical practice.

PUBLISHED REPORTS—DID DESIGN AFFECT YOUR CONCLUSION?

The RN in our clinical case is trying to understand how D.M.'s psychosocial needs might best be addressed. Additionally, he wonders how he might help D.M.'s adolescent son adjust to learning that his father's accident was alcohol-related. The RN in our clinical case has begun to understand that nurses do not have much evidence on what interventions facilitate the psychosocial needs of ICU patients. Additionally, the RN is aware that we understand more about substance abuse issues, but adolescents whose parents have a substance abuse issue represent a unique cultural group. From this perspective, the research designs are beginning to make sense. The school-based support group article (Gance-Cleveland, 2004) (Appendix A-8) is an example of a qualitative ethnographic study, while the feeling safe article (Hupcey, 2000) (Appendix A-7) found by the RN in this chapter is an example of qualitative grounded theory. Neither of these researchers used an experimental design, but there was also little known about the phenomenon of interest to these researchers. However, the researcher in the school-based support group article was interested in a unique cultural group, and the researcher in the feeling safe article was interested in social process. From this perspective, the researcher's method selection seems reasonable and appropriate.

While most evidence-based studies focus on research in the form of clinical trials, this gold standard can be used only when we know enough about a topic to use a true experimental design. **Clinical trials** refer to studies that test the effectiveness of a clinical treatment, and some researchers would say that a clinical trial must be a true experiment. For many problems in clinical practice, however, there have been only a few true experimental studies, so it is not uncommon to see clinical trials defined more broadly.

Given the nature of the question and the evidence from the studies, the RN concludes that D.M.'s psychosocial need for safety should be a dominant focus of his care planning. Additionally, the RN realizes that he may not need to worry quite so much about the negative impact on a feeling of safety because the patient's family is away, and the research showed that family can sometimes actually increase a patient's feeling unsafe. The RN also is more comfortable about dealing with the needs of the patient's son and feels that, if possible, he could recommend that the son find a school-based support group to help in his adjustment.

CRITICALLY READING THE DESCRIPTION OF THE STUDY DESIGN IN A RESEARCH REPORT

In Box 9-4, you will find questions that you can use to critically read about the design of a research study. Often the study design is part of the methods section of a research report, but since we have discussed designs in a separate chapter, we will also address questions to ask about designs as a separate component to consider when reading a report of research. The first question asks "Did the report include a clearly identified section describing the research design?" The RN reading the feeling safe study did find a clear statement of the study design; however, some research reports may fail to identify the type of design, making it necessary for you as a reader to try to classify that design based on other information in the report. If you read a report and are uncertain about the study design even after reviewing the complete method section, then it may be that the researchers failed to have a systematic plan for their study, and that would affect your trust of the total study.

The second question to ask is "Does the design make this a quantitative, qualitative, or a mixed method study?" The answer to that question allows you as a critical reader to evaluate the fit of the design to the procedures and measures used in the study. A misfit between design and actual measures would suggest that the researcher(s) may have implemented a less than consistent and systematic study and would cause you to wonder about the usefulness of the results of that study for practice. For example, if a research report indicates the study design is ethnography and then indicates that data were collected using a series of written scales, we would have

---

Box 9-4 How to Critically Read the Description of Study Design in a Research Report

Does the report answer the question "How were those people studied—why was the study performed that way?"

1. Did the report include a clearly identified section describing the research design?
2. Does the design make this a quantitative, qualitative, or a mixed method study?
3. Does the report address approaches taken to assure study rigor, internal validity, and/or external validity?
4. Do I think that the researcher(s) should have designed the study differently in order to answer my clinical question?

---

to wonder about the quality of the study, as this type of measurement does not fit with a qualitative design.

A third question to ask as you critically read about a study design is "Does the report address approaches taken to assure study rigor, internal validity, and/or external validity?" In order to answer this, you must be familiar with these concepts and will have to critically read the description of the implementation of the study. Finally, you will want to ask yourself "Do I think that the researcher(s) should have designed the study differently in order to answer my clinical question?" For example, the RN in our clinical case wants to assist D.M. in his psychosocial adjustment while in the ICU. As he reads the study about feeling safe in the unit, he recognizes that his clinical question is one about patient experiences and perceptions, and therefore, the qualitative design used is appropriate and will give him useful evidence on which to base his practice.

The RN realizes that without the research findings contained in the article that he read, his care may have been different and perhaps not nearly as effective in improving his patient's health. The results also suggest the importance of the nurse's role in both contributing to the patient's feelings of safety and, in some cases, being the cause of the patient feeling less safe. These are things that the charge nurse did not mention to the RN, who is glad that he chose to read the study. The RN wonders why the researchers were so concerned about the psychosocial needs of ICU patients. To answer that question, he will have to read the beginning of the article that describes the background for the study as well as the research problem.

Clearly, then, the type of research design used in a study affects the usefulness and meaningfulness of the results for clinical practice. The language of research design is complex and confusing at times because several terms are used in different ways in different contexts.

Nevertheless, it is possible to acquire a good general understanding of the meaning of most of the terms so that this important aspect of a research study can be understood and interpreted as related to the applicability of the study to clinical practice.

OUT-OF-CLASS EXERCISE

How to Set the Stage for a Study

At the end of Chapter 8, you were asked to develop some ideas for a research design in order to study the effects of nursing school attendance on well-being. We have discussed in this chapter some possible designs that you may have considered and the need to have a better idea of what is already known before you can settle on a design. Chapter 10 discusses the background and statement of the research problem sections of research reports. It is this first part of a research report that provides the rationale for a study as well as information about previous research. Before reading Chapter 10, write one or two paragraphs that describe why a study of nursing students' well-being and the effect of attendance in nursing school are important enough to warrant a research study. If you were going to conduct such a study, what would you need to describe at the beginning to set the stage? After you have written your case for studying the nursing students' well-being, you are ready to begin Chapter 10.

References

Bond, A. E., Draeger, C. R. L., Mandleco, B., & Donnelly, M. (2003). Needs of family members of patients with severe traumatic brain injury: Implications for evidence-based practice. *Critical Care Nurse, 23*(4), 63–72.

Brush, B. L., & Capezuti, E. (2001). Historical analysis of siderail use in American hospitals. *Journal of Nursing Scholarship, 33*(4), 381–385.

Colaizzi, P. F. (1973). *Reflection and research in psychology: A phenomenological study of learning.* Dubuque, IA: Kendall/Hunt.

Gance-Cleveland, B. (2004). Qualitative evaluation of a school-based support group for adolescents with an addicted parent. *Nursing Research, 53*(6), 379–386.

Giorgi, A. (1971). Phenomenology and experimental psychology: II. In A. Giorgi, W. Fischer, & R. von Eckartsberg (Eds.), *Duquesne studies in phenomenological psychology* (Vol. I). Pittsburgh, PA: Duquesne University Press.

Glaser, B. G., & Strauss, A. L. (1967). *The discovery of grounded theory: Strategies for qualitative research.* New York: Aldine.

Hupcey, J. E. (2000). Feeling safe: The psychosocial needs of ICU patients. *Journal of Nursing Scholarship, 32*(4), 361–367.

Leininger, M. (1991). *Culture care diversity and universality: A theory of nursing.* New York: National League for Nursing Press.

Parse, R. R. (2001). *Qualitative inquiry: The path of sciencing.* Sudbury, MA: Jones and Bartlett Publishers and National League for Nursing Press.

Spiegelberg, H. (1976). *The phenomenological movement* (Vols. I and II). The Hague: Martinus Nijhoff.

Spradley, J. P., (1979). *The ethnographic interview.* New York: Holt, Rinehart & Winston.

Strauss, A., & Corbin, J. (1994). Grounded theory methodology: An overview. In N. K. Denzin & Y. S. Lincoln (Eds.), *Handbook of qualitative research* (pp. 273–285). Thousand Oaks, CA: Sage Publications.

van Kaam, A. L. (1966). Application of the phenomenological method. In A. L. van Kaam (Ed.), *Existential foundations of psychology.* Pittsburgh, PA: Duquesne University Press.

White, C. L., Mayo, N., Hanley, J. A., & Wood-Dauphinee, S. (2003). Evolution of the caregiving experience in the initial 2 years following stroke. *Research in Nursing & Health, 26,* 177–189.

Wyatt, G. K., Donze, L. F., & Beckrow, K. C. (2004). Efficacy of an in-home nursing intervention following short-stay breast cancer surgery. *Research in Nursing & Health, 27*(5), 322–331.

Zalon, M. L., (2004). Correlates of recovery among older adults after major abdominal surgery. *Nursing Research, 53*(2), 99–106.

Resources

Denzin, N. K., & Lincoln, Y. S. (Eds.). (1998). *Collecting and interpreting qualitative materials.* Thousand Oaks, CA: Sage Publications.

LoBiondo-Wood, G., Haber, J., & Krainovich-Miller, B. (2002). Overview of the research process. In G. LoBiondo-Wood & J. Haber (Eds.), *Nursing research: Methods, critical appraisal, and utilization* (5th ed.). St. Louis: Mosby.

Pedhazur, E. J., & Schmelkin, L. P. (1991). *Measurement, design, and analysis: An integrated approach.* Hillsdale, NJ: Lawrence Erlbaum Associates Inc.

Polit, D. F., & Beck, C. T. (2003). *Nursing research: Principles and methods* (7th ed.). Philadelphia: Lippincott Williams & Wilkins.

CHAPTER

10

BACKGROUND AND THE RESEARCH PROBLEM

Why Ask That Question— What Do We Already Know?

LEARNING OBJECTIVE:

The student will relate the background and the research problem to the research methods, results, and conclusions.

Sources of Problems for Research

Background Section of Research Reports

Literature Review Sections of Research Reports
   Directional and Nondirectional Hypotheses
   Null and Research Hypotheses

Linking the Literature Review to the Study Design

Published Reports—Has the Case Been Made for the Research Study?

Common Errors in Reports of the Background and Literature Review

Critically Reading Background and Literature Review Sections of
   a Research Report

KEY TERMS

Conceptual framework	Peer review	Secondary sources
Deductive knowledge	Primary sources	Specific aim
Directional hypothesis	Research hypothesis	Theoretical framework
Inductive knowledge	Research purpose	Theory
Literature review	Research problem	
Nondirectional hypothesis	Research question	

CLINICAL CASE

The RN from the clinical case in Chapter 9 continues to work with D.M. and, on the third night in the ICU, D.M. becomes very disoriented and tries to get out of bed. While attempting to settle and soothe D.M., the RN is struck in the face by one of D.M.'s flailing arms, and his nose is broken. As the RN recovers at home over the next couple days, he finds himself experiencing a number of feelings, including anxiety about returning to work, anger, and guilt, especially that he did not handle the situation in a manner that prevented any injury. He realizes that no one has ever discussed the impact of physical injury on nurses, neither during his education nor since his graduation, and wonders if his reactions are common or unusual. He decides to do a literature search to see if there has been any research about how nurses react to physical injury caused by a patient. The RN is surprised when he finds an integrative review and metasynthesis study titled "Non-somatic effects of patient aggression on nurses: A systematic review" (Needham, Abderhalden, Halfens, Fisher, & Dassen, 2005) (Appendix A-9). The RN wonders what kinds of research have been done about this problem and why the researchers decided to do a metasynthesis on this topic. Table 10-1 summarizes the RN's clinical question for this clinical case.

SOURCES OF PROBLEMS FOR RESEARCH

We started this book by discussing knowing and knowledge and why research is an important source of knowledge. This led us to recognize the need to understand and intelligently use research in nursing practice. As we moved through discussions of the different sections of most reports of research, we ended each chapter with a "why" question: Why did the researcher come to that conclusion? Why did the researcher use those patients and those measures? Why did the researcher plan the study in that way? We are now ready to discuss the beginning of research reports, in which the most important "why" question of all is asked: Why do this study? This is the most important "why" question because if there is no good rationale or basis for a research problem, then the rest of the study and report becomes trivial.

A good **research problem** represents a knowledge gap that warrants filling and can be addressed through systematic study. Research problems are derived from several sources, but two general sources of research problems exist. They are (1) problems derived from practice and (2) problems derived from theory. Figure 10-1 illustrates how research, practice, and theory can be viewed as one large braid because they wind together to develop knowledge.

We have focused on research questions that directly relate to practice, and practice is one of the major sources for identification of gaps in knowledge that must be researched. Nursing practice is broad and is a rich source of questions and problems for which we currently do not have answers. Examples of some of the questions that must be answered include:

- What are the best ways to support physiologic functioning in acutely ill patients?
- How can we facilitate individual and family growth through the stress of health crises?
- How can we assist patients in making major adjustments associated with chronic illness?
- How can we facilitate and promote positive healthy living, and what makes for a positive and healthy balanced life?
- What allows some people to adapt or cope with illness when some cannot?
- What makes some people more vulnerable to health and illness problems?
- How can we facilitate individuals and families during the transition from life to death?

TABLE 10-1

Statement of Clinical Question from the Clinical Case

What is known about the impact on a nurse of physical injury caused by a patient?

The *Who*	Nurses
The *What*	Response to physical injury
The *When*	After the injury
The *Where*	At home and at work
Key search terms to find research-based evidence for practice	Post-trauma
	Effects
	Nurses

These questions are broad and cannot be directly tested in a research study, but they do demonstrate the diversity of research areas that arise from nursing practice. Research problems derived from practice may be based on experiences in the practice arena, may be problems derived from mandated evaluation or accrediting requirements, or may reflect social issues as they affect practice.

Theory is another source of research problems. A **theory** can be defined as an abstract explanation describing how different factors or phenomena relate. In Chapter 8, we discussed theoretical definitions of variables, saying that this type of definition describes a variable conceptually rather than concretely. It is the conceptual or abstract nature of the ideas that, by definition, make something theoretical. Lazarus's theory of stress, used in several previous examples, provides an abstract explanation for how individuals and their environments interact to lead to stress (Figure 9-5). Nursing theories studied in other courses provide an abstract explanation of how nursing, persons, environment, and health all interrelate. Any

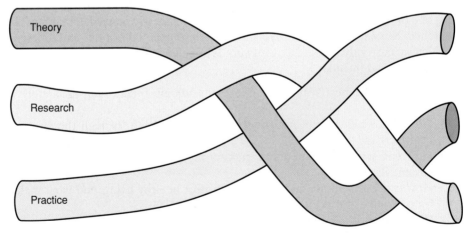

FIGURE 10-1 • The woven, or braided, relationships between theory, research, and practice.

theory can be a source of research problems because theory and research are closely intertwined: Theory is based on and guides research, whereas research tests theory to generate new knowledge.

In general, knowledge can be developed inductively or deductively. **Inductive knowledge** is developed by pulling observations and facts generated through research together to generate theory. Inductive knowledge development starts with pieces to build a whole theory. That theory is then used to suggest further observations that might be expected, which are then used to refine the theory. **Deductive knowledge** is developed by proposing a theory regarding a phenomenon of interest. It starts with the whole and breaks down the parts of the theory, seeking observations and facts to support the abstract relationships proposed in that theory. Observations that support or refute a theory's predictions of relationships are used to revise or refine the theory, which then undergoes further testing. In nursing, many of the observations for either inductive or deductive knowledge development arise from research studies as well as from practice, hence, the intertwining relationships among practice, research, and theory that are illustrated in Figure 10-1.

Although practice and theory are the major sources of research problems, much more is required to develop a specific narrow research problem than just identifying a broad question from either source. In the background section of a research report, we should be able to follow the trail of thinking that has led from a relatively general research problem to a specific, narrowly stated research purpose.

The first sections of most research reports are labeled "Background," "Introduction," "Problem," "Theoretical Framework," "Literature Review," or some combination of these. In all cases, these first sections of a research report should (1) provide the broad context or rationale for the problem, (2) define the problem, and (3) summarize what is already known about the problem. These three purposes are not always discrete and distinct because one purpose also may relate to another purpose. Therefore, information about what is known about a problem also may help to define it, or the context or rationale for a problem also may include what is or is not known about it. However, after reading the introductory sections of a research report, we should have a general understanding of these purposes. The purposes of context and definition are often discussed in the introduction or background section of a research report, whereas a section titled "Literature Review" often specifically describes the current state of knowledge about a problem. Our discussion will follow this division.

BACKGROUND SECTION OF RESEARCH REPORTS

To provide a context for a research problem, most study reports start with a broad and general description of a health concern derived from theory or practice. This description of the concern can be based on national health statistics; the costs of an important health problem; the goals or agenda of an organization that supports health, such as the American Nurses Association (ANA); or an emerging health crisis. For example, the beginning of the report of the study "Complex physical and mental health needs of rural incarcerated women" (Kane & DiBartolo, 2002) (Appendix A-2) states that the number of incarcerated women has nearly doubled since 1990. It goes on to point out that there have only been a few studies examining the health needs of this population, despite evidence that this is a highly underserved population. The "Motherhood in the context of maternal HIV infection" research report (Sandelowski & Barroso, 2003) (Appendix A-1) starts by pointing out that initially HIV/AIDS was viewed largely as a disease of men; thus, there was little research regarding the unique experiences of women with HIV. In both of these research reports, however, the authors set the stage by providing the context for the specific problem that they are going to study and the reason why they believe it matters.

Providing the context for a specific research problem also often establishes the relevancy of the problem for health care, in general and, possibly, nursing specifically. That HIV is a major health problem affecting many women, and that these women's experiences in dealing with this illness are unique, give us a clear idea of why a study should be aimed at understanding the experience of motherhood for women with HIV infection. However, the study does not directly connect the problem to nursing. Some research reports include a subsection at the beginning that specifically addresses the relationship between the research problem and nursing. More often, the potential nursing implications of the problem are addressed indirectly as the research problem is framed and refined.

The RN in our clinical case wants to understand what led the researchers to do a systematic review about the effects of patient aggression on nurses. He knows that this is a problem that he neither had experienced personally until now, nor had been taught anything about it in his basic education. He is surprised to discover that patient violence is considered to be a long-standing problem in some clinical settings and also is surprised to learn that the reported rates of physical injury in nursing range from 2% to 16%, although serious injuries occur less frequently (Needham et al., 2005). Both of these pieces of information provide him with a beginning understanding about why the researchers implemented a systematic review of research in this area.

In addition to setting a broad context for a research problem that may also define the clinical relevancy of that problem, the background section of a report should narrow and refine the research problem. General problems, such as low birth weight and differences in vulnerability in rural and urban settings, are not specific enough to be easily examined using research. Even with qualitative research methods, a specific phenomenon, an aspect of a cultural group, or social interaction must be refined and delineated as the focus of the study to guide data collection and analysis.

Research problems are usually refined either through reference to existing literature about the problem or through theoretical frameworks. Existing literature used to refine a research problem may include scholarly papers, research studies, or clinical case studies. The focus of the literature when refining the research problem is on the aspects of the problem that have been recognized, what is known about these aspects, and how they may relate. Although the background section refers to existing literature, that literature will be relatively general and address the overall research problem. Often, a background section is followed by a literature review section, in which the literature referenced is usually more focused on the particular research problem than the literature in the background section, which usually differs from the more extensive literature review because the former is relatively general and addresses the overall research problem. The literature review section often addresses the research problem after it has been refined. The background and literature review sections of a research report, then, might fit together to develop a story. The background gives us the general scene and characters, perhaps including the relationships among the characters, and it ends by presenting a specific conflict or problem among selected characters. The literature review continues the story and gives us a much more complete description of the central characters specifically relevant to that problem.

Another approach that may be used to refine a research problem, either by itself or in combination with literature, is application of a theory, theoretical framework, or conceptual framework to the research problem. A **theoretical framework** is an underlying structure that describes how abstract aspects of the research problem interrelate based on developed theories. A **conceptual framework** also is an underlying structure, but it comprises concepts and the relationships among them. We have said that a theory is an abstract explanation describing how different factors or phenomena relate. In the purest sense, these three different terms have different meanings, but understanding those meanings is not essential to intelligently use research because they all describe proposed relationships among abstract concepts.

CORE CONCEPT 10-1

Theory, theoretical frameworks, and conceptual frameworks all provide a description of the proposed relationships among abstract components that are aspects of the research problem of interest.

We must be clear that we are not talking about theoretical definitions of specific variables at this point. As shown in Figure 10-2, abstractions such as theory and theoretical definitions of variables are connected with different sections of the research report. The word *theory* does refer to something that is abstract, so theoretical definitions of variables are abstract definitions of specific variables to be studied and may derive from a specific theory or framework. However, before we can narrow in on specific variables, we must refine the research problem to a point that it can be systematically studied. As Figure 10-2 indicates by the hourglass shape, in the background section of a report, we expect that a broad and general concern, such as the health of incarcerated women, will be narrowed to a

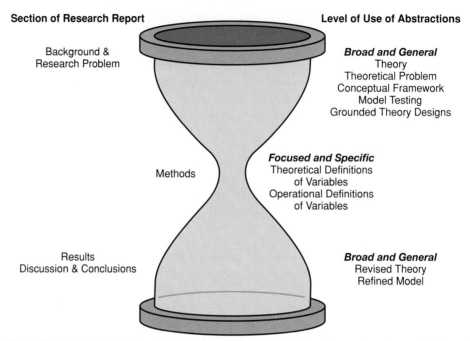

Section of Research Report   **Level of Use of Abstractions**

Background &
Research Problem
                                                    Broad and General
                                                    Theory
                                                    Theoretical Problem
                                                    Conceptual Framework
                                                    Model Testing
                                                    Grounded Theory Designs

                                                    Focused and Specific
                                                    Theoretical Definitions
                            Methods   of Variables
                                                    Operational Definitions
                                                        of Variables

Results
Discussion & Conclusions
                                                    Broad and General
                                                    Revised Theory
                                                    Refined Model

F I G U R E   1 0 - 2 • Relationship between sections of a research report and use of abstract language.

specific research purpose. The **research purpose** is a clear statement of factors that are going to be studied to shed knowledge on the research problem. These factors may also be referred to as the variables to be studied. In general, we expect the research purpose to identify the major variables. Abstract descriptions of these more narrow concepts are then included in the methods section. The discussion and conclusion sections once again use broad and more general abstractions as the results of a study are connected back to the original theory or conceptual framework.

In Chapter 8, we discussed the study "Efficacy of an in-home nursing intervention following short-stay breast cancer surgery" (Wyatt, Donze, & Beckrow, 2004) (Appendix A-6). That study used a conceptual framework to develop the intervention, and the report describes the four life domains in that model as part of the background section. These domains were "biological, social, psychological, and spiritual/existential" (Wyatt et al., 2004, p. 324) (Appendix A-6). The use of this conceptual framework provides a rationale and support for the components of the intervention that the researchers plan to test. This study does not actually test that model or framework directly; rather, it identifies four specific research questions at the end of the introduction section. However, when the intervention is found to impact social/family aspects of quality of life, the authors in their discussion of the results comment that these results support the conceptual framework that was the foundation of the intervention (Wyatt et al., 2004).

Similarly, the study found by the RN in the clinical case for this chapter used a conceptual framework suggested by Lanza (1992) in an early published report that addressed nurses as victims of patient assaults, in order to categorize the many factors found in their systematic review of multiple research studies (Needham et al., 2005) (Appendix A-9). The authors indicate that Lanza did not elaborate on the four categories, so the authors themselves provide us with theoretical definitions for each category. Specifically, they state "the following conceptualizations are employed in this review:

- Bio-physiological effects refer to non-visible somatic responses in a physiologically involuntary fashion.
- Emotions are sentiments not associated with any kind of psychological or psychiatric pathology but rather are common or 'normal' feelings.
- Cognition is defined as a non-emotive mode of perceiving, including perception of self or referring to a person's system of beliefs or convictions.
- Social interaction refers to interpersonal exchange." (Needham et al., 2005, p. 285) (Appendix A-9).

In this quote, the authors are narrowing and refining four abstract concepts in order to clearly and consistently categorize the findings from their review. Before this, the authors cite a number of research studies to set the stage for the specific focus of their systematic review. Specifically, they point out that many studies have focused more on physical injury rather than on psychological issues, despite that there are studies indicating significant psychological and emotional problems that continue over time for staff who have been victims of assault. This background leads the researchers to establish the aim of completing a systematic review in order to identify and categorize the predominant nonsomatic effects of patient assault on nurses. Thus, the authors take the broad problem of nurses' responses to violence, use existing research to identify a gap in knowledge related to the nonphysical or nonsomatic effects of this violence, and then employ a theoretical categorization that had been previously described in order to narrow and define the categories used in their study.

A third example of using literature and a conceptual model to refine a research problem into a research purpose is found in "Correlates of recovery among older adults after major abdominal surgery" study (Zalon, 2004) (Appendix A-3) used in Chapter 3. The author of this research report indicates that nursing needs to increase our understanding of the nature of recovery from surgery in order to better accomplish this in the context of shortened hospital stays after surgery. She indicates that three factors have been examined in the research with older adults in residential care—depression, pain, and fatigue—but that these have not been examined in relation to general abdominal surgery in community-dwelling older adults. The author further narrows and refines the research problem by describing a conservation model by Levine (1991) as a conceptual framework for understanding how the three factors of pain, depression, and fatigue may be interrelated to impact recovery. The author continues by reviewing the major research to date about each of the three factors and ends with a specific research question: "What is the relation of pain, depression, and fatigue to recovery, as measured by functional status and self-perception of recovery in older adults who have had major abdominal surgery?" (Zalon, 2004, p. 100) (Appendix A-3). Thus, the broad problem of recovery from surgery has been narrowed down using previous research and a conceptual framework to a research question about the connections between three specific factors to two specific outcomes.

In the previous three examples, we have referred to a *study aim* and a *research question*. These terms and several others refer to the specific focus of the research study that is being reported. Two other terms also used refer to the specific focus of a research study are *research purpose(s)* and *research objective(s)*. All of these terms mean essentially the same thing: They refer to a statement of purpose of the research and identify the variables that will be studied.

Often, the research purpose (or question, **specific aim**, or objective) also will include language that defines the type of question being asked in the research—whether the question is descriptive, relational, or predictive. The research purpose for the recovery from surgery study used the term *relation* in the research question (Zalon, 2004) (Appendix A-3), thus clearly identifying that it is asking a question about relationships or connections. The nonsomatic effects review uses the terms *to identify* and *categorize*, clearly indicating a purpose of description (Needham et al., 2005) (Appendix A-9), whereas the efficacy of an in-home intervention study asks in all four research questions about whether there are "any differences among the groups," indicating a purpose of differentiating or predicting (Wyatt et al., 2004) (Appendix A-6).

CORE CONCEPT 10-2

The terms research purpose, research question, study, or specific aim(s) or research objective(s) all refer to the statement of the variables to be studied that are related to the broad research problem.

In summary, the background section of a research report has two major purposes: (1) to establish the context for the research problem and (2) to refine that problem to a specific research purpose. The section of the report that we are referring to as *background* may simply be the beginning of the report without any title, may be titled "Introduction," or may be titled "Background." Information that provides the broad context for the research problem may include issues from either practice or theory and may reflect societal concerns, health care policy changes, or major health concerns. Refining the research problem may be accomplished using literature, theory, or both. In either case, the goal is to move from the general problem to a specific purpose or question that identifies the variables to be included in the study and often the type of question being asked.

LITERATURE REVIEW SECTIONS OF RESEARCH REPORTS

We said earlier that the use of literature to refine the research problem is not necessarily the same as the formal literature review. A **literature review** is a synthesis of the literature that describes what is known or has been studied regarding the particular research question or purpose.

Much of the literature review consists of a synthesis of existing published research, but some scholarly and theoretical work that is not actual research also may be included in the review. The literature review is more than a listing or summary of relevant research; it entails the combination of several elements or studies to provide a different or new focus on the research problem. For example, the literature review—titled "Review of the Literature"—in the health of incarcerated women report from Chapter 1 (Appendix A-2) points out that data from studies show that women who are incarcerated often previously lived in environments of deprivation, violence, and chronic chaos and, therefore, are a unique vulnerable population. The new perspective created in this initial paragraph is supported by a number of references. In a later paragraph, the authors state, "Only a few studies have explored the physical health issues ... [and these] have focused on pregnancy, pregnancy outcome and sexually transmitted diseases" (Kane & DiBartolo, 2002, p. 212) (Appendix A-2). This sentence is followed by references to six different studies. Thus, the authors have summarized the focus of research into physical health of incarcerated women addressed in six studies into one sentence. A recitation of all of them would be monotonous and useless. However, it is useful for the reader to know that most previous research looking at physical concerns have addressed traditional women's health issues, rather than broader more general health problems. Box 10-1 summarizes the purposes for literature reviews.

CORE CONCEPT 10-3

The literature review is guided by the variables that have been identified in the research purpose and aims to give the reader an overview of what is known about those variables, how those variables have been studied in the past, and with whom they have been studied.

The RN in our clinical case has found a report of a systematic review that the authors in their description of their study aim call a "literature review" (Needham et al., 2005) (Appendix A-9). In this case, the purpose of the authors' research is to review systematically existing research literature in order to distill the findings from that literature so that it can be used to guide future research. We mentioned earlier that authors use other literature to establish and support their specific aim. However,

Box 10-1 Specific Purposes of the Literature Review

• Description of what is known about the variables for the study
• Description of how the variables have been studied in the past
• Description of with whom the variables have been studied

they do not provide a formal review of the literature because that is what they have identified as the gap in knowledge that must be addressed to develop further understanding about care of nurses who are victims of violence.

To assure us that the literature review reflects the state of the science, the author must include current or recent studies. Usually, we would expect that most of the literature cited in a literature review has been published within 3 to 5 years of the date of the study or the publication of the report. However, sometimes little research has been conducted on selected variables, there has been a gap in time since the problem was addressed, or some important or classic studies may have been done more than 5 years ago. In these cases, we may appropriately see literature cited that was published more than 5 years ago. We care about how current the literature cited is because we want to know that the researcher is building on the most current knowledge related to the problem of interest.

Another way of ensuring that a study, either proposed or reported, is based on current knowledge is its use of primary sources. **Primary sources** are the sources of information as originally written. To be accurate and current, it is important that the researcher has read and synthesized the actual research reports or scholarly papers that are relevant to the study. A **secondary source** is someone else's description or interpretation of a primary source. For example, Wyatt et al. (2004), in the efficacy of intervention in short-stay breast cancer surgery study (Appendix A-6), states in her literature review that "Burke, Zabka, McCarver, and Singletary (1997) found that most patients had no problems with drain or incision care and were prepared to leave the hospital on the first post-operative day" (p. 323). This is an example of using a primary source because Wyatt et al. must have read Burke et al.'s study, and reported on what they read. However, suppose that another researcher named "Smith" wanted to study postoperative recovery, had read Wyatt et al.'s research report, and then stated in the literature that "Burke, Zabka, McCarver, and Singletary (1997) found that most patients had no problems with drain or incision care and were prepared to leave the hospital on the first postoperative day" (Wyatt et al., 2004, p. 323) (Appendix A-6). In this case, Smith would be citing a secondary source: She has not read the Burke et al. study, only Wyatt et al.'s description of it. We know this because Smith tells us the names of the authors who reported the original study, then references different authors, in this case, Wyatt et al., as the source of the information.

One problem with secondary sources is the potential for inadvertent error or distortion of the findings of a study. Think about the childhood game of telephone, in which six or seven children sit in a circle, and one child starts a message around the circle by whispering it into the ear of the child next to him or her. That child then whispers the message that he or she heard into the next child's ear. As we all know, by the time the message gets around the circle, it is likely to have changed significantly from what was originally stated. The same problem can occur with reports of research or other scholarly work. The greater the number of times that the work is interpreted beyond the original, the greater the possibility that the actual results will be distorted or changed.

The second reason that we expect a researcher to use primary sources is that we look to the researcher to do some discriminating in terms of the quality of the sources used to support his or her current research study. If we depend on Wyatt et al.'s sentence about Burke et al.'s study, we are also depending on Wyatt et al.'s judgment about the quality of that study related to the recovery from abdominal surgery study. Once we read the report of Burke et al.'s study, we might decide that it is not relevant to the proposed study of health behaviors in pregnant women.

In addition to the use of current and primary sources, the RN in the clinical case should expect to see literature that has been published in referred or peer-reviewed journals. We mentioned in Chapter 1 that the quality of information acquired on the World Wide Web must be carefully evaluated because anyone can create a Web site and claim to be an authority on a subject. Similarly, there is variety in the quality of published literature. A standard that ensures a published report has been carefully scrutinized for quality is the use of peer review. **Peer review** means that the manuscript for the published report has been read and critiqued by two or more peers before being accepted for publication. *Refereed* is another term that means that there was critical review of manuscripts before being accepted for publication. Manuscripts that are peer reviewed are intentionally sent to individuals who have expertise in the manuscript's topic. Therefore, the reviewers' comments are likely to reflect current and well-established knowledge. Not all sources of reports on research are peer reviewed or refereed. You can find out whether a particular publication is refereed by checking the author's guidelines for a journal—often available on a Web site, and always in the journal itself.

All of the studies used as examples in this text are from peer-reviewed journals. However, not all of the citations listed when doing a search using search programs such as CINAHL will be from peer-reviewed publications. As an intelligent user of research for clinical practice, you should consider not only the content of the research study, but also the type of publication. When you read research published in refereed journals, you know that the published report has been reviewed by several individuals with expertise in the research area, giving you some assurance about the quality of the study before you read it.

Part of what assures us of the quality of a literature review and, therefore, the knowledge on which the study was based, is that the literature cited was from refereed publications. Therefore, the RN in our clinical case will read the background literature and the systematic review expecting that recent literature, from primary sources and peer-reviewed journals, will give him information about what is known about nurses' nonphysical responses to being victims of patient violence.

The "Needs of family members of patients with traumatic brain injury" report (Bond, Draeger, Mandleco, & Donnelly, 2003) (Appendix A-5) used in Chapter 6 provides a good example of a review of the literature. If we look at the literature cited, we see a range of publication dates from 1975 to 2002. Most of the literature was published after 1996, and when we look at the 1975 citation, we see that it is part of a description of the historical development of understanding and measurement of family needs when in crisis. This is an example of a "classic" or an important historical element related to the topic. Further, the references cited are all studies published in major nursing journals that are peer reviewed.

The literature review content gives us background about the development of nursing knowledge with regard to family needs when in crisis. This includes research studies and use of selected measures, and the authors identify the populations that have been studied in the past, such as ICU patients and their families. The authors also identify that there have been contradictory findings in a number of studies and conclude their literature review by citing selected researchers who have indicated that use of a single measure to understand and work with families in crisis is not appropriate. This brings the authors to the purpose of their study, "to explore the needs of patients' families through individual interviews during the course of the patients' stay in the ICU" (Bond et al., 2003, p. 65) (Appendix A-5). The authors' synthesis of this literature focuses on existing literature that suggests we do not fully understand the complexity of family needs when in crisis and thus set the stage for a qualitative study that seeks to understand the unique experiences of this population.

In contrast to the report of the study about needs of family members, the literature review in the efficacy of an in-home nursing intervention article focuses on research that examined the benefits and barriers to short-term stays for women following breast surgery (Wyatt et al., 2004) (Appendix A-6). Again, most of the literature is current, although some is older because the researcher used a measure that has been used in research for a long time. The publications are all from peer-reviewed journals. The authors give us a description of the literature that has shown benefits to short-term stays as well as the literature that has argued against short-term stays. They then summarize existing research about outcomes of short-stay surgery for breast cancer. They conclude that little research has focused on the needs of patients once they return home, thus setting the stage for their intervention study.

As the RN in our clinical case reads the background literature review that is the basis for the systematic review regarding nonsomatic effects of violence, he gains an increased understanding about the problem and about what has been studied in depth in the past. The authors use this background to support the need for a systematic review of literature about nonphysical effects.

Therefore, the literature review should provide focused information about the specific variable(s) to be examined in a study. The review should provide some understanding of what is known about the variables, how they have been studied in the past, and with whom they have been studied. This should logically support the design and methods for the research study reported. Returning to our earlier analogy, by the time the literature review is completed, the major plot and subplots for the story should be clear. For those plots to make sense, we must understand the characters and their past "relationships" or stories.

After the literature review, some research reports include detailed research questions or hypotheses. Not all reports do so because not all research studies have detailed questions or hypotheses. In particular, we do not expect such information in a study using a qualitative approach because the emphasis should be on understanding the whole of an experience or a phenomenon, rather then breaking it down and studying its discrete parts. We also do not expect detailed research questions or hypotheses from quantitative studies whose purpose is general description. However, studies that test theory and predictions from theory or attempt to test the effect of manipulation usually have focused detailed research questions or hypotheses.

The language of research can be confusing at this point. We said earlier that a research problem is broad and general, while a research purpose is narrowly stated, may also be called a research question, and will specify the factor(s) or variable(s) to be examined. Now, we are talking about "detailed" research questions. Another way to think about these questions is as subquestions to the narrow and specific question or purpose of the study. For example, the efficacy of an in-home nursing intervention study from Chapter 8 (Appendix A-6) states, "Therefore, based on these issues, a nursing intervention was developed and piloted to address the following research question: can a focused nursing intervention that targets the needs of women following short-stay breast cancer surgery improve the outcomes of physical functioning, QOL, and anxiety in a cost-effective manner?" (Wyatt et al., 2004, p. 324) (Appendix A-6). This sentence clearly identifies the independent variable as the nursing intervention, and the dependent variables as being physical functioning, QOL, and anxiety. Yet, at the end of this same section, the authors state

> The study's specific research questions were as follows: (1) were there any differences among three groups in the post-surgery outcomes of functional status or activities of daily living (ADLs), QOL, and anxiety; (2) were there differences among groups in changes over time on the outcome variables?" (Wyatt et al., 2004, p. 324) (Appendix A-6).

Notice that these questions break down the larger research purpose into two more detailed and specific questions. The questions include not only the specific variables of interest in the study but also the specific relationship to be tested and the time frame for that testing. As an intelligent reader and user of research, you should understand that it is important to know that most reports of research studies start with a general problem, move to a more refined research purpose or question, and then, if appropriate, develop specific measurable questions or hypotheses, as illustrated in Figure 10-3. The research problem, purpose, and question are descriptions of the knowledge sought by the study that differ in their depth and specificity, but content from one may overlap with another at times. They also may differ in the actual terms used, such as the research purpose being called a specific aim or the research questions being written as objectives. However, a research report should include at least two, and often three, levels of depth and specificity of statements about the knowledge being sought in the study. These levels are differentiated by the specificity of the statements, with the problem being general, the purpose stating the variables for the study, and the questions or hypotheses stating specific measurable predictions or relationships.

In Chapter 5, we defined a hypothesis as a prediction regarding the relationships or effects of selected factors on other factors. We now know that the factors in a study are called *variables*. A research question and a **research hypothesis** are often opposite sides of the same coin because they both state predictions about relationships among variables. A **research question** puts the predictions in the form of a question, whereas a hypothesis puts the predictions in the form of a

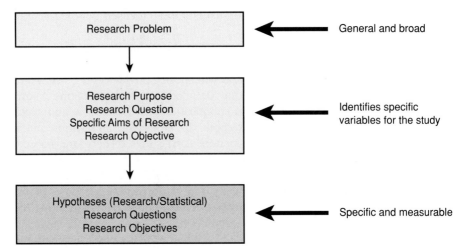

FIGURE 10-3 • Levels of development of the statements of the knowledge sought by the study.

statement. There are two types of research hypotheses and questions: directional and nondirectional.

Directional and Nondirectional Hypotheses

A hypothesis may predict whether there will be a relationship between two variables, or it may state the nature of the relationship between them. When we speak about the nature of a relationship, we are referring to whether the relationship is positive or negative; another word for this is the *direction* of the relationship. We talked about negative and positive relationships in Chapter 6, when we discussed correlations. A positive relationship exists between two variables if one increases as the other increases and vice versa. A negative relationship exists if one variable increases as the other variable decreases. Figure 10-4 illustrates a positive relationship between

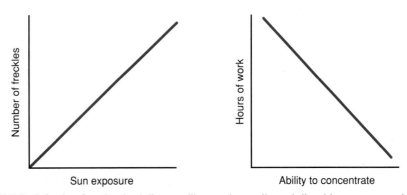

FIGURE 10-4 • Graphs depicting positive and negative relationships among variables.

number of freckles and sun exposure and a negative relationship between hours of work and ability to concentrate. A **directional hypothesis** predicts that two variables will be related and as well predicts the direction of that relationship. It will predict, for example, that as the score for one variable increases, the score for a second variable will increase. A **nondirectional hypothesis** predicts that two variables will be related but does not predict the direction of that relationship.

Research questions can also be directional and nondirectional. If a researcher asks "Is there a relationship between sun exposure and number of freckles?," this would be a nondirectional question. If a researcher asks "Do the number of freckles increase as the amount of sun exposure increases?," this would be a directional research question. Whether a hypothesis or research question is directional or not depends on the current level of knowledge about the variables of interest or the extent to which theory has been developed about the variables. A well-developed theory proposes not only relationships among factors but also the direction of those relationships. Therefore, a study using such a theory would be more likely to have directional hypotheses.

If we look at the report of the efficacy of in-home nursing intervention (Wyatt et al., 2004) (Appendix A-6), we find that the authors had four specific research questions. This is logical because the efficacy of an in-home nursing intervention tests a specific intervention based on a conceptual model. All of the questions in this study were nondirectional, asking simply if there were differences among the groups rather than predicting that one group would have better outcomes than another group. An example of a directional research question might have been "Does receipt of the in-home intervention improve the quality of life and functional status of patients after short-stay breast surgery?" This question includes a proposed direction for the effect of the intervention—that is, the intervention is proposed to positively affect QOL.

Null and Research Hypotheses

In addition to hypotheses being directional or nondirectional, there are two forms for hypotheses: the null and research forms. We described research and null hypotheses in Chapter 5. The research hypothesis predicts relationships or differences in variables, whereas the null hypothesis states that there will be no relationship or differences among variables. Remember that the null hypothesis is developed for statistical purposes and represents the assumption made in inferential statistics that most relationships or differences that may be found in any particular sample might have occurred by chance alone. Only when a difference or relationship among variables found in a sample is so large that it would only occur by chance in fewer than 5% of samples can the null hypothesis or statistical hypothesis be rejected. Usually, when a study has a null hypothesis, an alternate hypothesis also is stated, and that alternate hypothesis will predict both a relationship and a direction to that relationship. The idea of a "null" form is not applied to research questions, only to predictions in the form of statements.

Because we did not have any examples of use of null hypotheses in the studies that we have read for the previous chapters, let us think about a study examining pregnancy behaviors to predict pregnancy outcomes using statistical hypotheses. Suppose that the purpose of the study was "to describe and compare the patterns of health-related behaviors, including smoking, alcohol use, use of prenatal care, exercise, and nutrition among women in rural and urban settings, and to test the relationship among these behaviors and the outcomes of low birth weight and premature birth." Two sets of possible hypotheses could be stated:

H_0: There will be no differences in the pattern of tobacco use among pregnant women from urban and rural settings.

H_1: Women from rural settings will use tobacco more when pregnant than will women from urban settings.

H_0: Timing and regularity of use of prenatal care will not be related to birth weight among rural and urban samples.

H_1: Earlier and more regular use of prenatal care will decrease the incidence of low birth weight infants in both the rural and urban samples.

The symbol "H_0" represents the null hypothesis, and "H_1" represents the alternate hypothesis. You can see that the null hypothesis is a neutral or negative prediction, written primarily to support the assumptions of inferential statistics. A study that is using research hypotheses without null hypotheses also may use the symbol of an uppercase "H," but they will be numbered consecutively as H_1, H_2, H_3, and so on. A researcher should only include hypotheses at the beginning of a study if there is some basis for the predictions from either previous research or theory, and the literature review should include the information from theory or research that supports the hypotheses.

LINKING THE LITERATURE REVIEW TO THE STUDY DESIGN

When we first discussed the literature review, we said that it should give us an overview of what is known about the study variables, how they have been previously studied, and with whom they have been studied. We have discussed the quality of the literature review and mentioned that the research questions or hypotheses are specific predictions that should be supported by the literature review. The final aspect of the literature review that is important is the support it should provide for the study design.

The literature review should provide a synthesis of what is known but also should synthesize the approaches that have been taken to develop knowledge in this area. In this way, a literature review not only synthesizes but also critiques existing research about a problem. A true critique identifies strengths and weaknesses, and this is what we should expect to see in the literature review section of a research report. The strengths and weaknesses of previous research should serve as the basis for the study currently being described. The researcher should tell us at the beginning of the report how the results of this study will fit within the overall structure of knowledge about the problem. For example, the needs of incarcerated women study (Kane & DiBartolo, 2002) (Appendix A-2) identifies in the literature review that while there is research into the physical and mental health needs of incarcerated women, the complexity and multiplicity of these needs has not been demonstrated empirically. This information supports a descriptive design because it identifies that we lack knowledge about the complexity of the multiple health needs of this population. The authors also state that the results of this study are intended to develop appropriate strategies and services to meet the health needs of incarcerated women. Thus, the authors indicate how the findings from their study could fit with and increase existing knowledge.

Similarly, Zalon (2004) (Appendix A-3) tells us in the literature review that, although fatigue as a factor in postoperative recovery has been studied, the measures used have often been untested for reliability and validity, and most have not examined the relationship of fatigue to functional status. She also tells us how an existing model, Levine's Conservation Model, suggests that there should be a relationship between fatigue and functional status, providing a justification for a correlational design in her study.

A literature review may specifically address problems in study design from previous research or limitations of past samples. The literature review also may synthesize and critique the existing literature without directly addressing design and sampling issues. However, in either case, one of the purposes of the literature review is to identify the rationale for the design used in the study. Like a well-written story, each section or chapter should build a foundation for the next section or chapter. Choices of research design should be based on approaches taken in the past, with the goal of improving on or expanding on previous knowledge.

In summary, the background and literature review sections of a research report set the stage for the remainder of the study. The background gives the broad context for the research problem and an overview of factors relevant to that problem. This overview may present an abstract set of concepts and their relationships to one another called a *theory, conceptual framework,* or *theoretical framework.* The background usually ends with a statement of a research purpose or questions that specify the variables to be studied. The literature review starts with the purpose and describes the current state of the science in relation to the study variables. To do so, the literature review must be current and use mostly primary sources from peer-reviewed journals. The literature review should include what is known about the variables and how and with whom they have been studied. It establishes the basis for the design of the study and may end in specific research questions or hypotheses.

PUBLISHED REPORTS—HAS THE CASE BEEN MADE FOR THE RESEARCH STUDY?

We began this study wondering why the authors of the nonsomatic effects of patient aggression on nurses study (Needham et al., 2005) chose to do a systematic review.

If we examine the literature review, we find that several studies in the past have examined the physical effects of being a nurse who has experienced aggression or violence. The authors' critique of these past studies is that they have focused on the physical, rather than psychological and emotional, even though it is known that such effects can interfere with working and normal life for some period of time after an event. The information about findings from previous studies and the limitations of previous studies set the stage for the authors' systematic review, using clearly identified inclusion and exclusion criteria in order to organize and categorize findings about nonphysical effects.

After reading the introduction of the Needham et al. report, the RN in our clinical case has more information to use in understanding the findings from the systematic review. He understands the general problem that the study is attempting to address as well as the specific aim of the review. He also understands why the authors of the review chose to only include nonsomatic effects. He decides that he is not alone in the feelings he is experiencing and that he will read the results of the systematic review in some detail in order to better understand what he might expect for himself.

At the end of Chapter 9, you were asked to make a case for why a study of nursing students' well-being should be implemented. After reading this chapter, you should have a clearer idea about how you might have developed that rationale and why it can be an important part of a research report. The background and literature review set the stage for the rest of the research report by giving us a general setting for the study in terms of the problem; the specific purpose of the study, including the study variables; and an understanding of how this study will fit with current theory and research-based knowledge.

COMMON ERRORS IN REPORTS OF THE BACKGROUND AND LITERATURE REVIEW

One of the first errors that may occur in the background and literature review sections of a research report is a failure to develop a consistent link between the research problem, the research purpose, and any specific hypotheses or questions. The fictional article that describes the study of nursing students' choices of practice after graduation (Appendix B) gives a good example of a background that does not directly link the problem, purpose, and research questions. The introduction to that report discusses the general problem of the nursing shortage and the need for workforce planning. It then states that in addition to the sheer number of students, we must consider choice of practice in workforce planning, indicating that specific sites for practice will have greater needs for nurses in the future. International differences are mentioned, but there is no further mention of international aspects through the rest of the report. The next section, titled "Background," continues with the thread that students who will choose the most severe shortage sites should be targeted for recruitment to schools of nursing and concludes with a research purpose to "examine the relationships among nursing students' demographic characteristics and their choices for practice following graduation." At this point, the connections become weak. After the research purpose, the author lists three specific questions, the first of which addresses specific demographic variables (age, gender, race, and marital status), but the second and third introduce new variables, students' well-being and students' experiences that relate to their choices of practice, that have not been mentioned at any point in the preceding section. This is like an author of fiction placing an entirely new character into the middle of a story without connecting that character to anything or anyone in the previous part of the story.

The example in the fictional article is somewhat extreme, and what makes it an even poorer example is that no literature review is included. Consequently, we have no idea of what research has been done with students and choice of practice, what methods were used to conduct the research, or what types of students were studied. Published research reports vary in the consistency and links that they draw between the research problem, purpose, and specific measurable questions. If, as an intelligent reader of research, you finish the background and literature review section and still do not know what is going to be studied and why, one explanation may be that connections between the problem, purpose, and research questions have not been clearly or consistently identified in this section of the report.

A second problem that can occur is a failure to provide the information needed to fulfill the important purposes for these sections. For example, a literature review may provide a thoughtful synthesis of what is known about the variables of interest in the study but may fail to connect it to the purpose of the study being reported. This can leave us uncertain concerning the basis for the researcher's selection of research design and approach to measurement or how the study will fit with current knowledge.

Another problem that can occur is a failure to adequately reference statements. If the author of a research report makes a statement about the variables of interest that reflects knowledge that is not common and does not provide a reference, then we are left wondering how much we can trust the statement. We must wonder whether the statement is simply the opinion of the researcher, some stray fact that was found on the World Wide Web, or a well-documented research-based piece of knowledge. Occasionally, the number of references imbedded in a sentence in a literature review can almost be distracting from the meaning of the sentence, but those references assure us that the information is well founded and accurate.

The last potential problems with background and literature review sections of research reports are those we have discussed: the use of secondary sources and out-of-date references. The point of these beginning sections is to give us a clear and accurate picture of the state of knowledge about the research problem and to develop a coherent set of connections between that knowledge and the specific research purpose and questions. Secondary sources and references that are all more than 5 years older than the date of publication of the study do not give us much confidence that the study will fit well with current levels of knowledge.

CRITICALLY READING BACKGROUND AND LITERATURE REVIEW SECTIONS OF A RESEARCH REPORT

There are seven questions that you can ask yourself as you read the background and literature review sections of a research report, and these are listed in Box 10-2. We will take these one by one and examine each more closely. First, and most obvious, is "Does the report include a clearly identified background and/or literature review section?" Several of the reports that we have read in previous chapters do not clearly identify the background or literature review; they simply start with a statement of a problem or concern and then describe literature relevant to that problem, eventually concluding with a research question or purpose. The lack of specific headings may or may not interfere with your understanding about why a study was implemented. You will have to judge whether this is a problem.

A second question is "Do I think the background discusses aspects of my clinical question?" The RN in our clinical case selected the report of a systematic review because he wanted to have a better understanding of what he was experiencing. If the background had focused on the workforce impact of patient aggression, he might have quickly decided that the study was not going to be relevant to his clinical question. A third question that is related is "Does the literature help me understand why the research question is important to nursing?" In all but this last clinical case, we have asked patient care questions relevant to direct nursing care, and even

---

Box 10-2	**How to Critically Read the Background Section of a Research Report**

Does the report answer the question "Why ask that question—what do we know?"

1. Does the report include a clearly identified background and/or literature review section?
2. Do I think the background discusses aspects of my clinical question?
3. Does the literature help me understand why the research question is important to nursing?
4. Is the majority of the literature cited current (less than 5 years old) or very important to understanding the research question?
5. If a nursing or other theory was presented, does it connect to my clinical question?
6. Is the specific research question/problem/hypothesis connected logically to the literature and/or theory presented in the background section?
7. Is the specific research question/problem/hypothesis relevant or related to my clinical question?

in the last clinical case, we are asking a question that will affect a nurse's ability to deliver patient care. So, one aspect that we would expect to find in the literature review, sometimes explicitly and at other times implicitly, is identification of the relevance of the research question to nursing.

The next question to ask yourself is "Is the majority of the literature cited current (less than 5 years old) or very important to understanding the research question?" Some reports may include literature that is dated and neither seems relevant nor addresses the stated problem for the research. For example, while most of the report of the systematic review by Needham et al. is logical and connected (Appendix A-9), the last sentence in the introduction seems to be giving us information that is not immediately relevant to the research aim that follows. Specifically, the researchers indicate that "On an organizational level, Richter notes that the effects of psychological sequelae for the organization cannot be estimated (Richter, 1998)" (Needham et al., 2005, p. 284) (Appendix A-9). Yet, in no place before or after this do the authors discuss the effects of violence on organizations, and indeed their systematic review is about the effects of patient assault on nurses. Therefore, after critically reading this introduction, we might conclude at least that this last statement does not seem that important to our understanding of the research aim.

The fifth question, "If nursing or other theory was presented, does it connect to my clinical question?," also addresses congruency and logical building of content in a background and literature review. If you read any research report and find in it a description of a theory that is not later connected to the purpose or question addressed in the research, you should wonder why it was included at all. As we stated earlier, theory can be a very important source of research problems, and often a background section describes a theoretical framework or conceptual model to support the approach taken to a clinical problem. But if that theoretical framework or conceptual model does not seem to be relevant to your clinical question and is not used in a specific manner to establish the research study, then it is superfluous and detracts from the reader's understanding of a study.

The sixth and seventh questions are related—"Is the specific research question/problem/hypothesis connected logically to the literature and/or theory presented in the background section?" and "Is the specific research question/problem/hypothesis relevant or related to my clinical question?" Thus, these questions critically examine the specific research purpose or question or hypotheses and ask if these flowed from the background and literature review, providing a specific focus for the research study that addresses the clinical question of interest. Remember the analogy of these sections resembling a story. If this story concludes with an unrelated ending, we clearly recognize that it is not a very good story. Similarly, if the specific research question, problem, or hypothesis is not connected to the background and literature review "story" that has preceded it, the quality of those sections have to be questioned. Moreover, if the specific research question, problem, or hypothesis does not seem relevant to the clinical question of interest, then reading and understanding the rest of the report will not be particularly useful.

OUT-OF-CLASS EXERCISE

Pulling It All Together

We have now completed the second section of this book. We have looked at the entire research report, starting with the conclusions and moving forward to the background and literature review. As we discussed the sections, we also focused on selected aspects of the research process. The last two chapters return to the traditional approach to discussing research: starting at the beginning of a study or report and moving to the end. We discuss how the research process is related to the published research report and to the nursing process itself. We also examine the history of nursing research and how evidence-based practice and quality improvement relate to the research process. To prepare you for these chapters and to help you pull together the different sections of a research report, write an abstract that describes a research problem addressed by the in-class exercise. Decide on one question that you think could have been answered by that study. Then, in approximately 250 words (one page, double spaced), write an abstract that includes (1) background, (2) objective or purpose, (3) methods, (4) results, and (5) conclusions. If you have had the opportunity, you may be able to use real results generated in your class. If not, make up the results. The point of the exercise is to write a concise description of a research study using the specific language of research. Go back and read some of the abstracts of the research reports that we have used in this book, or find some published research of interest to you to serve as examples of what your abstract should look like. Remember that abstracts are organized differently in different journals, but for this exercise, try to use the five headings listed in this paragraph.

If you did not have an in-class study, you may want to take the fictional article from Appendix B and think of another question that might be addressed, given the variables in that study, or at least rewrite the abstract for the study using the headings listed in the previous paragraph. After you have completed this exercise, you are ready to move on to Chapter 11.

References

Bond, A. E., Draeger, C. R. L., Mandleco, B., & Donnelly, M. (2003). Needs of family members of patients with severe traumatic brain injury: Implications for evidence-based practice. *Critical Care Nurse, 23*(4), 63–72.

Burke, C. C., Zabka, C. L., McCarver, K. J., & Singletary, S. E. (1997). Patient satisfaction with 23-hour "short-stay" observation following breast cancer surgery. *Oncology Nursing Forum, 24,* 645–651.

Kane, M., & DiBartolo, M. (2002). Complex physical and mental health needs of rural incarcerated women. *Issues in Mental Health Nursing, 23,* 209–229.

Lanza, M. L. (1992). Nurses as patient assault victims: An update, synthesis, and recommendations. *Archives of Psychiatric Nursing, 5,* 163–171.

Levine, M. E. (1991). The conservation principles: A model for health. In K. M. Shaefer & J. B. Pond (Eds.), *Levine's conservation model: A framework for practice* (pp. 1–11). Philadelphia: F. A. Davis.

Needham, I., Abderhalden, C., Halfens, R. J. G., Fischer, J. E., & Dassen, T. (2005). Non-somatic effects of patient aggression on nurses: A systematic review. *Journal of Advanced Nursing, 49*(3), 283–296.

Sandelowski, M., & Barroso, J. (2003). Motherhood in the context of maternal HIV infection. *Research in Nursing & Health, 26,* 470–482.

Wyatt, G. K., Donze, L. F., & Beckrow, K. C. (2004). Efficacy of an in-home nursing intervention following short-stay breast cancer surgery. *Research in Nursing & Health, 27,* 322–331.

Zalon, M. L. (2004). Correlates of recovery among older adults after major abdominal surgery. *Nursing Research, 53*(2), 99–106.

Resources

LoBiondo-Wood, G., Haber, J., & Krainovich-Miller, B. (2002). Overview of the research process. In G. LoBiondo-Wood & J. Haber (Eds.), *Nursing research: Methods, critical appraisal, and utilization* (5th ed.). St. Louis: Mosby.

Polit, D. F., & Beck, C. T. (2003). *Nursing research: Principles and methods* (7th ed.). Philadelphia: Lippincott Williams & Wilkins.

THE RESEARCH PROCESS

How Is the Research Process Related to a Published Research Report?

LEARNING OBJECTIVE:

The student will relate the process of research to the sections of published research reports and to the nursing process.

KEY TERMS

Aggregated data
Assumptions
Codebook
Dissemination
Pilot study

CLINICAL CASE

In Chapter 8, our clinical case concerned an RN who worked in home health and cared for patients who had short-stay breast cancer surgeries. Shortly after altering her care based on the evidence from research, the RN was invited to participate in a new research group. The goal of the group is to develop and implement a study of patient and staff relationships as a predictor of rehospitalization of women who have had surgery for breast cancer. The RN is considering returning to school to earn her master's degree and decides that this group will provide a good opportunity to increase her knowledge about the research process. The research group is being led by a professor from the school of nursing affiliated with the RN's hospital and an oncology clinical nurse specialist (CNS) who has a joint appointment with the RN's hospital and the school of nursing.

In the last eight chapters, we learned about the different sections of a research report and discussed the process of doing research, but we have not yet focused on the research process itself. Now that we are comfortable with much of the language of research and with some of the aspects of the research process that are reflected in a research report, it is time to look at the research process as a whole. This chapter describes the research process from beginning to end, links that process to the research report, and discusses the relationship between the research process and the nursing process.

THE RESEARCH PROCESS

In Chapter 2, we briefly described the five steps of the research process:

1. Define and describe the knowledge gap or problem.
2. Develop a detailed plan to gather information to address the problem or gap in knowledge.
3. Implement the study.
4. Analyze and interpret the results of the study.
5. Disseminate the findings of the study.

A process, whether it is the research process, the nursing process, or the critical thinking process, is, by definition, fluid and flexible. All of these processes refer to steps because certain parts of the process are necessary before one can successfully move to the next part. However, the steps do not always follow one another in a step-by-step manner: At times, the results of a step in the process leads to returning to the preceding step, or possibly two steps occur at the same time.

CORE CONCEPT 11-1

The steps of the research process are not always linear: They may overlap or be revisited during the research process.

For example, a refined research purpose is necessary before beginning to develop a detailed research plan, but it is possible that as a plan is developed, the research purpose may be revisited and refined further. Similarly, a research plan is needed before a study is implemented, but it is possible that as the study is implemented, the plan will be revised. In fact, in most qualitative methods, the methods are expected to change as the study progresses. Therefore, although this chapter discusses the steps of the research process in order, the process may be more fluid and flexible in action.

Define and Describe the Knowledge Gap or Problem

The RN in our clinical case, who is beginning to participate in a research group, finds that when she attends the first meeting of the group, it is starting the first step in the research process. The CNS begins by describing a question that she has developed based on her work on the surgical unit. She has noticed that in some patient cases, the ICU staff and the patients and family develop warm and interactive relationships, whereas in other cases, the patient–staff relationship is poorly developed, with limited communication and contact. The CNS wonders why this difference occurs and how the differences in relationships may affect patients. Another member of the research group states her belief that when the staff has better communication with patients and their families, the patients have shorter hospitalizations and are rehospitalized less frequently. Other members of the group begin talking about reasons why they believe that relationships between patients and staff differ: Some focus on characteristics of patients, some on nursing staff, and some on medical staff. Then, another member of the group suggests that length of hospitalization itself is an important factor in both what kind of relationship is established between staff and patients and rehospitalization. The RN in our clinical case suggests that the staff:patient ratio and whether a woman is admitted on the weekend also affect nurse–patient relationships and hospital outcomes.

It is obvious to the RN that at this point in the group's process, there is no agreement about the knowledge gap that must be addressed. Creating a flowchart of all the ideas that have been discussed is suggested. Figure 11-1 illustrates the results that might have come from this effort. Once the group sees all its ideas in a flowchart, it begins to identify some of the areas that it must explore further. For example, the group identifies that it must find out what is known about staff–patient relationships. Relationships and communication are recognized as two separate but connected concepts. The group agrees that it will focus on the relationships between nursing staff and patients but will consider how physician–patient relationships may be a factor in the nurse–patient relationships. Beyond looking for information about nurse–patient relationships within surgical units, the group agrees that it needs to look for information about the effects of relationships on health care outcomes as well as information about factors that may affect relationships, such as staff:patient ratio and nurse and patient characteristics. The members of the group divide the list of various ideas they have discussed and agree to conduct a literature review focusing

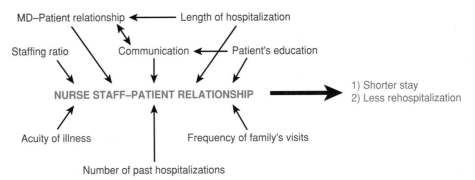

FIGURE 11-1 • Possible flow chart developed during brainstorming about a research problem.

on a particular subset of ideas, returning in 2 weeks to share what they have found. The process described in this hypothetical situation illustrates aspects of the first step in the research process.

The information required for this first step will be acquired from existing theory and research to identify what is known about the problem and the relevant factors related to the problem. This step also requires thoughtful analysis because rarely does theory or past research easily blend into an obvious research purpose. At this point in the research process, often what is needed is an explosion of ideas and information, all of which then must be thoughtfully analyzed and synthesized to develop a refined purpose. The brainstorming session that our RN experienced may be the first of several sessions in which many ideas are explored, validation and information about those ideas are sought and digested, and new ideas are generated. This step can be both exciting and frustrating: exciting because of the amount to be discovered about a problem of interest and frustrating because of the amount to digest and integrate to develop a refined research purpose.

For example, our hypothetical research group may find a great deal of information about nurse–patient communication, primarily with adult patients. However, perhaps little has been done examining nurse–parent communication in short-term surgical settings with patients who have cancer. Perhaps the focus primarily has been on communication rather than on the broader concept of relationships. The group does find theory about the concept of relationship formation in general, which certainly includes the concept of communication as well as characteristics of the participants in a relationship. The group recognizes that several of the nurse theorists have focused on nurse–patient relationships and have identified a range of concepts that are important to their development. They also found several studies that conclude by recognizing the importance of the relationship between staff and patients of breast cancer patients. Yet, they find few research studies that link nurse–patient communication or relationships to long-term outcomes, such as length of hospitalization or rehospitalization. Finally, nothing exists in either theory or literature about structural factors, such as overall staff:patient ratio or timing of admissions during weekends versus weekdays and nurse–patient relationships. Despite this lack of literature, the RN believes from her experience that when patients are admitted on the weekends, they and their families often do not establish as good a relationship with the weekend staff as do patients who come in during the week with the regular weekday staff.

All of these findings leave the group with even more information than they compiled when they brainstormed and with no immediately obvious connections between all the possible factors that it might consider. This is what was meant by an explosion of information: As ideas are analyzed in this step of the research process, they sometimes explode into multiple new ideas to explore.

Despite the potential explosion of information, notice that our hypothetical group has now acquired a foundation of knowledge about what is known, has been theoretically considered, or has been studied in the past. Developing that foundation of knowledge is the goal of the first step of the research process. That foundation of existing knowledge should include existing research, practice experience, and any appropriate and relevant theory. The challenge then becomes synthesizing the existing knowledge; critically examining practice experience, theory, and past research; and identifying a research purpose that includes specific factors or variables to be studied. Notice also that the foundation of knowledge found strongly supports the relevancy of the problem that this group has identified for nursing practice.

In addition to establishing a foundation of knowledge about the research problem, another part of this first step entails identifying assumptions that are imbedded in the approach to the problem and the purposes being considered. **Assumptions** are ideas that are taken for granted or viewed as truth without conscious or explicit testing. Assumptions can be difficult to identify because they are ideas that we "just know" or "all understand" and are usually unspoken. However, assumptions can sometimes color how a research problem is viewed so that the approach to knowledge development is limited in some way. Several assumptions are often made in nursing research, and one researcher studied reports of research to describe some of these. Williams (1980) identified 13 assumptions that are commonly present in nursing studies. Included were assumptions that stress is something to avoid, that health is a priority for most people, and that people operate on the basis of cognitive information. Identifying the assumptions imbedded in a study can be helpful because we may realize that the assumptions must be researched and confirmed before we can move forward in knowledge development.

In the hypothetical study that we are discussing, there is an assumption that relationships between patients and staff can be viewed as "good" or "bad." There is a second assumption that patients' experiences in the surgical unit will affect their health afterward. Because of these assumptions, the research group is not considering exploring whether the terms *good* and *bad* apply to relationships; it is beginning with looking at factors that make relationships good or bad. Perhaps this approach is too simplistic and there are only different types of relationships, some of which are more or less helpful in promoting positive health outcomes for the patients. If so, the study of factors that make relationships good or bad may miss some important types of relationships.

As the research problem is refined into a specific purpose, the types of questions that will be addressed and the approach likely to be taken are often beginning to be identified. We previously discussed how research questions that address prediction or examine the effects of manipulation of a variable require a relatively large amount of background or foundational knowledge. It becomes increasingly clear to our hypothetical research group that not enough research or theory about factors affecting nurse–patient relationships or the effects of these relationships on outcomes exists to make predictions or to plan to manipulate any factor. Because the researchers cannot find studies and theory that convince them to predict that a certain variable will have a desired outcome, they realize that they must consider questions about relationships between variables in the nurse–patient relationship or questions that describe the nurse–patient relationship.

The group also begins to consider whether a qualitative, quantitative, or mixed method approach is most logical as it begins to refine the general problem of nurse–patient relationships. Some of the group argues that because so little has been studied regarding the patients' experiences in their interactions with nursing staff, the first study should be phenomenological. Others suggest that a grounded theory approach might be taken, broadly based on Peplau's theory of interpersonal relations (1952). A grounded theory approach based on Peplau's theory would aim to develop concepts and links that are grounded in nurses' and patients' experiences of developing and maintaining relationships. Others believe that nursing theory and existing theory about relationships in general as well as past research about nurse–patient communication provide a set of relevant factors that can be measured and tested to see how they affect nurse–patient relationships in women having short-stay breast cancer surgery. These members think that a correlational study is what is needed. Everyone agrees about the need to discover whether staff–patient relationships can be linked to outcomes, such as a shorter total hospitalization or fewer rehospitalizations.

It is not uncommon that during the first step of the research process several potential research studies are identified that are relevant to the problem. Refining a problem clarifies the nature of the gaps in knowledge as well as the factors relevant to the problem. In many cases, the problems of interest to nursing are too complex to address in a single study. Let us assume for now that after several meetings, substantial discussion, and review of theory and the literature, the hypothetical group in our clinical case agrees on a tentative purpose: to identify and examine factors that affect nurse–patient relationships in the short-stay surgical settings and the role that these relationships have in patient outcomes. This purpose tells us that the variables in this study will be unspecific "factors," nurse–parent relationships, and patient outcomes. This purpose will probably need further refining, which will occur as the group moves into the second step of the research process. In this next step, the group takes the purpose it has identified and develops a specific research plan that includes the research design and methods of measurement and sampling.

Develop a Plan to Gather Information

As the purpose for a study is refined, ideas about gathering information about the problem being studied also begin to generate. As researchers review past research studies regarding the problem, they consider not only the findings from that research, but also the methods and samples used. This helps to clarify gaps in knowledge and identifies measures and approaches that previously have been successful in addressing the problem. For example, our hypothetical research group has found that most studies of nurse–patient communication have been conducted with adults who were the primary medical care recipients rather than with adults who have just had a major surgery and are being discharged home within 48 hours. They also found that many of the communication studies have used videotaping as a method of data collection, with analysis of discrete episodes of communication as the focus of study. Because this group is interested in more than isolated episodes of communication, it knows that it needs a different research method.

The second step of the research process is complex and involves many considerations and decisions. This step includes deciding on the general approach to be taken to the study and a specific research design; identifying and developing plans for the study sample or participants; and planning the measurement process, including specific techniques, measures, and timing. Finally, at the end of this step, an institutional review board proposal must be written and submitted in preparation for implementation of the study.

The group in our clinical case intentionally left its preliminary statement of a research purpose broad because it had not reached an agreement about whether this research needed to develop further knowledge about nurse–patient relationships or describe how factors that it has found in the literature and from practice affect that relationship. The group eventually decides that a mixed method approach makes the most sense, beginning with a grounded theory study of the relationships between nursing staff and breast cancer patients in the short-stay surgical unit. It plans to follow this with a descriptive correlational study about how the factors they have identified from research and practice affect length of hospitalization and rehospitalization within the following month. These factors include history of hospitalization, stage of cancer, educational level, timing of initial admission, and average staff–patient ratio during hospitalization as well as any factors that are identified from the grounded theory study that can reasonably be included. Following this overall decision about the study, the group is able to refine their purpose: to describe the perceptions of nurses and patients of their relationship during the hospitalization for short-stay breast cancer surgery, including their perceptions of how that relationship does or does not impact health outcomes, and to describe how nurse, patient, and hospital unit factors impact length of hospitalization and need for rehospitalization within a month after discharge.

The refined purpose described reflects several decisions that have been made by the research group. It has decided that a grounded theory method is a better design for its purpose than a phenomenologic design because it is examining interactions, has a general theory in Peplau's psychodynamic nursing theory, and wants to develop knowledge about relationships. The group has ruled out doing a true longitudinal study, as it did not find strong research evidence about factors relevant to staff–patient relationships or the effect of factors on the outcomes of interest. A longitudinal study requires more time and resources than a cross-sectional correlational study, and the group members believe that they do not have the knowledge base to justify that effort at this time. The group has also settled on two outcomes—length of hospitalization and occurrence of rehospitalization within a month of discharge—partly for pragmatic reasons. They know that administration and insurance companies are interested in shortened hospitalization and avoiding unnecessary rehospitalization, so they expect that they may be able to get support for this study from the hospital. Also, these two outcomes are easily measured. Other outcomes that the group discussed included patients' sense of control and efficacy, rate of recovery, and rate of complications. These are all still considered relevant by the group, but it agreed that potential difficulties with measurement precluded examining them in this study.

Thus, the second step of the research process requires critical thinking and decision making. Researchers must consider what is known, what has been shown to work, and what is feasible. The last consideration includes issues of time, cost, established measures or approaches, and other resources, such as space or access to samples. We will discuss these further when we discuss factors that affect research.

Decisions about the best possible methods for implementing the chosen study designs must also be made during this part of the research process. In the case of the grounded theory phase of the hypothetical study, for example, researchers must make decisions about methods of data collection, such as interviews, observations, or use of journaling, as well as the timing for the data collection. Similarly, to implement the descriptive correlational phase of the study, researchers will have to make decisions about measures, such as chart audits, and the use of a questionnaire or a structured interview. The issues of rigor, validity, and reliability that we discussed in Chapters 8 and 9 are central to making these decisions about methods and measurement.

Another important part of the second step is deciding on the sample for the study and approaches to the process of sampling, as discussed in Chapter 6. For example, the surgical unit sees patients at different stages in their breast cancer treatment. Although the group plans to measure severity of illness during the second phase of the study, it recognizes that the stage of cancer, whether or not this is the first admission for the cancer, and individual physician practices all also will affect length of hospitalization. The grounded theory phase of the study will benefit from researchers' talking with several patients, including those who have experience with the surgical unit and those who do not. After some discussion of normal patient census and the most common types of patients seen, the research group decides to limit the study to women newly diagnosed with breast cancer. This decision is based on the experience of our RN and several other group members who suggest that patients who have already had treatment such as chemotherapy for their cancer have different needs and outcomes than those who have just been diagnosed and the surgery is their first treatment.

In addition to deciding who will participate in the study, the group in our clinical case must consider how comfortable patients will be talking about their relationships with nursing staff and how nursing staff might change regarding their relationships with patients when they know there is a study in progress. This would be an example of the Hawthorne effect described in Chapter 9. Patients might be concerned about repercussions on their care if they express any negative feelings, and staff might be concerned about negative effect on their performance evaluations. These issues could lead to a threat to internal validity from testing and to researcher effects threatening external validity. The research group decides to use individuals who are not associated with the surgical unit in any way as data collectors and to put extra effort into ensuring anonymity of participants and subjects to address this concern.

The hypothetical group in our clinical case will make other specific decisions as it moves through the second step, and the details of these decisions could probably

---

Box 11-1 Considerations Affecting the Development of the Detailed Research Plan

- Methods and samples used in previous research
- Potential setting(s) for the study
- Experience and knowledge of the researcher(s)
- Resources available, such as time and money
- Subject safety and rights
- Rigor, reliability, and validity

---

fill several chapters. Overall, this process is based on a further exploration of past research to identify research designs and methods that have been used, measures that are available, and sampling considerations. This research literature, along with the realities of the specific setting for the research, the knowledge and experience of the researchers, and resources such as time and money, all will be considered in developing a detailed plan to gather information about the research purpose. Box 11-1 summarizes these and other considerations affecting the development of the research plan.

Once a detailed plan is developed, the last part of this second step is to ensure the protection of human subjects and to acquire the resources needed for the study. We discussed informed consent and the role of IRBs in Chapter 7. The type of study we are discussing in this chapter would likely have to receive IRB approval from the hospital board as well as from the university board. This will require two written proposals describing the study background, purpose, literature review, design, and measures and how the rights of subjects will be assured. Developing this type of IRB proposal often helps a researcher or research group to tighten the details of their plan of study but also takes time and must be considered when planning a time line for a research study. In addition, many studies cannot be implemented without acquiring some outside resources to support the time and materials needed. Depending on the complexity of the proposed study and the resources inherent in the study site, researchers often must write and submit proposals for funding before they can implement it. Again, the writing, review, and receipt of funding can take weeks to months. However, both the review of IRB proposals and the funding proposals provide outside input into the plans for a research study and often significantly improve those plans before the study is implemented.

Implement the Study

The third step in the research process is to implement the study. This is when the advance planning and decisions can pay off and when unexpected issues can arise. One of the biggest responsibilities of the researcher during implementation is to maintain meticulous documentation of the sampling and data collection process. This documentation allows the researcher to later clearly identify any points in the study at which plans were changed and the rationale for decisions made during the implementation process. Areas that may need to be addressed and documented during this step include data about numbers and characteristics of those who were approached to be in the study but declined or later dropped out, any revisions in sampling criteria, any changes in the timing or the measurement process, and any anecdotal or incidental data that become relevant during the study implementation.

In Chapters 6 and 8, we discussed things that can go wrong with sampling and measurement and how important it is to consider those aspects when deciding on the usefulness of research for practice. The careful documentation kept by researchers during the study implementation is the basis for reporting information that will allow us to evaluate the sampling and measurement process. In addition, incidents or occurrences that are unexpected may have a big effect on the meaning of results of a study. For example, suppose that patients who had one particular physician all declined to be in our hypothetical study. Or, suppose that as the study is implemented, patients start approaching the research staff and ask to participate before they have been recruited. Either of these observations suggests that there may be some underlying factor at work during the process of study implementation. In the first case, that factor may be a physician who has told parents not to participate because he is unhappy about the study, thus eliminating data about relationships with a provider who is controlling. In the second case, the underlying factor might be that patients have a strong need to talk about their experiences, which this study is meeting. This unmet need may be important to consider when gaining understanding about staff–patient relationships. One could speculate about the meaning of either observation, but what is important is to document the observation for future consideration as the results of the study are analyzed.

During the study implementation, the steps of the research process may be particularly fluid, moving back and forth between this step and the previous step of planning or to the next step of analysis and interpretation. As we discussed in Chapter 8, in the implementation step, qualitative methods depend on a spiraling process of data collection followed by data analysis and interpretation that informs the next round of data collection. Sometimes during the study implementation, the plans for sampling prove to be unrealistic, perhaps because criteria are too strict or because the desired subjects for the study are not willing to participate. The researchers will then have to revise their sampling plan to implement the study. Or, perhaps data collectors note that all subjects are confused and have difficulty answering some part of a questionnaire. The researchers will have to use this information to decide whether to change their measures in the middle of their study or to continue with a measure that may have problems with reliability. These are just a few examples of the many kinds of problems that can be encountered during the study implementation. The process requires time, care, consistency, and ongoing monitoring.

Analyze and Interpret the Results

The fourth step of the research process involves the analysis and interpretation of study results. As we indicated, this step may be interwoven with the step of implementation in a qualitative study. In contrast, most of the data analysis in a quantitative study is usually reserved until the entire data collection process is complete. This difference reflects the differences in philosophy behind the two types of approaches. A qualitative method uses data as it is generated to build additional data, with the goal of arriving at information that is dense and thick to inform our understanding of a phenomenon. Quantitative methods strive to control and isolate phenomena to understand each discrete element. Therefore, quantitative methods defer analysis of most of the data until the collection process is complete to avoid contaminating the data collection process with ideas generated from the analysis. The exception to this is in analysis of sample characteristics. A purposive sample or a matched sample, as discussed in Chapter 6, requires the analysis of subject characteristics during the study implementation to effectively implement the sampling plan.

Data analysis, whether carried out in a qualitative or quantitative study, requires the same level of meticulous care and documentation that is needed during the implementation step of the research process. In qualitative research, this is accomplished through the audit trail and notations within the software programs that are often used during data analysis. In quantitative research, decisions about data analysis are often documented in a codebook. In research, a **codebook** is a record of the categorization, labeling, and manipulation of data about variables in a quantitative study. It includes information about how each of the variables in the study was measured; how the data from the study were reviewed and transferred into computer files; and all decisions made regarding the management of problems, such as incomplete responses or confusing responses. Like an audit trail, a codebook provides a detailed description of how the data from a study were managed.

Qualitative data are often collected in an interview, so the first thing that must be done is to transcribe the data into a word-processing program. Once transcribed, the data can be either loaded into a qualitative analysis program or printed and analyzed on hard copy. In either case, data management often includes careful reading and listening to interviews that have been transcribed to ensure that the transcription is accurate and complete. Similarly, quantitative data have to be entered into computer software programs to be analyzed. This can be done in several ways, including direct entry of numbers from quantitative measurement into a data file or use of an optical scanner that reads and records numbers off of a data collection measure into a data file. In either case, once it is in a data file, the data must be carefully examined for accuracy. Human error in keying numbers into a file or computer error in scanning answer sheets can significantly affect and even invalidate study results.

The researcher can proceed with the analysis and interpretation of the results once data have been put into a form that allows that process. As discussed in Chapters 4 and 5, data analysis is complex and challenging. It also is an exciting time in the research process because the researchers begin to find out what their study says about the research problem that started this whole process. In addition to information about data management, codebooks in quantitative data analysis often include information about decisions regarding analysis approaches and the mathematical manipulation of the data. For example, a researcher can decide to use a mean score of items from a measure of a variable in the analysis or to use a score that is just the sum of all the items. Alternatively, a researcher may decide to study all subjects as one large group who have differences on a variable of interest or to divide subjects into two groups that clearly differ on that variable. All of these types of decisions are usually documented in the codebook so that as the research progresses, the researcher can recall those decisions and the rationale behind them. Thus, both the audit trail and the codebook reflect documentation of data management and analysis, which are important aspects of the fourth step of the research process.

Interpretation is the last part of this step. Interpretation of the results of a study entails pulling the whole process together into a meaningful whole. The theory and research literature that served as a foundation for the study, the decisions made in the planning step of the process, and the decisions and observations that were made during the implementation step all must be considered and tied into the results of a study. At this point, the expertise of the researchers and their personal knowledge and experience are also used in interpreting results. For example, suppose that during the implementation of the hypothetical study of staff–patient relationships, subjects started hearing about the study and asking staff to be included. The research team will have to decide why this occurred and how it affected the data collected. The RN and research team in our clinical case may decide that this interest in participating in the study reflected a strong need on the patients' part to feel included in their care. Or, they might conclude that patients needed an avenue for expressing their feelings about the nursing staff and the care they receive. These are different interpretations and would have different meanings for the results of the study.

Disseminate the Findings

The last step of the research process brings us back to where we started in this book—to the research report. **Dissemination** of research findings refers to the spreading of knowledge and is an essential step in the research process because knowledge development is wasted unless it becomes known so that it can be used. The dissemination of research findings may be accomplished in several ways. Findings may be disseminated through a report of the research to the agency or organization that funded or hosted the study. This type of dissemination is targeted at the specific groups that were closely involved in the study. Often, the results of a research study also are reported back to participants in that study. In addition, findings from a study may be verbally reported in the form of presentations to agencies or funding groups or at scholarly and professional meetings. Findings from research are reported in published journals in both print and online formats. Finally, research findings are sometimes disseminated to the public through the lay press, television, or other medium. Each of these types of approaches to dissemination of findings targets different groups of potential users of the research, with the report to those closely involved in the study clearly reaching a much smaller group than a published article in a major professional journal.

Because research dissemination targets different groups, the depth and detail of the dissemination varies. However, in all cases, the goal of dissemination is to accurately share the knowledge gained from the research so that it is useful and meaningful to the targeted recipients of that knowledge. For example, a summary of a research study that is being sent out in a regional newsletter will probably focus on a brief description of the problem, the sample, and one or two key findings. A presentation of a paper reporting the findings of a study at a professional meeting will usually be limited to 15 or 20 minutes, allowing inclusion of more detail than a newsletter column but less than what would be included in a published report in a research journal. A published report in a practice-focused journal will probably include fewer specifics about the research process than a report appearing in a research journal. However, in all cases, the researcher must be sure that the findings of a study are clearly and accurately stated.

The other consideration that is important for all types of dissemination is ensuring the anonymity of subjects or participants in a study. This requires that data primarily are reported in the aggregate and that there is careful scrutiny of that data. **Aggregated data** means that the results from the study are reported for the entire sample rather than for individual members in the group. Usually, when data are aggregated, no specific result from the study can be attributed to any participant in the study. However, with a small sample, it is possible that even with aggregated data and elimination of any traditional identifiers, the anonymity of individual subjects might be lost.

For example, suppose that the hypothetical study of staff–patient relationships acquired a sample of 50 subjects in the descriptive correlational phase. One characteristic of subjects that will be reported is race, and perhaps only three subjects in the study were Asian. Further, suppose that there was one finding stating a difference in patients' perceptions of staff by race, with Asian patients reporting much more negative experiences with staff. The staff on the surgical unit could read those results and likely know immediately which patients reported negative experiences because they have so few Asian patients, thus eliminating the anonymity of those patients. In this type of circumstance, it is possible that a result may have to be withheld from dissemination to protect the rights of the subjects in the study. Given that the reason the results may breech anonymity is because the numbers of Asian patients was so small and, therefore, that the results may have happened by chance alone and must be confirmed with a larger sample, the withholding of such a result does not jeopardize knowledge development.

It should be noted that even at this last step in the research process, a researcher might revisit an earlier step. Sometimes only when writing up the findings of a study does a researcher discover the need to consider and report a specific descriptive result or conduct a particular statistical test. Sometimes after sharing findings from a study with others, suggestions are made for additional analysis that may shed further light on the research problem. Of course, the findings from a study often raise new questions or suggest new research problems, taking us back to the first step.

It should be clear from this description of the research process that it is complex, exacting, and challenging (Box 11-2). The dissemination product of that research often does not provide a full picture of all the thought and work that went into a research study. Throughout this book, we have discussed common errors that

Box 11-2 Characteristics of the Research Process	
• Systematic • Complex	• Exacting • Challenging

can occur in a research report. However, any report of research deserves to be read with respect because of the effort and risk taken by the researcher to implement the research process and then make public the results of his or her efforts. Few research studies are perfect, and research reports certainly vary in their completeness and usefulness to practice. However, reports of research reflect a substantial time commitment of one or more individuals to address a gap in knowledge through the use of the complex and often strenuous process of research. The next section looks more closely at how and why publications of research do not always fully reflect the research process.

RESEARCH PROCESS CONTRASTED TO THE RESEARCH REPORT

In Chapter 2, we discussed the relationship between the research process and the sections of a research report. This relationship is illustrated in Figure 11-2. Now that we have discussed the research process in more detail, a fuller comparison of the process to the research report is possible.

The first step of the research process of describing and defining the knowledge gap or problem is summarized in the background and literature review sections of a research report. These sections give us the context for a research problem and tell us about relevant theory and research regarding aspects of the problem. The information included in the report is a synopsis of the much more extensive information that was gathered and synthesized during the first step in the research process. The research purpose and specific questions or hypotheses that conclude the first sections of a report reflect the final refinement of the research problem into specific variables and a specific type of research question.

The second step of the research process is reflected in the methods section of a research report. The methods section tells us the study design, sampling plan, methods of measurement, and procedures. Again, all of the previous research, practicalities, and experience that enter into the decisions about settings for a study, the sample, and the measurement are distilled into a few paragraphs describing the final decisions that were reached about the study plan.

The third step of implementing the study is usually reflected in the results section of a research report because it is there that we learn who participated in the study. We also may see part of the implementation of the study reflected in the methods section if what occurred during the implementation process changed the sampling or

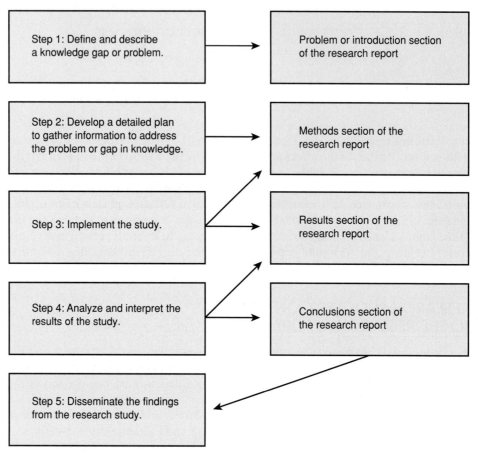

FIGURE 11-2 • The relationship between the research process and the sections of a research report.

measurement approaches taken. In either case, the information included in a report rarely reflects all of the details of a study's implementation.

The fourth step of analysis and interpretation of the results of a study are reflected in both the results and conclusions sections of a research report. Of all the steps of the research process, probably this one is most fully described in the report. However, even with this step, a great deal more goes into the process than is reflected in the results and conclusion sections of most reports.

Finally, the fifth step in the research process is the research report itself. However, developing and publishing a research study report also requires more effort than may be obvious when looking at the final product. The publication of a research study depends on several factors. These include the fit between the purpose of the study and the emphasis of journals that publish research, the relevance and quality of the research study, and the ability of the researcher to express clearly and succinctly all the pertinent elements that are needed to fully understand and use the research. The first two factors primarily affect the user of research because they affect what research is available through journals and online. Some research journals publish all types of research in each issue; others develop themes for different issues, limiting the types of studies that they will publish at any particular time. Other journals reflect specialties, such as obstetric nursing, and are only interested in research that is relevant to that specialty. Some journals do not want to publish research that is highly theoretical because they target readers who want practical and practice-focused information. To disseminate the study findings, a researcher first has to find journals that fit with the purpose of the completed study.

We mentioned in Chapter 10 that research reports from refereed or peer-reviewed journals are more respected because they have been reviewed and critiqued by experts in the area of the research. Some research is not published because problems with the quality of the research are identified during the review process that decreases the meaningfulness or validity of the study's results. This does not mean that the research was bad but simply that some flaw or aspect of the study creates enough doubt about the findings or meaning of the results to preclude its warranting publication.

Another factor that affects publication of research studies is the ability of the researcher to express in writing adequate information to accurately describe the entire research process. As you will recall, many of the common errors in research reports discussed throughout this book were errors of omission or lack of complete information. We have now seen how much more thought and work goes into the research process than can go into a research report. The challenge for a researcher, then, and for the reviewers and editors who contribute to the final publication, is to describe clearly and completely all the aspects of the research process that were relevant to the particular study. The goal is to provide the readers with enough information to allow them to fully understand the study and to make intelligent decisions about the usefulness and meaning of the research for practice. One way that this is accomplished is by using the language of research to limit the need to fully explain each study aspect. Yet, that very language of research may interfere with using research in practice because the practitioner may not be familiar with or understand that language.

FACTORS THAT AFFECT THE RESEARCH PROCESS

In the previous section, we discussed factors that affect the publication of research studies. What about factors that affect whether a research study is implemented? Potential barriers to the implementation of research include lack of knowledge; lack of resources, such as money, time, or both; and lack of methods or measures.

Occasionally, research is not implemented because those who see a problem do not have the knowledge or skill to carry out the research process. For example, an RN in practice may see an important problem but be unable to find others who have a similar interest with the skills to implement the research. Similarly, a community or a group of patients may see a problem that is not recognized as important by providers or by those who are prepared to implement research.

Research requires time and effort and is not without expense. Some research is not implemented because there are no resources to support the particular study. Expenses in research range from potentially small costs, such as copying, to potentially huge costs for sophisticated measures, such as ultrasounds or specialized laboratory testing. Costs are associated with the researcher's time and the time of others, such as data collectors or workers who enter data. Costs are associated with providing space and equipment needed for some research. As well, costs may be directly associated with subjects in the study, such as incentive payments or payments for travel or lodging.

Financial support for research can come from numerous sources, including individuals; local, regional, or national organizations; or the government. In almost every case, to receive financial support for a study, a researcher must prepare a proposal describing the study and identifying how the study will help to meet the goals of the funding source. Herein lies another limit or potential barrier to some research.

Sources of financial support for research usually have goals or initiatives that relate to the purpose of the group providing the support. Occasionally, these goals are specific, such as those of the National Alzheimer's Association, which are to support research into the mechanisms and treatment of Alzheimer's disease. Sometimes these goals are broad, such as the goal of the National Institute for Nursing Research (NINR) to support knowledge development in nursing. However, even the NINR, with its broad goal, has research priorities and target areas for research, such as studies with vulnerable populations, which may influence the success of a particular study in receiving funding. The Web site of a professional organization, such as Sigma Theta Tau or the NINR, usually publishes its research priorities. When developing a proposal for a research study, decisions about the study purpose, sample, or methods may be based, at least in part, on the goals and priorities of the potential funding source.

In addition to direct financial support for research, sources of indirect support also may affect the types of research implemented. In nursing, large health care organizations and nursing colleges in universities often employ individuals with the expectation that they will implement research as part of their role. These organizations pay for part of the time a researcher spends on research because the results of research fit with the mission of the organization. A nurse researcher in a large metropolitan medical center, for example, may not need to find financial support for his or her time but may need to limit the types of research implemented to problems directly relevant to delivery of tertiary health care.

Another factor that affects the implementation of research is the availability of safe and tested methods and measures to study what we are interested in studying. For example, we may be interested in predictors of pancreatic cancer because it is so lethal but have no effective way to identify the dependent variable of interest— pancreatic cancer—until an individual is so ill that it is no longer feasible to implement measurement of selected biologic or psychosocial parameters. Or, a researcher may be interested in a concept, such as empathy, but find that no instruments have been developed that can be used to measure empathy. Sometimes it is unethical to implement a study using what might be the best design validity because of the need to protect the rights of human subjects, as discussed in Chapter 7.

One approach that researchers can take to address some of the limits related to measures and methods is to implement a pilot study. A **pilot study** is a small research study that develops and demonstrates the effectiveness of selected measures and methods. Occasionally, this type of study is used to demonstrate the potential importance of a selected factor to a research problem. At other times, it is used to demonstrate the reliability or validity of selected measures in a unique situation or sample. A pilot study also may be used to demonstrate the ability of the researcher(s) to implement a study. Because knowledge development regarding any particular gap in knowledge is a process that takes time and usually requires multiple studies, pilot studies can be an important first step in building a research program.

GENERATING KNOWLEDGE CAN BE FUN!

We started this book by stating that the goal was not to make you a researcher but to give you the knowledge and tools needed to understand and use research intelligently. However, we do not want to end this chapter with an emphasis on how complex and arduous the research process can be or the many potential barriers there can be to both implementing and publishing research. The research process is a wonderful and exciting challenge. It is like a giant interactive puzzle because as each piece is solved and fit into place, the rest of the pieces change and must be addressed in their new form, given what has already been completed. Fitting each piece into the puzzle can be extremely satisfying, and finishing small sections of the puzzle through completion of a research study can be rewarding.

Part of the reason the research process is fun is because it is a continuous learning experience for those involved. When one is trying to develop new knowledge, the challenges of planning and implementing a valid and meaningful study always require problem solving and creative solutions, so the opportunity to learn and create can be immense. More and more, we are recognizing that most research is best approached by using teams with members from different backgrounds and disciplines. This allows the knowledge brought to bear on a research problem to be wide ranging and to enhance the potential for a high-quality product.

It is the authors' hope that as you read and use research, you will develop an interest in and excitement about the process of research as well as for the problems that it addresses. Although the baccalaureate nurse is not expected to plan and implement research, there are several roles for nurses in the research process, such as participation in planning a study or in subject recruitment and data collection.

We started this chapter with the RN joining a newly formed group seeking to address a research problem. We talked about the process employed by this group and how that process relates to the research report. As we discussed the research process, you may have noticed some similarities between it and the nursing process. For one thing, both are processes, and both have been broken down into steps. In the broadest sense, the nursing and research processes are similar because they are used to solve problems. Both a research problem and a patient care problem (whether the patient is an individual, family, or community) can be viewed as a complicated puzzle, where often only some of the pieces are available at any time point.

Both types of problems are initially addressed through gathering information. In the nursing process, this gathering of information is referred to as assessment, and in the research process, it is referred to as describing and refining the knowledge gap or problem. However, in both cases, we are collecting information to guide us in understanding the problem and formulating a plan.

The second, third, and fourth steps of the nursing and research processes also initially may appear similar, although they differ in some major ways. Although the second step of the nursing process is planning and the second step of the research process is developing a detailed plan, the two processes differ because they have fundamentally different purposes. The purpose of the nursing process is to provide informed, scientifically based nursing care for human responses to potential or actual health problems. The purpose of the research process is to develop or validate knowledge. The goal of the nursing process is action to promote the established outcome of improved health. The goal of the research process is to acquire new knowledge, and the outcomes for that new knowledge cannot be known until the knowledge is established. Therefore, the second and third steps of the nursing process address planning and implementing care, whereas the second and third steps of the research process address planning and implementing acquisition of new information. As a result, the fourth steps of these two processes have different focuses because evaluation in the nursing process is concerned with outcomes, whereas data analysis and interpretation are concerned with understanding. Table 11-1 summarizes the similarities and differences between the two processes. We discuss the roles of nursing in research more in the next chapter.

Although there are some similarities and differences in the processes of nursing and research, it is essential that there be a strong relationship between the two. The research process should provide knowledge that is the basis for the nursing process. This is why this entire book focuses on understanding and intelligently using research in practice. In addition, the nursing process will often be the source of problems that need to be addressed using the research process. As we plan, implement, and evaluate nursing care, we often find problems or face questions about the best

TABLE 11-1

Comparison of the Research Process and the Nursing Process

	Research Process	**Nursing Process**
Similarities	A process with steps A form of problem solving Complex "puzzle"	A process with steps A form of problem solving Complex "puzzle"

Differences	Purpose is to develop
	  knowledge
	Plans and implements
	  knowledge acquisition
	Analysis and interpretation
	  concerned with knowing
		Purpose is to provide scientifically
		  based care
		Plans and implements delivery
		  of care
		Evaluation concerned with
		  outcomes

ways to achieve our outcome of improved health. The nursing and research processes differ in purpose, but they are closely linked and together ensure the growth and development of nursing as a profession.

CORE CONCEPT 11-2

While different in purpose, the nursing process shares several steps and skills with the research process.

PUBLISHED REPORTS—WHAT DO YOU CONCLUDE NOW?

We have used nine research study reports in this book as examples of how research can be used and related to clinical practice. In several cases, the studies examined a research problem from the two different approaches of qualitative and quantitative methods. None of the studies that we examined could be called perfect, and to expect them to be so is unreasonable, but each made a meaningful contribution to our knowledge about patients and patient care. No one study, however, gave us the full answer to our clinical questions and often had clear limitations in trying to apply the findings to our RN's clinical case. This is often a frustration for nurses in practice. With a better understanding of the research process, it should be clearer now why usually no one study fully answers a clinical question. Clinical questions are usually too complex, and too many variables and factors must be considered and examined for any one study to provide a complete answer. However, as research studies about a particular study accumulate, we should see answers begin to unfold. Evidence-based practice, which is discussed in Chapters 1 and 12, explicitly recognizes the need for an accumulation of knowledge regarding a problem to ensure the best and safest delivery of health care.

Therefore, what do you conclude now about the needs of the RN from Chapter 1, who is facing complex planning for her incarcerated, HIV-positive, substance-abusing patient? What do you conclude about how the RN from Chapter 3 is taking care of C.R. with her abdominal aortic aneurysm should intervene with the patient's ambulation needs? What should the RN in Chapter 4 do differently in caring for the stroke patient and her husband? How should the RN plan protocols that address family caregiver needs? You should now be able to accomplish the following tasks and answer five questions as you read the research we have reviewed. As you look at these questions, realize how much you have learned and how much you now know regarding research.

- You can read and understand the background and literature review of a report to find out *"Why was the research question asked—what do we already know?"*
- You can read the design and methods sections of a research report to find out *"How were those people studied—why was the study performed that way?"*

- You can read the sampling section of the research report to find out *"To what types of patients do these research conclusions apply?"*
- You can read the results and conclusions sections of the report to find out *"Why the authors reached their conclusions—what did they actually find?"*
- Finally, you can use the answers from the above four questions to decide *"What is the answer to the question—what did the study conclude?"*

You also now know that finding the "answer" to your question will only be the beginning, and that it may give you new knowledge and insight into patient care, but may also leave you asking even more questions.

OUT-OF-CLASS EXERCISE

Critiquing the Whole

Before starting the last chapter of this book, exchange your abstract with another student. Read the abstract and critique it, giving at least two positive statements about it and at least two constructive suggestions for improvement. You may focus on the connections and links among the different parts of the abstract, how well each component was succinctly stated, the creativity of the abstract, or its usefulness for knowledge development. Return the abstracts to each other, and see how well your effort to organize an abbreviated research report was understood. In Chapter 12, we discuss how nursing research has developed over time. We will examine the links between research, practice, and education, and we discuss evidence-based practice and quality assurance as two concrete areas where research is explicitly used in practice.

References

Peplau, H. E. (1952). *Interpersonal relations in nursing: A conceptual frame of reference for psychodynamic nursing.* New York: G. P. Putnams' Sons. [Reprinted 1991, New York: Springer].

Williams, M. A. (1980). Editorial: Assumptions in research. *Research in Nursing & Health, 3*(2), 47–48.

Resources

LoBiondo-Wood, G., Haber, J., & Krainovich-Miller, B. (2002). Overview of the research process. In G. LoBiondo-Wood & J. Haber (Eds.), *Nursing research: Methods, critical appraisal, and utilization* (5th ed.). St. Louis: Mosby.

Locke, L. F., Silverman, S. J., & Spirduso, W. W. (1998). *Reading and understanding research.* Thousand Oaks, CA: Sage Publications.

Polit, D. F., & Beck, C. T. (2003). *Nursing research: Principles and methods* (7th ed.). Philadelphia: Lippincott Williams, & Wilkins.

Tomey, A. M. & Alligood, M. R. (2002). *Nursing theorists and their work* (5th ed.). St. Louis: Mosby.

12

THE ROLE OF RESEARCH IN NURSING

LEARNING OBJECTIVE:

The student will relate nursing research to the development of the professional practice of nursing.

History of Nursing Research
Linking Theory, Education, and Practice With Research
Evidence-Based Practice: Pros and Cons
Quality Improvement: Framed Within the Research Process
Where Are We Going? Roles of Nurses in Research
Finding Answers Through Research
Fictional Article: What Would You Conclude?

KEY TERMS

Quality improvement
Research utilization

CLINICAL CASE

S.J. is in the last semester of an RN-to-BSN program. One of her courses is nursing leadership. She has been assigned to present a review of a relevant research study on the nursing shortage in her next class. Of course, she also has several big papers due the same week!

S.J. notices the fictional article entitled "Demographic characteristics as predictors of nursing students' choice of type of clinical practice" (Appendix B) in her nursing association district newsletter. The article begins by addressing the nursing shortage. Because the article is research, S.J. decides that it will fulfill her assignment for the nursing leadership class. She decides to read the article, using the five questions that organize this text.

Knowledge development through research is a core element in the development of the overall nursing profession. In this chapter, we step back to consider the history of nursing research and how nursing research relates to nursing practice, education, and theory. We move beyond the individual nurse's use of research in practice to consider the more structured process of evidence-based practice. Also, we examine how research is used and reflected in quality improvement studies. We finish by considering the future of nursing research and returning to how we started this book: considering the use of research in patient care.

HISTORY OF NURSING RESEARCH

History helps us to understand the past and its continuing influence on the future. Nursing research started slowly, but it has evolved at an ever-increasing and progressive rate. Figure 12-1 provides a time line highlighting some major events in nursing research.

It is widely accepted that the history of nursing research begins with Florence Nightingale and her studies of environmental factors that affected the health of soldiers in the Crimean War. During the last half of the 19th century, nurses, particularly in public health, continued to refine Nightingale's findings published in *Notes on Nursing* (1860). Little is known, however, of any nursing research during that time.

Between 1900 and 1940, nurses conducted research, but the larger focus was the preparation of nurses. During those years, the *American Journal of Nursing* began publication, baccalaureate nursing programs increased, and the first doctoral program in nursing opened at Teacher's College, Columbia University. Each of these developments helped to promote an increase in nursing research.

In the infancy of nursing research, we tended to study ourselves. In the 1940s and 1950s, it primarily focused on studying characteristics of nurses and nursing education. This occurred probably because nursing was relatively new to the university system, and most doctoral-prepared nurses had education degrees. Despite this focus, nursing research made significant progress during this time, as evidenced by the publication of the journal *Nursing Research*.

During the 1960s, nursing began to recognize the need for theoretical foundations to its practice and research. Research also shifted away from the study of nurses toward the study of the clinical care provided by nurses. Within nursing education, nursing faculty began to teach the research process in baccalaureate nursing programs.

By the 1970s, nursing research examining clinical practice had increased significantly, as evidenced by the publication of three additional journals to disseminate research: *Research in Nursing & Health, Advances in Nursing Science,* and *Western Journal of Nursing Research*. Doctoral nursing programs continued to emerge, leading to steady growth in nurses who were specifically prepared to be researchers. The emphasis in nursing research during this time was traditional quantitative methods, often testing theories borrowed from other fields. Despite this emphasis, nursing theory also was growing during this period, and qualitative methods were increasingly used.

The steady increase in both research itself and nurses prepared to do research reached a critical level in the 1980s, culminating in the establishment in 1986 of the National Center of Nursing Research at the National Institutes of Health. The

Historical Development	Research Focus of Development
• 1860	Environmental factors that affect health
Florence Nightingale	
• 1900–1940	Nursing preparation
Goldmark Report 1923	
American Journal of Nursing published	
First doctoral program in nursing	Characteristics of nursing education and nursing students
• 1940s–1950s	
Publication of *Nursing Research*	
• 1960s	Research about clinical practice
Development of theory in nursing	
First research process classes taught	
• 1970s	Theory-based research
Publication of three more research journals in nursing	
Development of multiple doctoral programs in nursing	
• 1980s	Development of programs of research
National Center for Nursing Research started at NIH 1986	
• 1990s	Priorities for research developed
National Institute of Nursing Research starts in 1993	Qualitative methods gain recognition

FIGURE 12-1 • Time line showing important developments in the history of nursing research.

national recognition of nursing as a science, warranting funding for its own research agenda and center, was a major milestone. Nursing was now acknowledged as an important player among other "big" players, such as the National Institute for Medicine and the National Institute of Mental Health. In 1993, 7 years after its establishment, the National Center for Nursing Research became the National Institute of Nursing Research. This change placed nurses on equal footing with colleagues in medicine and other health-related fields. In addition, during the 1980s and 1990s, five more major nursing research journals were published, and priorities for nursing research were developed. Nursing research had come of age.

At the beginning of the 21st century, nursing research continues to grow exponentially. Nurses preparing at the doctoral level, sources and opportunities for funding of nursing research, and diversity of topics examined in nursing research all have increased steadily. Since the 1990s, when qualitative approaches became recognized and respected as appropriate methods of scientific inquiry, nursing has been implementing mixtures of quantitative and qualitative methods for study design and analysis that fit the unique research problems of the field.

Probably most important, as nursing research has grown, the body of nursing knowledge also has developed. As nurses, we have expanded our horizons to consider outcomes research, international research, and traditional laboratory research. We have replicated and expanded on previous findings. Our researchers have completed multiple studies all related to the same problems, allowing us to truly build knowledge and to find real answers to complex questions. As a result, we now have Centers for Research housed in various universities, where groups of nurses with research expertise in specific areas (such as health-promoting behaviors) can work and build their research together to achieve a better-connected and deeper knowledge. Nurses also have recognized their limits as well as their strengths, moving increasingly toward the creation of and participation in interprofessional teams of researchers, capitalizing on the strengths inherent in the blending of many different disciplines.

LINKING THEORY, EDUCATION, AND PRACTICE WITH RESEARCH

Although nursing research has made great strides, it still has a long way to go. The journey is linked with the past development of nursing education, practice, and theory, and these connections will continue in the future. In Chapter 10, we discussed the intertwining braid of theory, research, and practice. In fact, that "braid" contains four strands, the last of which is nursing education. Historically, nursing education occurred in an apprenticeship format, mostly within hospital schools of nursing. Only as nursing has moved into university education and has begun to claim a unique body of knowledge have nurses started considering independent research. Nursing education has fostered nursing research, partly through the demand for faculty with credentials equivalent to those of other faculty in university settings and partly through the preparation of nurses who expect to use, participate in, and conduct nursing research. Doctoral preparation in nursing has given nurses the training and skills needed to become researchers. The existence of clinically based nursing has led to the education of nurses to use research in practice. Therefore, education has been, and remains, integral to the development and use of nursing research.

The four-stranded braid of nursing theory, research, education, and practice represents the future of the nursing profession (Figure 12-2). Nursing theory must

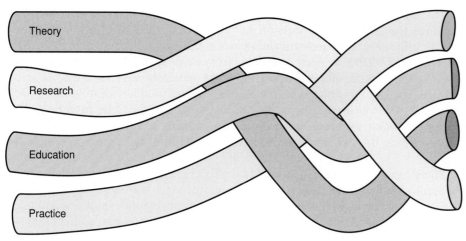

FIGURE 12-2 • Four-stranded braid of theory, research, education, and practice.

be based on and applicable to nursing practice. Nursing research must test and refine nursing theory for practice. Nursing education must teach both theory and research as they relate to practice and develop in nurses a commitment to the understanding and use of research as evidence for practice. Nursing practice must be based on an ever-developing body of knowledge derived from research and theory. Nurses must be educated to have an open, skeptical, and critical view of their practice to identify areas for using and problems to be addressed by nursing research.

The four-stranded braid is not without its symbolic "knots." As indicated within the discussion of the history of nursing research, early studies focused on nurses themselves and were not useful for direct practice. As practice-based research began, a real gap developed between nursing theory and nursing research. Nursing theory was highly conceptual and broad, focusing on the entire practice of nursing. Conversely, nursing research often was problem focused, addressing narrow and specific clinical situations. The two did not go hand-in-hand, and, as nursing research studies were completed, there often were no or few follow-up studies to build on the initial knowledge developed. We have seen that it is unusual for a single study to fully answer a clinical question. Yet, at times, nursing has produced several single isolated clinical studies that failed to contribute to a coherent body of knowledge. One reason for this was the failure to use and to build theory relevant to the clinical problems of interest to nursing. Another problem has been limits in the dissemination of research. A third problem has been lack of funding for ongoing research programs. Finally, a gap has existed between researchers and practitioners of nursing. This gap occasionally has resulted from nurse researchers' limited connections with practice and occasionally from practicing nurses' discomfort with using research.

The gap between research and practice has been of particular concern to nursing. Since the 1970s, the profession has made a significant effort to facilitate research utilization. **Research utilization** means the use of research in practice. Several research studies have been completed to examine specifically whether research is assimilated into nursing practice. The results generally have been discouraging, although the extent to which research innovations are used has improved over time (Ketefian, 1975; Coyle & Sokop, 1990). Because studies continue to indicate that nursing often fails to use research in practice, nursing has looked closely at what may be causing this "knot" in the intertwining relationship between research and practice.

Many factors have been identified that affect research utilization, including limited applicability of some research to practice, resistance within health care organizations to make changes based on research, and difficulty understanding and using research among practicing nurses. The goal of this entire book is to address that last factor. Nursing has responded to the gap between findings from research and clinical practice by developing several different projects to increase the use of research findings in daily practice. Overall, the projects have demonstrated that research utilization can happen if the research relates directly to practice and is communicated broadly in ways that practicing nurses can understand and use (Horsley, Crane, Crabtree, & Wood, 1983).

One response in nursing to the problem with research utilization has been to develop models to describe and explain the process of using research. These models define phases or steps that may facilitate research utilization and include the Stetler model (1994), the Rogers (1995) theory of research utilization, and the Iowa Model of Research-Based Practice (Titler et al., 1994). Any of these models may help you to understand and to organize your use of research in practice. Rather than starting with an entirely new model, however, you may want to begin by using the five questions organizing this text.

This text presents the contents of a research report by starting at the end and moving forward. Now that you have a better understanding of the language and process of research, it will be easier to read reports starting from the beginning and moving to the end. To use research in practice, start by using your understanding about how to search for research as described in Chapter 1. Then, use the five questions that organize the content of this text while reading the research you have found. As you do so, ask yourself:

- Why ask that question—what do we already know?
- How were those people studied—why was the study performed that way?
- To what types of patients do these research conclusions apply—who was in the study?
- Why did the author(s) reach that conclusion—what did they actually find?
- What is the answer to my practice question—what did the study conclude?

As you ask and answer these questions, always be openly questioning and critically reading the study design, methods, sample, results, and conclusions. Doing so will help you to answer the questions identified in Chapter 2 that allow you to critique each section of the research report. Figure 12-3 contains the six inter-related sets of questions for critiquing a research report, which we have talked about as we discussed each section of a research report. The answers to these questions will help you answer the overall question of how convincing the study is as evidence to use in practice. To help you read research, the end of this text includes a glossary, which provides definitions of terms and the page(s) in the book that describe them. It is hoped that this glossary will be a resource for you as you develop your skills at reading and understanding research. Using your understanding and knowledge about the language and the process of research, you will be able to make intelligent decisions about the use of research in practice.

In summary, we have examined the history of nursing research and how that has led to today's interacting relationships between theory, research, education, and practice. We have identified that although the relationships are essential to the ongoing development of nursing as a profession, there is still much to improve on in the relationships. We have also seen that one of the biggest concerns in nursing has been and continues to be the dissemination of research results into practice. In the next section, we will explore resources for evidence-based practice that are currently used within nursing to strengthen the link between research and practice.

EVIDENCE-BASED PRACTICE: PROS AND CONS

At the beginning of this book, we defined *evidence-based nursing (EBN) practice* as the term used to describe the process used by nurses to make clinical decisions and to answer clinical questions. We stated that EBN has four approaches to answer questions:

1. Reviewing the best available evidence, most often the results of research.
2. Using the nurse's clinical expertise.
3. Determining the values and cultural needs of the individual.
4. Determining the preferences of the individual, family, and community.

The phrase *evidence-based practice* (EBP) originated in the field of medicine. The concept often is considered to have been established by Dr. Archie Cochrane, a physician and epidemiologist. Cochrane was the developer of the "Cochrane Reviews," an electronic database similar to CINAHL, which consists of systematic reviews in various health care fields (French, 2002). If you search for topics in this database, you will find a short, focused systematic review, along with a list of relevant primary sources. Remember that a systematic review is the product of a process that includes asking a clinical question, conducting a structured and organized search for theory and research related to the question, reviewing and synthesizing the results, and reaching conclusions about the implications for practice.

Another important source for systematic reviews is the *Online Journal of Knowledge Synthesis in Nursing* (OJKSN) (Sigma Theta Tau International [STTI], 1993). The purpose of this recently developed online journal is to present "synthesized knowledge to guide nursing practice and research." A third source for systematic

---

How to Critically Read the Background Section of a Research Report

Does the report answer the question:
"Why ask that question—what do we already know?"

Did the report include a clearly identified background and/or literature review section?
Do I think the background discusses aspects of my clinical question?
Does the literature help me understand why the research question is important to nursing?
Is the majority of the literature cited current (less than 5 years old) or very important to understanding the research question?
If a nursing or other theory was presented, does it connect to your clinical question?
Is the specific research question/problem/hypothesis connected logically to the literature and/or theory presented in the background section?
Is the specific research question/problem/hypothesis relevant or related to my clinical question?

How to Critically Read the Description of Study Design in a Research Report

Does the report answer the question:
"How were those people studied—why was the study performed that way?"

Did the report include a clearly identified section describing the research design?
Does the design make this a quantitative, qualitative, or a mixed method study?
Dose the report address approaches taken to assure study rigor, internal validity, and/or external validity?
Do I think that the researcher(s) should have designed the study differently in order to answer my clinical question?

How to Critically Read the Methods Section of a Research Report

Does the report answer the question:
"How were those people studied—why was the study performed that way?"

Did the report include a clearly identified section describing methods used in this study?
Do the methods make this a quantitative or a qualitative study?
Do I understand what my patient population would be doing if they were in this study or a study using similar methods?
Do the measures and procedures in this study address my clinical problem?
Do I think that the measures used in this study would provide helpful and useful information when used with my patient population?
Do I think what the researcher collected and the method of collection was the best way to address the clinical question?
Do I think that the researcher(s) should have planned the study differently in order to answer my clinical question?

(continued)

FIGURE 12-3 • Questions for critically reading research reports.

reviews that is focused on the health professions is the Joanna Briggs Collaboration (available at http://www.joannabriggs.edu.au). This collaboration is a coordinated effort by a group of centers from around the world to promote evidence-based health care, education and training, the conduct of systematic reviews, the development of Best Practice Information Sheets, the implementation of EBP, and the conduct of

---

How to Critically Read the Sample Section of a Research Report

Does the report answer the question:
"To what types of patients do these research conclusions apply—who was in the study?"

Did the report include a clearly identified section or paragraphs about sampling?
Did the report give me enough information to understand how and why this sample was chosen?
Is there enough information about the sample to tell me if the research is relevant for my clinical population?
Was enough information given for me to understand how rights of human subjects were protected?
Would my patient population have been placed at risk if they had participated in this study?
Can I identify how information was collected about the sample?

How to Critically Read the Results Section of a Research Report

Do the results answer the question:
"Why did the authors reach these conclusions—what did they actually find?"

Did the report include a clearly identified results section?
Were the results presented appropriately for the information collected?
Were descriptive versus inferential results identifiable if this is a quantitative study?
Were themes or structure and meaning identifiable if this is a qualitative study?
Were the results presented in a clear and logical manner?
Did the results include enough information about the final sample for the study?

How to Critically Read the Conclusions of a Research Report

Do the conclusions answer the question:
"What is the answer to my practice question—what did the study conclude?"

Did the report include a conclusions section?
Did the conclusions section assist me with my clinical problem?
Did the conclusions assist in a general manner or provide specific information about my clinical problem?
Did the conclusions section include limitations of the study?
Did the limitations diminish my ability to use the conclusions in practice?
Do the conclusions seem reasonable or warranted based on the results of the study?

FIGURE 12-3 • *(continued)*

evaluation cycles and primary research arising out of systematic reviews. There are currently more than 20 collaborating centers covering the disciplines of nursing, midwifery, physiotherapy, nutrition and dietetics, podiatry, occupational therapy, aged care, and medical radiation.

The Cochrane Reviews, the OJKSN, and the Joanna Briggs Collaboration all serve an important function in improving the use of research in practice because they pull together disparate studies into an easily accessible and organized form. This allows the nurse to find multiple studies on the same clinical question already synthesized into a single review that ends with recommendations for practice. Clearly then, systematic reviews address the issues of access to research and, to some extent, applicability of research to practice.

Use of systematic reviews for EBN has limits as well as strengths. Just as a researcher implementing a traditional research study must make decisions about methods and sample, the author(s) of a systematic review must make decisions about what research to include. This raises the question of what constitutes the "best" evidence. As demonstrated in "Non-somatic effects of patient aggression on nurses: A systematic review" study (Needham, Abderhalden, Halfens, Fischer, & Dassen, 2005) from Chapter 10 (Appendix A-9) often the standard set for appropriate studies to include in a review is that they be *empirical*, a term used for studies using quantitative approaches. Although there is no question that studies using a quantitative approach are important and useful for answering some questions in nursing, many problems in nursing do not lend themselves to the level of quantitative study. Therefore, an overdependence on systematic reviews of clinical research may limit both the types of problems that practitioners consider appropriate for research utilization and the dissemination of important knowledge acquired using other research methods.

Systematic reviews as a type of research have an important place in EBN. Reading and understanding systematic reviews should be conducted using the same five questions mentioned throughout this book and keeping the same openly questioning, critical mind. The difference in reading and understanding systematic reviews is that you must answer the five questions at two different levels, rather than just at one level. For example, when considering the question "How were those people studied—why was the study performed that way?," you must consider the methods for the different studies included in the review. However, you also must consider the rationale for use of a systematic review approach to this clinical question. Probably the toughest two-layered question will be "To what types of patients do these research conclusions apply—who was in the study?" To answer, you must consider the samples in the different studies in the review as well as the sample of "studies" that comprise the review. The second layer becomes "Why did the reviewer include those studies and not others?" Table 12-1 provides an overview of how one might apply the five questions to a systematic review.

Systematic reviews are an important source of evidence for practice, but they are not the only evidence, and they are not even the only source of research evidence. We have looked at a number of studies throughout this book that used a qualitative approach to knowledge development, and the knowledge they yield can be useful EBN. As an intelligent reader and user of nursing research, you must find how the use of evidence in the form of systematic reviews can be most useful to you in your clinical practice.

QUALITY IMPROVEMENT: FRAMED WITHIN THE RESEARCH PROCESS

Although systematic reviews are an important form of research that can be used in practice, quality improvement is a process that resembles, yet differs, from the

TABLE 12-1

Five Research Questions Applied to Systematic Reviews and Quality Improvement Reports

Guiding Question	Application to Systematic Reviews	Application to Quality Improvement Reports
Why ask that question—what do we already know?	What do we already know that suggests the need for a systematic review?	What is the basis for the standard or outcome to be examined?
How were those people studied—why was the study performed that way?	Why was a systematic review used? Why were the studies that were included in the review performed that way?	Why was the study done that way? What was the justification for the approach taken?
To what types of patients do these research conclusions apply—who was in the study?	What types of studies were included as evidence in the review? What types of samples were used in the studies reviewed?	What types of practices, settings, and patients are reflected by the information collected for the study?
Why did the author(s) reach that conclusion—what was found?	Why did the review reach its conclusions? What did the studies find?	Why did the report reach its conclusions? What was found about practice?
What is the answer to the research question—what did the study conclude?	What is the answer to the clinical question?	Were the standards or outcomes met? What does the report tell us about why or why not?

research process. **Quality improvement** is a process of evaluation of health care services to see if they meet specified standards or outcomes of care and to identify how they can be improved. As discussed in Chapters 1 and 2, quality improvement often is based on research, and the process and product resemble the research process. The questions in quality improvement are whether a certain set of actions is occurring and how desirable outcomes can be facilitated. This is a form of a descriptive research question. The standard or outcome itself usually is based on earlier research that indicates the set of actions or outcome that can and should be achieved. Standards of care change as research findings suggest better approaches to and potential outcomes of care.

In addition to asking a descriptive question about the presence or frequency of a set of actions or outcomes, quality improvement studies also often examine relationships among factors that may affect the outcome or actions of interest. Just as we want to know what factors may influence a clinical problem of interest, we want to know what factors influence the consistency of achievement of standards or outcomes.

The usefulness of a quality improvement study can be understood using the same five questions discussed throughout this book. Table 12-1 outlines how they might be applied. We can consider why the standard or outcome was established— what is the evidence for that standard? We can ask about the manner by which the study was implemented because various methods can be used to implement quality improvement, including chart review, observation, interviews, and questionnaires. Various approaches can be taken to the "sample" for a quality improvement study, including convenience, random selection, and purposive sampling. Similarly, data from a quality improvement study can be handled and analyzed in several ways, making the fourth question about what was actually found appropriate to consider. The last question of what the study concluded is obviously also relevant to quality improvement studies. Just as an accurate and meaningful research study can inform clinical practice, an accurate and meaningful quality assurance study can evaluate and strengthen practice. Findings from a quality improvement study that indicate standards are being met support continuation of existing practices. Findings indicating that standards are not being met should guide revision of existing practices to improve care. As with traditional research, findings from a quality improvement study may lead to the need for another study to further clarify issues that may relate to meeting standards or outcomes.

In such ways, traditional research often serves as the basis for quality improvement standards. Moreover, many of the methods used in research directly apply to the process of evaluating quality. Finally, gaps in quality of care may indicate fresh areas requiring research as well as needs for changes in practice.

WHERE ARE WE GOING?
ROLES OF NURSES IN RESEARCH

This text has focused on the baccalaureate-prepared nurse's role in understanding and using research in EBN practice. It also has suggested some other ways that research may be part of the role of the baccalaureate nurse. For example, nurses may be asked to use research as the basis for decisions about the development of clinical programs. They may be asked to participate in some step of the research process, particularly in acquiring informed consent and in collecting data. Equally important, as the nursing profession recognizes the need for clinically relevant and informed research, baccalaureate nurses may be asked to participate in all phases of a research study, from development and refinement of the purpose to interpretation of the results. For example, one of the hallmarks of hospitals that have the highest retention of nurses and quality of patient care—that is, hospitals that have received the American Nurses Credentialing Center (ANCC) Magnet Recognition Program status—is the inclusion of nursing research development and application in the clinical setting.

We began this book by saying that it was not the goal of this text to give you the tools to implement research independently. Doctoral-level nurses are expected to be the experts in the research process. Nurses prepared at the master's level are expected to be sophisticated consumers of research, who are able to critically evaluate and actively participate in research. Nevertheless, baccalaureate-level nurses often are the foundation from which research is developed and are absolutely the focus for research utilization. Your understanding of the language and the process of research, coupled with your clinical experience, will allow you to be a contributor

to a research team, should the opportunity arise. One hospital that perhaps best epit-
omizes the full extent of the potential role of the baccalaureate-prepared nurse in
research is housed on the grounds of the National Institutes of Health. Every patient
there participates in at least one research study, and the hospital employs only baccalaureate-prepared nurses. The nurses there not only participate in research but
also can develop their own cooperative research projects, with support from
researchers with advanced preparation. Baccalaureate-level nurses can be members
of Institutional Review Boards as well, bringing their knowledge of patients and
patient care to assist in assuring that the rights of patients are protected.

Nursing not only has a role in research that directly addresses questions generated within the profession, but it also addresses larger questions in health care. We
mentioned that nursing has moved increasingly to interprofessional teams to
address research problems. Nurses also are being sought increasingly to participate
in research teams led by researchers from other disciplines. Nursing's unique understanding of health as it affects the whole person, family, and community is a perspective that often contributes important ideas to research studies. Nurses are good
at working with people. Thus, researchers from other disciplines often find that
nurses can implement sampling plans effectively, with little subject loss.

Beyond generating and participating in research, nursing has an important role
in formulating the national research agendas regarding health. The research supported and generated through the National Institute of Nursing Research at the
National Institutes of Health has earned the respect of other, more established
research disciplines. That development has contributed to ensuring that health concerns particularly focused on nursing have become part of national agendas for
health-related research. Nursing research has made great progress since the days of
Florence Nightingale, and we can be proud not only of our heritage of research but
also of our current and future contributions to meaningful research that improves
the care of our patients.

FINDING ANSWERS THROUGH RESEARCH

What have we learned about reading and using research to answer questions about
clinical practice? First, we have acknowledged that turning to research is not always
the easiest way to get answers. We have identified that the language of research is
unique. We have described how to find research and have examined each section of
a research report in some detail. We have also considered the research process and
how it is reflected in and relates to the nursing process, EBN, and quality improvement. Throughout the previous chapters, we have identified 34 core concepts,
which are the foundation of ideas that can help nurses to understand and use
research in practice. These concepts are summarized in Table 12-2. Together, these
core concepts form the backbone of your knowledge about the language and process
of research.

One important idea that we have discussed throughout this text is the differences and relationships between qualitative and quantitative research approaches.
Traditional science and medicine primarily have used and supported the quantitative

TABLE 12-2	
Core Concepts Summarized According to Chapter	

Chapter 1	Nursing research is the systematic gathering of information to gain, expand, or validate knowledge about health and responses to health problems. Abstracts from research reports can be helpful in narrowing or focusing on the appropriate research to acquire and to read. They cannot, and should not, be depended on to provide a level of understanding to support clinical decision-making. An effective clinical question for EBN includes a concern that someone else has studied, focuses on a concern that can be measured or described, and is a concern relevant to nursing. The question also addresses *Who, Where, What,* and *When* in terms of the clinical concern.
Chapter 2	What distinguishes conclusions in a research report from those in other reports is the expectation that they contain either new knowledge or confirmation of previous knowledge. The differences between results and conclusions is that results are a summary of the actual findings or information collected in the research study, whereas conclusions summarize the potential meaning, decisions, or determinations that can be made based on the information collected. Most research attempts to gather information systematically about a subset, or small group of patients or people, to gain knowledge about other similar patients or people. Many research methods are aimed at ensuring that what happens in the subset or sample studied is as similar as possible to what would happen in other larger groups of patients or people. Many terms used in research have a range of meanings rather than a single, discrete locked-in meaning.
Chapter 3	The summary of findings in the discussion section of a research report contains only selected results from the study. It does not give the reader a complete picture of the results found in the study but does give information about some key or important results. The discussion section of a research report contains a debate about how the results of the study fit with existing knowledge and what those results may mean.
Chapter 4	Research results that only describe or explain cannot be used to predict outcomes or to directly identify the cause of the findings. Measures of central tendency and distribution are univariate statistics that summarize information about a variable.
Chapter 5	Inferential statistics are used to report whether the results found in a specific study are likely to have happened by chance alone. Statistical significance is not an absolute guarantee that the values are really different or related in the real world. Rather, statistical significance means that there is less than a 5% chance that the amount of relationship or difference happened by chance. Whether the report includes *p* values or confidence intervals, the authors are telling you how likely it is that the results from the study happened due to chance and, therefore, how likely it is that these results can be used to infer similar results in future similar situations. Researchers use different types of statistics to test for the same kind of relationship depending on the form of the data collected. The research report may tell you why a particular type of statistical test was applied. A correlation between two variables tells us only that they are connected in some way and are not the cause of that connection.

TABLE 12-2

Core Concepts Summarized According to Chapter (*continued*)

	The size of the sample, or number of cases in a study, affects the likelihood that the study will find statistical significance.
	Statistical significance does not directly equate with clinical meaningfulness.
Chapter 6	A researcher may define the population of interest for a study in one way but end up with a sample that differs from that defined population.
	Sampling strategies in qualitative and quantitative research differ in their goals and approaches, even when they are using a similar strategy.
Chapter 7	It is unethical and illegal to implement a research study using animal or human subjects without approval of an institutional review board.
	The goal of research with human subjects is always to minimize the risks and to maximize the benefits.
	The five human rights in research are first and foremost the responsibility of the researcher(s).
Chapter 8	The measures in a quantitative study should reflect the specific variables under study.
	Operationalizing variables is similar to translating a phrase from one language to another. The researcher translates an abstract and theoretical variable into a concrete measure or set of measures.
	Consistent measurement is reliable measurement. Accurate or correct measurement is valid measurement.
	In a quantitative study, every variable should have an operational definition that specifies how the variable was measured.
Chapter 9	The type of research question being asked affects the type of research design that will and can be used.
	Studies with problems in internal validity automatically will have problems with external validity. Having internal validity, however, does not guarantee that the study will have external validity.
	The labels for quantitative research designs usually are a combination of words or terms that define the design according to function, use of time, and use of approaches to provide control.
Chapter 10	Theory, theoretical frameworks, and conceptual frameworks all provide a description of the proposed relationships among abstract components that are aspects of the research problem of interest.
	The terms *research purpose, research question, study or specific aim(s),* or *research objective(s)* all refer to the statement of the variables to be studied that are related to the broad research problem.
	The literature review is guided by the variables that have been identified in the research purpose and aims to give the reader an overview of what is known about those variables, how those variables have been studied in the past, and with whom they have been studied.
Chapter 11	The steps of the research process are not always linear; they may overlap or be revisited during the research process.
	Whether a research problem or question has been identified from practice or from theory, the first step in developing a research study requires thoughtful and informed exploration of the problem to arrive at a refined purpose for the study.

approach. As a result, nursing initially heavily emphasized quantitative approaches. Qualitative approaches, however, have been receiving steady recognition as being important to knowledge development in nursing. This text has attempted to present you with balanced information about both approaches so that you can read and understand research from both as well as research that uses mixed methods.

Using research in EBN practice has several advantages. The most obvious is that when research is used in practice, that practice is based on a clearly identifiable knowledge base. Using research in practice can open nurses to new ideas that are challenging and exciting to explore and to implement. It also can help nursing grow as a profession to achieve the broadest goal of promoting the health of patients. Using research in practice also has some disadvantages. First, time and effort are necessary to read and understand research reports. Like any skill, the more one does it, the easier it becomes. Nonetheless, going to research to answer a question definitely necessitates more effort than does asking someone (assuming that he or she has the correct answer when you ask). Another potential disadvantage to using research in practice is that accessing research may not always be easy. Again, this problem is steadily becoming less important as more journals become available online. Nevertheless, for some nurses in rural settings, even online access to a system (such as a university library) may be difficult. The third disadvantage is the potential resistance to change that is inherent in the adoption of new or revised practices. Change, however, is both needed and inevitable in all aspects of life. Facing some resistance initially may simply be part of practicing as a professional nurse.

FICTIONAL ARTICLE: WHAT WOULD YOU CONCLUDE?

The clinical case at the beginning of the chapter provides an opportunity to take one final look at the fictional article from Appendix B that is discussed throughout the book. As S.J. reads that article, she starts by asking "Why ask that question—what do we already know?" She finds that the background section of this report is brief. It provides a broad context for the problem of varying extents of shortages in different fields of nursing. It also makes a somewhat limited case for targeting student recruitment efforts in a way that may increase the numbers of new graduates who will enter fields of nursing that are expected to have the greatest shortages.

S.J. finds that the purpose of the study is stated clearly and that the author gives three specific research questions that identify variables. S.J. can identify that this study asks a question about relationships. She finds, however, several major gaps in the background section of the report. In particular, there is no literature review, so S.J. has no idea what other studies have been conducted to look at predictors of field of practice or what methods might have been used. In fact, although the purpose of the study is clear, the second and third research questions bring in two new variables that have not been mentioned: students' well-being and their previous experiences. S.J. has a general answer as to why the study asked this question, but she also is somewhat confused about why it included the particular variables. She does not have a clear picture of what is already known.

S.J. proceeds to read the methods section and finds that almost nothing in it tells her about the study design. Reading the abstract for the report, she learns that the study is identified as "descriptive," and she knows a descriptive study fits logically with the type of questions the study is to address. She skips the sample section and focuses on the measures section to see if she can clearly answer the second question, "How were those people studied–why was the study performed that way?" The measures section describes a questionnaire that asks specific closed questions. S.J. recognizes that this is a quantitative approach to description that again fits with the types of questions addressed in this study. The report gives S.J. a clear picture of the measure used, including some information about the reliability and validity of one of the included scales. This report includes no real theoretical or operational definitions, but most of the variables studied seem concrete. The exceptions are the two concepts—well-being and students' experiences—that also were not discussed in the literature review. Both are abstract; although the report is clear about their measurement, S.J. still is unclear about why they were included and why the author decided to add a more qualitative piece to the end of this questionnaire.

S.J. now returns to the sample section to try to answer "To what types of patients do these research conclusions apply?" This section answers her question relatively clearly. S.J. finds that a convenience sample was used. She knows that such a sample opens the door to several potential threats to the validity of the study. She finds a clear description of the type of nursing program and students from which the sample was taken, giving her a good idea about both the strengths and the limits associated with those who participated. S.J. finds that the sample is small for a descriptive study. She notes that some effort was made to ensure the confidentiality of the students as subjects; however, there is no mention of informed consent. The sentence indicating that subjects were told that the questionnaire was part of efforts to plan future programs suggests that students were, in fact, not fully informed of the purpose of the study, which concerns S.J. She believes that she has a clear answer to the question about who was in the study, but she also has some serious reservations about the ethics of this study.

The fourth question that S.J. wants to answer is "Why did the author reach the conclusions—what was actually found?" Reading the results section, she finds univariate statistics telling her the characteristics of the sample, which are also the variables included in the study. The variables in the analysis are the same as those discussed in the measures section, so a logical fit exists between these two sections. The report clearly tells S.J. the students' choices for fields of practice. The report then indicates that the nine fields identified in the table were categorized as either acute or nonacute; however, the report does not tell S.J. which fields were in each category. Although intensive care is obviously acute, she wonders if the author counted obstetrics as acute or nonacute, given that women often deliver and go home the same day. S.J. understands from the results that despite a small sample, which decreases the chance of statistically significant findings, there were differences in age and health rating that would have occurred fewer than 5% of the time by chance alone. Also, S.J. knows that regression means the author examined how a combination of more than two variables explained choice of acute and nonacute setting.

The results section starts with analysis that S.J. clearly recognizes as reflecting a quantitative approach to knowledge development. When the report starts to discuss "subjective findings," however, she notes language that reflects a qualitative approach. The report discusses themes and gives some specific examples derived from students' answers to the open question about their experiences. S.J. realizes that this study used a mixed methods approach, although this never was stated explicitly.

Finally, S.J. reads the discussion section considering the question "What is the answer to the research question—what did the study conclude?" She finds that the summary of findings is clear. The report provides some interpretation or debate about the meaning of the results, suggesting that age may relate to well-being and to type of experience, thus connecting findings that were separate before. Because no literature was at the beginning of the report, however, the author does not relate the findings to previous studies or to any existing theory. Therefore, although the ideas suggested in the discussion interest S.J., she realizes that they must be considered as informed speculation. She concludes that there is some limited evidence that older students particularly may be more likely to choose nonacute settings for practice after graduation than younger students. She also concludes that health self-rating may be a relevant factor in setting choice. S.J. understands, however, that this report has several limitations, and, as best as she can tell, the study itself had several limitations as well. Therefore, she concludes that she would not make any recommendations based on the results except that further research should be done.

S.J. has been able to read and understand this fictional example of a research report and to trust her interpretation of the study using the five questions that organized this text. As she answered these questions, she kept a critically open and questioning mind, looking for both strengths and weaknesses that might be important in her decision about whether and how to use the study in the real world.

Reading and understanding research can be a positive and exciting challenge. The reality is that research, especially single research studies, almost never provides absolute and complete answers to real clinical questions, mainly because those types of questions have no simple and absolute answers. In practice, nurses must make decisions about what to do for each patient as problems arise. Nurses do not have time to examine the research literature at the moment that they are delivering care. Nevertheless, the research literature and the theory derived from and based on it comprise the foundation for daily clinical decisions. Reading and using research in practice is the hallmark of a professional nurse. The hope is that this text has given you a good start in your journey into the professional practice of nursing.

References

Coyle, L. A., & Sokop, A. G. (1990). Innovation adoption behavior among nurses. *Nursing Research, 39,* 176–180.

French, P. (2002). What is the evidence on evidence-based nursing? An epistemological concern. *Journal of Advanced Nursing, 37*(3), 250–257.

Horsley, J., Crane, J., Crabtree, M., & Wood, D. (1983). *Using research to improve nursing practice: A guide.* New York: Grune & Statton.

Ketefian, S. (1975). Application of selected nursing research findings into nursing practice. *Nursing Research, 24,* 89–92.

Needham, I., Abderhalden, C., Halfens, R. J. G., Fischer, J. E., & Dassen, T. (2005). Non-somatic effects of patient aggression on nurses: A systematic review. *Journal of Advanced Nursing, 49*(3), 283–296.

Nightingale, F. (1859). *Notes on nursing.* London: Harrison & Sons.

Rogers, E. M. (1995). *Diffusion of innovations* (4th ed.). New York: Free Press.

Sigma Theta Tau International (STTI). (1993). *Manuscript guidelines for The Online Journal of Knowledge Synthesis for Nursing.* Retrieved August 10, 2002, from http://www.nursingsociety.org/library.

Stetler, C. B. (1994). Refinement of the Stetler/Marram model for application of research findings to practice. *Nursing Outlook, 42,* 15–25.

Titler, M. G., Kleiber, C., Steelman, V., Goode, C., Rakel, B., Barry-Walker, J., et al. (1994). Infusing research into practice to promote quality care. *Nursing Research, 43,* 307–313.

Resources

LoBiondo-Wood, G., Haber, J., & Krainovich-Miller, B. (2002). Overview of the research process. In G. LoBiondo-Wood & J. Haber (Eds.), *Nursing research: Methods, critical appraisal, and utilization* (5th ed.). St. Louis: Mosby.

Polit, D. F., & Beck, C. T. (2003). *Nursing research: Principles and methods* (7th ed.). Philadelphia: Lippincott Williams & Wilkins.

APPENDIX

A

Research Articles

The nine articles in Appendix A are discussed in various chapters throughout the text. Although an article may be mentioned in several chapters, it primarily corresponds to topics specific to one or two chapters. The following table lists the articles and the chapters in which they are discussed.

Appendix Article	Corresponding Chapter(s)
A-1. Motherhood in the Context of Maternal HIV Infection	1. Evidence-Based Nursing: Using Research in Practice 2. The Research Process: Components and Language of Research Reports
A-2. Complex Physical and Mental Health Needs of Rural Incarcerated Women	1. Evidence-Based Nursing: Using Research in Practice 2. The Research Process: Components and Language of Research Reports
A-3. Correlates of Recovery Among Older Adults After Major Abdominal Surgery	3. Discussions and Conclusions
A-4. Evolution of the Caregiving Experience in the Initial 2 Years Following Stroke	4. Descriptive Results 5. Inferential Results
A-5. Needs of Family Members of Patients with Severe Traumatic Brain Injury	6. Samples
A-6. Efficacy of an In-Home Nursing Intervention Following Short-Stay Breast Cancer Surgery	8. Data Collection Methods
A-7. Feeling Safe: The Psychosocial Needs of ICU Patients	9. Research Designs: Planning the Study
A-8. Qualitative Evaluation of a School-Based Support Group for Adolescents with an Addicted Parent	9. Research Designs: Planning the Study
A-9. Non-Somatic Effects of Patient Aggression on Nurses: A Systematic Review	10. Background and the Research Problem

Motherhood in the Context of Maternal HIV Infection

Margarete Sandelowski, Julie Barroso

Abstract: *Metasummary and metasynthesis tech-niques were used to integrate findings pertaining to motherhood in 56 reports of qualitative studies con-ducted with HIV-positive women. Motherhood in the context of maternal HIV infection entailed work directed toward the illness itself and the social conse-quences of having HIV infection in the service of two primary goals: the protection of children from HIV infection and HIV-related stigma and the preservation of a positive maternal identity. Motherhood both intensified and mitigated the negative physical and social effects of HIV infection. HIV-positive mothers engaged in a distinctive kind of maternal practice— virtual motherhood—to resist forces that disrupted their relationships with and ability to care for their children, as well as their identities as mothers.*

In the early years of its emergence as a defined and significant disease entity, HIV/AIDS was depicted as a disease affecting largely gay White men. Women in HIV-related research were portrayed as either care-givers of others having the disease or as carriers of the disease to others (Bova, 2000; Cohan & Atwood, 1994; Treichler & Warren, 1998). Yet largely motivated by rising rates of HIV infection in women (Campbell, 1990; Centers for Disease Control, 2003), recognition of the extent to which ignoring or distorting women's unique circumstances contributed to their illness and death, and a desire to give voice to a typically margin-alized group of women, a spate of qualitative studies were conducted to explore women's own experiences of the illness. In this article we present an integration of one set of findings from these studies in a topical domain of great significance to women's health and to HIV-positive and other chronically ill women themselves: motherhood.[1] Motherhood is a uniquely female experience that we surmised would permit us to draw conclusions about the unique, shared, and gendered (McMahon, 1995) aspects of HIV infection in women. Although motherhood and chronic illness each separately have been important topics of inquiry in health-related research, relatively few studies have been specifically directed toward examining mother-hood in the context of maternal chronic illness (Radtke & Van Mens-Verhulst, 2001; Thorne, 1990).

Research in Nursing & Health, 2003, Volume 26, pages 470-482.
Published online in Wiley InterScience (www.interscience.wiley.com)

METHOD

The research synthesis reported here was produced in the course of an ongoing methodological project to develop techniques to integrate the findings of qualitative studies. The set of studies we used to conduct this project included all qualitative studies conducted solely with women living with HIV infection in the United States of any race, ethnicity, nationality, or class. The first qualitative study of these women was published in 1991. The total sample consists of 114 reports of research studies, including 79 published reports (75 journal articles, two books, one book chapter, and one technical report) and 35 unpublished reports (4 master's theses and 31 doctoral dissertations). These works were retrieved between June 1, 2000 (when the project began), and December 31, 2002 (the end of the second phase of the project).[2]

---

[1]This article is the companion to "Toward a metasynthesis of qualitative findings on motherhood in HIV-positive women," published in *Research in Nursing & Health* and referred to in the text and in the reference list that follows as Sandelowski & Barroso (2003c). The previously published article focused on method, or the description, clarification, and illustration of techniques to create metasyntheses of qualitative research findings. This article focuses on results, or the metasynthesis itself. We split method from results because the primary result of the research project referred to in the text is method, and because space restrictions in most health science journals preclude extended presentations of both method and result. Accordingly, portions of the results used to illustrate the techniques featured in the method paper overlap with portions of the results featured in this paper. We have inserted quotations around material duplicated verbatim. To avoid further duplication, only a highly abbreviated description of method is presented in this article. In addition, the method article was written at the end of the first phase of our research project, when the total bibliographic sample size was 99, and the number of reports with motherhood findings was 45. This article was written after the end of the second phase of the project, when the final sample had grown to 114, and the final number of reports with motherhood findings had grown to 56. The addition of these references did not alter our interpretation of motherhood, but it did contribute to a more parsimonious rendering of findings.

[2]Further details concerning search procedures and inclusion criteria may be found in Barroso et al. (2003).

All the published articles as well as the sample characteristics and findings from the included books, theses, and dissertations were scanned into computer files (these latter works were too long to make scanning all their contents an efficient enterprise). The entire content of every report was then analyzed using a 14-item reading guide developed in the course of this study (Sandelowski & Barroso, 2002) that directs reviewers to extract information systematically about the background to, structure of, and findings of a study.

Focus on Motherhood

Of the 114 reports in the bibliographic sample, 56 contained motherhood findings, and these comprised the primary data for this report. Motherhood finding was defined as any data-based interpretation researchers offered pertaining to the decision to become a mother and the experiences of being a mother to minor children. Included in these 56 reports are 36 published and 20 unpublished works. As annotated in the reference list, in 35 of the 56 reports, one research project generated one report. But for 21 of these reports, one project generated at least two reports (usually a dissertation and one published article from that dissertation) and as many as four reports, with the findings contained in each report either unique to it or repeated in one or more other reports from the same parent research project. In the analyses of findings described later, duplicate findings were counted only once.

The primary authors' disciplinary affiliations (not counting multiple reports by the same authors and one report for which we could not discern affiliation) included nursing (n = 20), social work (n = 7), psychology (n = 7), public health (n = 4), behavioral medicine or science (n = 2), counseling (n = 1), education (n = 1), family and child development (n = 1), and sociology (n = 1). In 23 of the 56 research reports, the stated research purpose was specifically focused on motherhood. In the remaining 33 reports, motherhood findings appeared in the context of other stated research purposes, most notably, to describe the lived experience of women with HIV infection.

Sample sizes ranged from 3 to 159, with a total sample size across reports of 1,141, a mean sample size of 25, a median sample size of 15.5, and a modal sample size of 12 (counting reports with identical samples only once or the largest *n* in reports with overlapping samples). All the women were of reproductive age, and most were mothers or were pregnant. Of the women who participated in these studies 75% were from minority groups, with African-American women comprising 55% of the total sample of women across all studies.[3]

None of the studies featured in these reports was explicitly located in any theoretical orientation toward motherhood, and 26 reports contained no explicit reference at all to any theoretical orientation. Of the 30 reports with explicit theoretical orientations, seven referred to feminism or gender, and 23 referred to such nongender theoretical orientations as stigma and self-care. The stated methodology in 10 of the 56 reports was grounded theory; in nine reports, phenomenology or Heideggerian hermeneutics; in five reports, qualitative or naturalistic; in four reports, feminism or womanism; in three reports, narrative or discourse; and in one report ethnography. No methodology was specified in the remaining 24 reports.

Evaluation of Reports

Instead of excluding reports for reasons of quality, we conducted a posteriori analyses (Cooper, 1998) of the findings that were specifically directed toward determining how individual reports and reports stratified by type of finding (Sandelowski & Barroso, 2003a) contributed to the synthesis of the findings we produced. For example, by calculating how frequently findings occurred and noting in what reports they appeared, we could determine whether including unpublished reports made a difference to the strength of any finding. We found that whether we included all reports or only those published, the same seven findings (shown in Table 1) remained strongest, albeit with same variation in their order. We excluded reports when, as was the case in one dissertation, violations of the rights of human subjects had occurred in the course of the study and when reports contained no findings (or synthesis of data by researchers; Sandelowski & Barroso, 2003a). We excluded selected findings in included reports when they were not supported by data.

Metasummary and Metasynthesis

Both qualitative metasummary and metasynthesis techniques (Sandelowski & Barroso, 2003b,c) were used to lay the descriptive and conceptual foundation for the research integration that follows. The use of metasummary techniques (i.e., data extraction, data abstraction, and calculation of frequency effect sizes) resulted in a list of 67 statements representing a comprehensive empirical inventory of the findings across all 56 reports. The seven findings with the greatest frequency effect sizes are shown in Table 1. The use of metasynthesis techniques (i.e., taxonomic analysis, constant comparison, reciprocal translation and synthesis of in vivo concepts, and the use of imported concepts) resulted in a comprehensive conceptual inventory of the findings across all 56 reports[4] and in the conceptual renderings and translation and synthesis of segments of these findings, which are shown in Figures 1-4.

RESULTS

Motherhood for HIV-positive women entailed "love, toil, and trouble" (Brush, 1996). When they were contemplating whether to conceive or whether to continue or terminate a pregnancy, the toil of HIV-positive women entailed considering the likelihood they would transmit HIV infection to their children and justifying why they should have children. As mothers, they performed the labor of mothering. Their "mother troubles" (Hanigsberg & Ruddick, 1999) involved resolving the contradictions posed by HIV infection and motherhood.

Mother Work in the Context of Maternal HIV Infection

As shown in Figure 1, motherhood entailed work directed toward the illness itself and the social consequences of having HIV infection in the service of two primary goals: the protection of children (from contracting HIV infection and from HIV-related stigma) and the preservation of a positive maternal identity. Toward these ends, HIV-positive mothers engaged in: (a) surveillance and safety work to prevent the spread of HIV infection and HIV-related

---

[3]Further details on the women who participated in these studies may be found in Barroso & Sandelowski (2003).

[4]The full table of abstracted findings with frequency effect size calculations, and the full taxonomy are available from the first author by request.

TABLE A1-1

Motherhood Findings with Frequency Effect Sizes ≥ 20%

Findings	Effect Sizes
Mothers struggled with whether to disclose their HIV status to their children, worried about the effects of disclosure on child and maternal welfare and the mother-child relations, and engaged in strategies to disclose or to delay or avoid disclosing their HIV status to their children (Andrews et al., 1993; Armstrong, 1996; Arnold, 1994; Barnes et al., 1997; Bennett, 1997; Black & Miles, 2002; Caba, 1998; Ciambrone, 1999, 2002; Faithfull, 1992, 1997; Goggin et al., 2001; Gosling, 1995; Hackl et al., 1997; Hendrixson, 1996; Ingram, 1996; Ingram & Hutchinson, 1996b; 2000; Loriz-Lim, 1995; Marcenko & Samost, 1999; Moneyham et al., 1996; Palyo, 1995; Regan-Kubinski & Sharts-Hopko, 1995; Ross, 1994; Santacroce et al., 2002; Schrimshaw & Siegel, 2002; Semple et al., 1993; Smith & Russell, 1997; Tangenberg, 1998; Valdez, 1999, 2001; Walker, 1996, 1998; Winstead et al., 2002; Wright, 1995).	57%
Mothers had concerns over child care and/or placement, especially what would happen as their disease worsened and/or after their death (Andrews et al., 1993; Armstrong, 1996; Bonifas, 1994; Caba, 1998; Ciambrone, 1999; Faithfull, 1992, 1997; Frey, 1993; Goggin et al., 2001; Gosling, 1995; Hackl et al., 1997; Hendrixon 1996; Ingram, 1996; Ingram & Hutchinson, 1999a; Litwak et al., 1995; Loriz-Lim, 1995; Marcenko & Samost, 1999; Palyo, 1995; Regan-Kubinski & Sharts-Hopko, N., 1995; Semple et al., 1993; Valdez, 1999, 2001; Van Loon, 1996, 2000; Walker, 1996, 1998; Winstead et al., 2002; Wright, 1995).	44%
Children were the main reasons to live, fight, get off drugs, care for oneself, and avoid risky behaviors (Andrews et al., 1993; Armstrong, 1996; Bennett, 1997; Bonifas, 1994; Bunting & Seaton, 1999; Caba, 1998; Cameron, 2001; Ciambrone, 1999, 2002; Faithfull, 1992; Goggin et al., 2001; Gosling, 1995; Hutchison & Kurth, 1991; Ingram, 1996; Ingram & Hutchinson, 1999a, 2000; Kass & Faden, 1996; Loriz-Lim, 1995; Regan-Kubinski & Sharts-Hopko, 1995; Sankar et al., 2002; Valdez, 1999, 2001; Van Loon, 1996, 2000; Walker, 1996, 1998; Wesley et al., 2000).	40%
Whether their children were in or out of their care or custody, being a mother was central to women's lives: a source of self-esteem, strength, normalcy, inspiration, pride, hope, joy, sense of well-being, and sense of self as a whole woman (Andrews et al., 1993; Caba, 1998; Ciambrone, 1999, 2002; Faithfull, 1992; Goggin et al., 2001; Hutchison & Kurth, 1991; Kass et al., 1996, 2000; Walker, 1996, 1998; Wesley et al., 2000).	26%
Women had varying knowledge, concerns about, and interpretations of, and used various strategies to address, the risk of HIV transmission to fetuses and children (Bonifas, 1994; Ciambrone, 1999; Faithfull, 1992, 1997; Frey, 1993; Hackl et al., 1997; Ingram, 1996; Ingram & Hutchinson, 2000; Napravnik et al., 2000; Semple et al., 1993; Smith & Russell, 1997; Sowell & Misener, 1997; Tangenberg, 1998; Walker, 1996, 1998).	22%
Mothers worried about the negative impact of maternal HIV (the illness itself and/or its stigma) on their children, including their negative reactions to it and others' negative reactions to their children (Andrews et al., 1993; Armstrong, 1996; Barnes et al., 1997; Ciambrone, 1999, 2002; Hackl et al., 1997; Ingram, 1996; Ingram & Hutchinson, 1999b, 2000; Marcenko & Samost, 1999; Santacroce et al., 2002; Semple et al., 1993; Van Loon, 1996, 2000; Walker, 1996, 1998).	21%
Both HIV-related and -unrelated factors were involved in women's decisions to conceive, continue or terminate pregnancies, with the same or different morality, desires, risk assessments, or circumstances leading to the same or different decisions (Armstrong, 1996; Bonifas, 1994; Faithfull, 1992; Frey 1993; Hutchison & Kurth, 1991; Ingram, 1996; Ingram & Hutchinson, 2000; Kass & Faden, 1996; Siegel & Scrimshaw, 2001; Sowell & Misener, 1997; Walker, 1996, 1998; Wesley et al., 2000).	20%

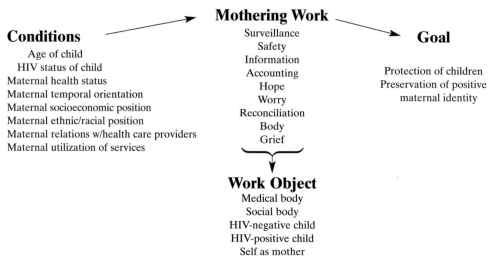

FIGURE A1-1 • Mothering work in the context of maternal HIV infection.

stigma to their children; (b) information work to make decisions and take action concerning themselves and their children; (c) accounting work to calculate the benefits and risks of disclosing their own and their children's HIV status to children and others, of adhering to antiretroviral therapy, and of utilizing health care services; (d) hope and worry work concerning their children's futures; (e) reconciliation, legacy, and redefinition work to establish, maintain, and preserve positive mother-child relations and maternal identity; (f) body work to manage the physical aspects of HIV infection and child care; and (g) grief work to anticipate and manage the death of HIV-positive children.

The work of mothering was directed toward five discrete work objects: (a) the medical body (or the physical manifestations and demands of HIV infection); (b) the social body (or the stigma associated with HIV infection); (c) the HIV-negative child; (d) the HIV-positive child; and (e) the maternal self. Factors that influenced maternal work included the age and HIV status of the child; the health status, ethnic/racial and socioeconomic position, and temporal orientation of the mother; and the mother's relations with health care providers. For example, mothers deemed their children either too young or old enough to learn of the HIV status of their mother. Whereas the central dilemmas for mothers of HIV-positive children involved the health and future of

those children, the central dilemma for mothers of HIV-negative children involved role reversal, that is, the worry or expectation that these children would assume adult roles (caring for their mothers or their HIV-positive siblings, performing household tasks, or serving as the lone source of emotional support). The preservation of their identity as good mothers was easier when they were not ill and did not appear to be so. HIV-positive mothers often focused their efforts on present concerns to avoid thinking of the future and their own deaths, even as they prepared for it. Minority and socioeconomically disadvantaged HIV-positive mothers were already marginalized—prior to infection with HIV—by virtue of their social positions. In addition, positive relations with health care providers tended to facilitate the use of services and treatments, while negative relations impeded their use.

Mother Troubles: Paradoxes of Motherhood in the Context of Maternal HIV Infection

As shown in Table 1, the research findings with the strongest presence encompassed HIV-positive mothers' struggles concerning disclosure of their HIV status to their children, their concerns over child care and child placement as their disease worsened or after their deaths, and the centrality of children and motherhood to their health, lives, and identities as women.

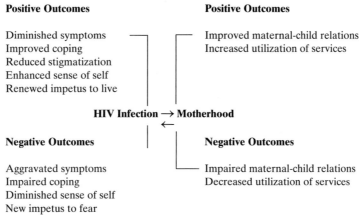

Positive Outcomes

Diminished symptoms
Improved coping
Reduced stigmatization
Enhanced sense of self
Renewed impetus to live

Positive Outcomes

Improved maternal-child relations
Increased utilization of services

HIV Infection → Motherhood
←

Negative Outcomes

Aggravated symptoms
Impaired coping
Diminished sense of self
New impetus to fear

Negative Outcomes

Impaired maternal-child relations
Decreased utilization of services

FIGURE A1-2 • Paradoxical mother-child and illness outcomes in the context of maternal HIV infection.

For the HIV-positive women who participated in the studies reviewed, the physical, emotional, and cognitive demands of caring for children were added to the physical, emotional, and cognitive demands of living with and fighting the mortal and stigmatizing effects of HIV infection. Motherhood aggravated the symptoms of the infection and intensified the stigmatization associated with it because HIV-infected mothers were seen to place "innocent" children at risk.

Moreover, by virtue of being mothers, being women with the ability to bear children, and being persons who often bore the sole responsibility for rearing children, these HIV-positive women were compelled to make both culturally loaded and morally charged decisions concerning disclosure of HIV, the care and custody of children, reproduction, the utilization of health care and social services, and the use of antiretroviral drugs in pregnancy. Indeed, one of the most important kinds of mother work in which they engaged was the accounting work of weighing the risks and benefits of the courses of action available to them.

Yet the findings in approximately half of the reports reviewed indicate that motherhood also had a highly salutary effect on HIV-positive women, providing them with social support, self-esteem, and most important, a reason to live and to fight HIV infection. Motherhood made it easier for women to cope with the physical manifestations of the disease and with the stigma associated with it. The findings in four reports featured the positive impact that having HIV infection had on mother-

hood, especially in women who had previously abused drugs, as it served as an impetus to be better mothers and to repair previously impaired relations with children.

Accordingly, the findings taken as a whole suggest, as illustrated in Figure 2, the dual and even paradoxical effects of motherhood in the context of maternal HIV infection. As motherhood added to the physical, emotional, and social burdens of HIV infection for women, it also reduced their load. The diagnosis of HIV infection—a mortal threat—often coincided with the diagnosis of pregnancy, an affirmation of life. Although often it was a pregnancy diagnosis that was the impetus for the testing for and subsequent diagnosis of HIV infection, making it possible for the women to be treated in a timely and appropriate fashion, the HIV diagnosis exposed women to stigmatization. Having children was a source of hope and esteem for women, but it was also believed to constitute a risk of disclosure, as the mothers often perceived children as unable to keep secrets. HIV infection, in turn, both enhanced women's motivation and impaired their capacity to be good mothers and both improved and impaired mother-child relations.

The duality of motherhood in the context of maternal HIV infection appeared to reside not only in the paradoxical effects that motherhood had on HIV infection and vice versa, but also in the contradictory effects of the same maternal action, and the common effects of opposing actions. For example, as illustrated in Figure 3, what complicated HIV-positive mothers' accounting work was that one action

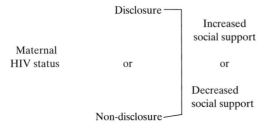

FIGURE A1-3 • Contrary decisions and contradictory outcomes.

(e.g., disclosing HIV status) could lead to either increased or decreased social support. Similarly, two contrary actions (e.g., disclosing and not disclosing HIV status) could result in the same outcome: either receiving or not receiving needed support.

Also contributing to the paradox of motherhood in the context of maternal HIV infection was that it simultaneously exemplified both normality and deviance. Although motherhood is typically the fulfillment of a cultural norm, for the HIV-positive women studied, it was deemed a deviant act that required justification. The stigmatizing effects of HIV infection were intensified because of the automatic association of HIV-positive women with drug use, promiscuity, and prostitution and because of the risk of transmission of the disease to "innocent" children. Whereas motherhood usually confers normality on women (as childlessness confers abnormality), motherhood exaggerated the deviant status of the HIV-positive women studied, placing them in a cultural "double bind" (Ingram, 1996; Ingram & Hutchinson, 2000).

Virtual Motherhood: A Discursive Countermove

To counter the mortal and social threats of HIV infection and the contradictions of Western motherhood embodied in being an HIV-positive mother, the HIV-positive mothers studied engaged in a distinctive kind of maternal practice (Ruddick, 1980)—virtual motherhood—aimed at both the preservation of children's lives and self-preservation as good mothers. As depicted in Figure 4, virtual motherhood is an integration of Goffman's (1963, p. 19) concept of "virtual identity" and the in vivo concepts of "eternal motherhood" (Barnes, Taylor-Brown, & Wiener, 1997), "defensive motherhood" (Ingram, 1996; Ingram & Hutchinson, 1999a, 2000), "la protectora," or protec-

tive motherhood (Van Loon, 2000), and "redefining treatment" (Santacroce, Deatrick, & Ledlie, 2002).[5]

Virtual motherhood encompasses both embodied and transcendent maternal practices focused on self-care and child care. Motherhood was a highly embodied practice when these mothers worked to stay alive and well for their children and to protect their children against the mortal and social threat that HIV infection posed. Yet the inability to meet the physical requirement of motherhood (in large part, because of the physical demands of the infection itself) caused HIV-positive mothers to conceive of motherhood as a disembodied and transcendent practice. Virtual motherhood was a discursive response to all the circumstances in which the HIV-positive mothers studied were, or anticipated being, physically incapacitated or separated from their children by illness, care and custody arrangements, imprisonment, or death. To bypass the physical requirements of motherhood, the HIV-positive mothers recast it as demanding oversight of their children, rather than necessarily demanding direct physical contact with them. Motherhood was defined not only as watching children (a direct embodied encounter) but also, in a more disembodied vein, as watching out for them.

In the physical absence of the mother, motherhood can only be accomplished "in the virtual sense: by proxy, remotely, or at a distance" (Sandelowski & Barroso, 2003c, p. 166). In the social presence of stigma, HIV-positive mothers' identities *as mothers* remain virtual as long as they are primarily viewed as diseased women. Accordingly, women sought to create mementos and memories to ensure that their children would forever remember them as present, healthy, and good. Even if not present in the flesh, they could always be present in the minds and hearts of their children. As we previously concluded (Sandelowski & Barroso 2003c, p. 166), virtual motherhood signifies visions of a "life and an afterlife" able to "transcend the mortal body and any presumed sins of the flesh," in which "children are never motherless, mothers are never childless, and mothers are always good." In virtual motherhood HIV-positive women found both "a reason to live and a way to live forever" (p. 166).

---

[5]Each of these concepts is fully described in Table 3 and on p. 166 in Sandelowski & Barroso (2003c).

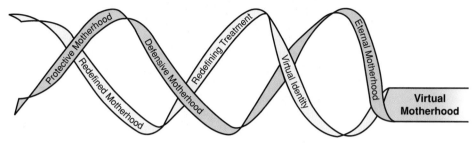

FIGURE A1-4 • Reciprocal translation and synthesis of key concepts.

Shared and Distinctive Features of Motherhood in the Context of Maternal HIV Infection

Motherhood was central to the identities and lives of HIV-positive women who participated in the studies reviewed, just as it is to most women who are mothers (McMahon, 1995). As we noted previously (Sandelowski & Barroso, 2003c, p. 162), the HIV-positive women studied were like most women and mothers "in their desire for motherhood, in the opportunities and constraints they perceived as integral to motherhood, and in the work they performed as mothers." As we concluded, "HIV infection posed a unique mortal and social threat to these mothers," but their experiences of motherhood clarified and "even dramatized what motherhood typically means and entails for any woman" (p. 162).

Like middle- and working-class mothers, the HIV-positive mothers studied loved their children, worked to protect their lives and to preserve their own capacities and identities as mothers, and found in motherhood an opportunity for self-transformation (i.e., to be better mothers and better persons; McMahon, 1995). Like motherhood for women who have been battered or are addicted to drugs, motherhood for the HIV-positive woman was a source of strength and esteem, an anchor in a turbulent life, and a refuge from and buffer against physical and social adversity (Hardesty & Black, 1999; Irwin, Thorne, & Varcoe, 2002). Like motherhood for battered women and women with other chronic illnesses and physical disabilities, however, motherhood for HIV-positive women entailed some impairment of their ability to perform the physical acts of motherhood and meant reliance on their children for instrumental and emotional support (Grue & Laerum, 2002; Thorne, 1990).

Yet unlike other chronic illnesses mothers may have, including potentially mortal and genetically transmissible ones, HIV often garners more condemnation than sympathy. Although HIV-positive women share with HIV-positive men the effects of having a stigmatizing illness (Barroso & Powell-Cope, 2000), paradoxically, in women these effects appear both intensified and diminished by motherhood. Unlike the primarily gay White men in the Barroso and Powell-Cope study, who found the meaning of their illness in and by themselves, the primarily heterosexual minority women participating in the studies reviewed here found that meaning in motherhood and caring for their children.

But motherhood itself positioned these women precariously between life as a normal woman and life as a deviant one. Referring to other studies of motherhood (Hays, 1996; McMahon, 1995; Thurer, 1994; Weingarten, Surrey, Coll, & Watkins, 1998), we concluded previously (Sandelowski & Barroso, 2003c, p. 167) that motherhood in the context of maternal HIV infection "exemplifies the cultural contradictions inherent in Western motherhood, whereby motherhood is both redeeming and damning." Like other marginalized mothers (e.g., those who are in prison, on welfare, or homeless), these HIV-positive women mothered against the odds and could not escape the prevalent idea that they were bad mothers and bad women for even desiring motherhood (Coll, Surrey, & Weingarten, 1998).

Like the mothers on crack cocaine portrayed by Kearney, Murphy, & Rosenbaum (1994) and the addicted mothers described by Hardesty and Black (1999), the HIV-positive mothers in the studies reviewed here sought to maintain their standards of mothering and to avoid becoming or being viewed as bad mothers. The Kerney et al. (1994) explanation of "defensive compensation" (p. 355) as the central process involved in "mothering on crack" shares with virtual motherhood women's desire not only to mother their children well, but also to redefine mothering in ways that preserve their identities as good mothers. For the mothers on crack cocaine, the relinquishing of children was considered a form of good mothering. In the same way, for the HIV-positive mothers, good mothering also was not dependent on being in close physical proximity to their children or providing them with direct care. For the addicted mothers in the Hardesty and Black study and the HIV-positive mothers in the studies reviewed, just thinking about their children and striving to become good mothers could be construed as good mothering. Although these mothers had sometimes relinquished the care of their children to others, they had not relinquished their claim to motherhood.

Like the physically disabled mothers in the Grue & Laerum (2002) study, the HIV-positive mothers studied found that the discourses of motherhood and of HIV infection were incompatible, the former a discourse of social approbation and inclusion and the latter a discourse of social condemnation and exclusion. Both physically disabled and HIV-positive mothers were not necessarily viewed or treated as mothers, but rather as disabled or infected women. Yet both these groups of mothers used the discourse of motherhood to negotiate their identities—to draw attention away from their "deviant" conditions toward themselves as mothers. Both of these groups of mothers worked hard to "pass" as mothers (Grue & Laerum, 2002, p. 678).

DISCUSSION

This integration of qualitative findings indicates that motherhood in the context of maternal HIV infection is an experience of contradiction, extraordinary by its very ordinariness and ordinary because of the extraordinary efforts women make (Cooey, 1999). Motherhood both intensifies and buffers the negative effects of HIV infection, and HIV infection both enhances and impairs maternal identity and mother-child relations. HIV-positive mothers engage in the embodied and discursive practices of virtual motherhood to resolve these contradictions.

The motherhood depicted in the studies reviewed here was performed in the context not only of maternal HIV infection but also of low material resources, minority status, and sometimes, drug abuse, all of which are themselves stigmatizing conditions.

This motherhood was also performed mostly before the advent and use of new drug therapies that have transformed HIV infection in the United States from a fatal to a chronic illness. Most of the studies reviewed were conducted before these new therapies could make their way into common medical practice or before their effects could make their way into the lives of these women and therefore the findings from these studies. As a response to the immediate mortal threat HIV infection once posed, virtual motherhood as a transcendent practice arguably may no longer be as relevant a concept for contemporary practice. Yet maintaining the relevance of the concept is the social threat HIV infection still poses, and marginalized women frequently have diminished access to the best health care. Virtual motherhood therefore also may embrace and have relevance for other situations in which motherhood must be practiced "distally" (Malone, 2003) because mothers cannot be physically or otherwise *there* for their children in ways typically associated with culturally prescribed mothering practices (Lupton & Fenwick, 2001). Virtual motherhood is a form of normalization (Joachim & Acorn, 2000) and of resistance (Parker & Aggleton, 2003) to forces (i.e., disease and stigmatization) that disrupt mothers' relations with and their ability to care for their children, undermine their identities as mothers, and contest their status as good mothers.

A Caveat

An important caveat to the metasynthesis presented here is that any synthesis of research findings is a synthesist's (or a team of synthesists') construction of researchers' constructions of the data they obtained from research participants, which are themselves constructed within the research encounter. The best access anyone has to experience-as-lived is via experience-as-told, and qualitative metasyntheses are at least three times removed from the lived experiences they are meant to faithfully represent. Accordingly, the research synthesis presented here can be read as an empirically grounded (albeit experientially distant) interpretation of the lived experiences of the women who participated in the studies reviewed. Or, in a more deconstructive vein, it can be read as a narrative or discursive product that reveals more about ourselves and the selves of the researchers (with whom we share disciplinary and methodological values and norms) whose work we reviewed than any truth about the lived experience of HIV-positive women.

Indeed, an alternative to a strictly "vertical reading" (Kvale, 1995, p. 28) of this metasynthesis is a narrative or discursive one, whereby the metasynthesis is not viewed as a data-based interpretation but rather as a historically and culturally contingent social product of a unique encounter between two readers (us) and the texts (56 reports) we reviewed (Sandelowski & Barroso, 2002). These texts in turn are viewed as historically and culturally contingent products of an equally irreplicable and inescapably social interaction among multiple participant and researcher selves (Collins, 1998). For example, competing with a conventionally data-oriented view of research participants as informants or reporters are views of them as identity and impression managers, narrative strategists, and producers and objects of discourse (Grue & Laerum, 2002; Riessman, 1990; Sandelowski, 2002). Competing with the data-oriented view of researchers and synthesists as interpreters and communicators of findings are views of them as members of narrative or discourse communities, purveying collective stories, disciplinary values, methodological norms, and political agendas (Thorne et al., 2002).

A thematic element across the reports we reviewed was researchers' desire to offset negative images of HIV-positive women and to give voice to women they viewed as voiceless. As motherhood is arguably integral to the identity of every woman (whether or not she is or desires to be a mother; McMahon, 1996), talking about motherhood can be seen as a vehicle of communication for women that can cross any race, class, or other dividing line that might impede communication among them. The research participants were women in largely marginalized social positions; the researchers were mostly women in mainstream positions. The women participants wanted to offset negative images of HIV-positive women and to present themselves in a positive light. Indeed, the importance of motherhood to these women was neither solely attributable to its importance to the researchers, whose purpose was to study motherhood, nor to most of the women in the 114 reports comprising the total bibliographic sample

being pregnant and/or mothers. Of the 56 qualitative reports of HIV-positive women with mothering findings, 33 did not have the study of motherhood as their research purpose at all. It was the women participants themselves who made motherhood salient, protecting the "spoiled identities" (Goffman, 1963) that emphasized their HIV status over their status as mothers. Those who conducted the reviewed studies, who primarily were nurses (and other caregiving professionals), also wanted to offset the negative stereotypes of HIV-positive women and to present themselves as good listeners and compassionate interpreters. And as we ourselves are women and nurses, we, in turn, wanted to present ourselves as competent interpreters and also to produce a metasynthesis that would not contribute to the further stigmatization of HIV-positive women. Motherhood talk allowed us all to achieve our goals (Grue & Laerum, 2002).

Accordingly, it is with caution that we offer this research integration as a foundation for evidence-based programs of care for HIV-positive women. Such programs would be based on the recognition of motherhood as (a) a cultural and identity position (Radtke & Van Mens-Verhulst, 2001) that like gender, race, and class, shapes women's experiences of illness in frequently contradictory ways; (b) a social and discursive practice; (c) a buffer against the sequelae of disease; and (d) a protest against stigmatization. Such programs of care would be directed toward acknowledging the centrality of motherhood—whether conceived empirically or discursively—to the very physical and social survival of HIV-positive women and toward maximizing the benefits and minimizing the burdens of motherhood both for HIV-positive women and for their children.

References

*References marked with an asterisk indicate reports included in the bibliographic sample of the metasynthesis project with findings pertaining to motherhood. References marked with a superscript 1, 2, or 5–7 are identical samples; those marked with a superscript 3 are identical overlapping samples (samples of 18 in samples of 20); those marked with a superscript 4 are identical samples, but with different investigators; those marked with a superscript 8 are identical overlapping samples (sample of 11 in a sample of 12); and those marked with a superscript 9 are identical reports counted as one report.

*Andrews, S., Williams, A. B., & Neil, K. (1993). The mother-child relationship in the HIV-1 positive family. *Image: Journal of Nursing Scholarship, 25,* 193–198.

*Armstrong, V. A. (1996). *The experience of the HIV-positive mother with an HIV-positive child: A descriptive study.* Unpublished doctoral dissertation, University of California at San Francisco.

*Arnold, M. A. (1994). *Women with HIV disease: Psychosocial issues.* Unpublished doctoral dissertation, Massachusetts School of Professional Psychology, Boston.

Atkinson, P. & Silverman, D. (1997). Kundera's immortality: The interview society and the invention of the self. *Qualitative Inquiry, 3,* 304–325.

*Barnes, D. B., Taylor-Brown, S., & Wiener, L. (1997). "I didn't leave y'all on purpose": HIV-infected mothers' videotaped legacies for their children. *Qualitative Sociology, 20,* 7–32.

Barroso, J., Gollop, C. J., Sandelowski, M., Meynell, J., Pearce, P. F., & Collins, L. J. (2003). The challenges of searching for and retrieving qualitative studies. *Western Journal of Nursing Research, 25,* 153–178.

Barroso, J. & Powell-Cope, G. M. (2000). Metasynthesis of qualitative research on living with HIV infection. *Qualitative Health Research, 120,* 340–353.

Barroso, J. & Sandelowski, M. (2003). Sample reporting in qualitative studies of women with HIV infection. *Field Methods, 15,* 386–404.

*Bennett, M. J. (1997). *Stigmatization experiences of HIV infected women: A focused ethnography.* Unpublished doctoral dissertation, Louisiana State University Medical Center, New Orleans.

*Black, B. P. & Miles, M. S. (2002). Calculating the risks and benefits of disclosure in African American women who have HIV. *JOGNN: Journal of Obstetric, Gynecologic, & Neonatal Nursing, 31,* 688–697.

*Bonifas, J. M. (1994). *The psychologic experience of women living with HIV/AIDS: A phenomenological study.* Unpublished doctoral dissertation, Union Institute, Union Graduate School, Cincinnati, OH.

Bova, C. (2000). Women with HIV infection: The three waves of scientific inquiry. *Journal of the Association of Nursing in AIDS Care, 11(5),* 19–28.

Brush, L. D. (1996). Love, toil, and trouble: Motherhood and feminist politics [review essay]. *Signs: Journal of Women in Culture and Society, 21,* 429–454.

*Bunting, S. M. & Seaton, R. (1999). Health care participation of perinatal women with HIV: What helps and what gets in the way? *Health Care for Women International, 20,* 563–578.

*Caba, G. (1998). *The struggle for meaning in the lives of HIV+ women.* Unpublished doctoral dissertation, University of Toledo, OH.

*Cameron, A. E. (2001). *Narrative voice and countering silence. Women talk about life with AIDS.* Unpublished doctoral dissertation, City University of New York.

Campbell, C. A. (1990). Women and AIDS. *Social Science & Medicine, 30,* 407–415.

Centers for Disease Control, HIV/AIDS Surveillance Report. Retrieved March 12, 2003, from http://www.cdc.gov/hiv/stats/hasr1302.pdf

*Ciambrone, D. A. (1999). *Mending fractured selves: Biographical disruption among women with HIV infection.* Unpublished doctoral dissertation, Brown University, Providence, RI.[1]

*Ciambrone, D. A. (2001). Illness and other assaults on self: The relative impact of HIV/AIDS on women's lives. *Sociology of Health & Illness, 23,* 517–540.[1]

*Ciambrone, D. A. (2002). Informal networks among women with HIV/AIDS: Present support and future prospects. *Qualitative Health Research, 12,* 876–896.[1]

Cohan, N. & Atwood, J. D. (1994). Women and AIDS: The social constructions of gender and disease. *Family Systems Medicine, 12(1),* 5–20.

Coll, C. O., Surrey, J. L., & Weingarten, K. (Eds.). (1998). *Mothering against the odds: Diverse voices of contemporary mothers.* New York: Guilford Press.

Collins, P. (1998). Negotiating selves: Reflections on unstructured interviewing. *Sociological Research Online, 3(3).* Retrieved April 14, 2003, from http://www.socresonline.org.uk/3/3/2.html

Cooey, P. M. (1999). "Ordinary mother" as oxymoron: The collusion of theology, theory, and politics in the undermining of mothers. In J. E. Hunigsberg & S. Ruddick (Eds.), *Mother troubles: Rethinking contemporary maternal dilemmas* (pp. 229-249). Boston: Beacon Press.

Cooper, H. (1998). *Synthesizing research: A guide for literature reviews* (3rd ed.). Thousand Oaks, CA: Sage.

*Faithfull, J. (1992). *HIV, reproductive decision-making, and mothering experiences.* Unpublished master's thesis, Smith College, Northampton, MA.[2]

*Faithfull, J. (1997). HIV-positive and AIDS-infected women: Challenges and difficulties of mothering. *American Journal of Orthopsychiatry, 67,* 144–151.[2]

*Frey, L. M. (1993). *The psychological and socio-political sequelae of HIV infection in women.* Unpublished doctoral dissertation, Antioch University, Keene, NH.

Goffman, E. (1963). *Stigma: Notes on the management of spoiled identity.* Englewood Cliffs, NJ: Prentice-Hall.

Goggin, K., Catley, D., Brisco, S. T., Engelson, E. S., Rabkin, J. G., & Kotler, D. P. (2001). A female perspective on living with HIV. *Health & Social Work, 26,* 80–90.

*Gosling, A. (1995). *Pain, courage, and wisdom: Stories of women living with HIV.* Unpublished doctoral dissertation, Virginia Polytechnic Institute and State University, Blacksburg.

Grue, L. & Laerum, K. T. (2002). "Doing motherhood": Some experiences of mothers with physical disabilities. *Disability & Society, 17,* 671–683.

*Hackl, K. L., Somlai, A. M., Kelly, J. A., & Kalichman, S. C. (1997). Women living with HIV/AIDS: The dual challenge of being a patient and caregiver. *Health and Social Work, 22,* 53–62.

Hanigsberg, J. E. & Ruddick, S. (1999). *Mother troubles: Rethinking contemporary maternal dilemmas.* Boston: Beacon Press.

Hardesty, M. & Black, T. (1999). Mothering through addiction: A survival strategy among Puerto Rican addicts. *Qualitative Health Research, 9,* 602–619.

Hays, S. (1996). *The cultural contradictions of motherhood.* New Haven, CT: Yale University Press.

*Hendrixon, L. L. (1996). *The psychosocial and psychosexual impact of HIV/AIDS disease on rural women: A qualitative study.* Unpublished doctoral dissertation, New York University, School of Education.

*Hutchison, M. & Kurth, A. (1991). "I need to know that I have a choice": A study of women, HIV, and reproductive decision-making. *AIDS Patient Care, 5,* 17–25.

*Ingram, D. A. (1996). *HIV-positive women: Double blinds and defensive mothering.* Unpublished doctoral dissertation, University of Florida, Gainesville, FL.[3]

*Ingram, D. & Hutchison, S. A. (1999a). Defensive mothering in HIV-positive mothers. *Qualitative Health Research, 9,* 243–258.

*Ingram, D. & Hutchinson, S. A. (1999b). HIV-positive mothers and stigma. *Health Care for Women International, 20,* 93–103.[3]

*Ingram, D. & Hutchinson, S. A. (2000). Living with chronic illness: The interface of stigma and normalization. *Canadian Journal of Nursing Research, 32(3),* 37–48.

*Irwin, L. G., Thorne, S. & Varcoe, C. (2002). Strength in adversity: Motherhood for women who have been battered. *Canadian Journal of Nursing Research, 34(4),* 47–57.

*Joachim, G. & Acorn, S. (2002). Living with chronic illness: The interface of stigma and normalization. *Canadian Journal of Nursing Research, 32(3),* 37–48.

*Kass, N. & Faden, R. (1996). In women's words: The values and lived experiences of HIV-infected women. R. F. Faden & N. E. Kass (Eds.), *HIV, AIDS, and childbearing: Public policy, private lives* (pp. 426–443). Oxford, UK: Oxford University Press.

Kearney, M. H., Murphy, S., & Rosenbaum, M. (1994). Mothering on crack cocaine: A grounded theory analysis. *Social Science & Medicine, 38,* 351–361.

Kvale, S. (1995). The social construction of validity. *Qualitative Inquiry, 1,* 19–40.

*Litwak, E., Sudit, M., Baker, S., Dobkin, J., & Fullilove, M. (1995). *Caregiving needs of HIV-positive minority women.* Arlington, VA: United States Department of Commerce, National Technical Information Service.

*Locher, A. W. (1995). *The lived experience of women who have perinatally infected their children with human immunodeficiency virus.* Unpublished master's thesis, Medical College of Ohio, Toledo.

*Loriz-Lim, L. M. (1995). *Women's explanations of living with HIV.* Unpublished doctoral dissertation, George Mason University, Fairfax, VA.

Lupton, D. & Fenwick, J. (2001). "They've forgotten that I'm the mum": Constructing and practicing motherhood in special care nurseries. *Social Science & Medicine, 53,* 1011–1021.

Malone, R. E. (2003). Distal nursing. *Social Sciences & Medicine, 56,* 2317–2326.

*Marcenko, M. O. & Samost, L. (1999). Living with HIV/AIDS: The voices of HIV-positive mothers. *Social Work: Journal of the National Association of Social Workers, 44,* 36–45.[7]

McMahon, M. (1995). *Engendering motherhood: Identity and self-transformation in women's lives.* New York: Guilford Press.

McMahon, M. (1996). Significant absences. *Qualitative Inquiry, 2,* 320–336.

*Misener, T. R. & Sowell, R. L. (1998). HIV-infected women's decisions to take antiretrovirals. *Western Journal of Nursing Research, 20,* 431–447.[5]

*Moneyham, L., Scals, B., Demi, A., Sowell, R., Cohen, L., & Guillory, J. (1996). Experiences of disclosure in women infected with HIV. *Health Care for Women International, 17,* 209–221.

*Morrow, K., Costello, T., & Boland, R. (2001). Understanding the psychosocial needs of HIV positive women: A qualitative study. *Psychosomatics, 42,* 497–503.

*Napravnik, S., Royce, R., Walter, E., & Lim, W. (2000). HIV-1 infected women and prenatal care utilization: Barriers and facilitators. *AIDS Patient Care and STDs, 14,* 411–420.

*Palyo, K. (1995). *Lived experience of women with HIV within a self-care framework.* Unpublished master's thesis, Medical College of Ohio, Toledo.

Parker, R. & Aggleton, P. (2003). HIV and AIDS-related stigma and discrimination: A conceptual framework and implications for action. *Social Science & Medicine, 57,* 13–24.

Radtke, H. L. & Van Mens-Verhulst, J. (2001). Being a mother and living with asthma: An exploratory analysis of discourse. *Journal of Health Psychology, 6,* 379–391.

*Regan-Kubinski, M. J. & Sharts-Hopko, N. (1995). Illness cognition of HIV-infected mothers. *Issues in Mental Health Nursing, 16,* 327–344.

*Richter, D. L, Sowell, R. L., & Pluto, D. M. (2002). Attitudes toward antiretroviral therapy among African American women. *American Journal of Health Behavior, 26,* 25–33.

Riessman, C. K. (1990). Strategic uses of narrative in the presentation of self and illness: A research note. *Social Science & Medicine, 30,* 1195–1200.

*Ross, T. L. (1994). *The lived experience of hope in young mothers with human immunodeficiency virus infection: A phenomenological inquiry.* Unpublished doctoral dissertation, Adelphi University, NY.

Ruddick, S. (1980). Maternal thinking. *Feminist Studies, 6,* 342–367.

Sandelowski, M. (2002). Reembodying qualitative inquiry. *Qualitative Health Research, 12,* 104–115.

Sandelowski, M. & Barroso, J. (2002). Reading qualitative studies. *International Journal of Qualitative Methods* [online journal], 1(1), Article 5. Available at http://www.ualberta.ca/~ijqm/english/engframeset.html

Sandelowski, M. & Barroso, J. (2003a). Classifying the findings in qualitative studies. *Qualitative Health Research, 7,* 905–923.

Sandelowski, M. & Barroso, J. (2003b). Creating meta-summaries of qualitative findings. *Nursing Research, 52,* 226–233.

Sandelowski, M. & Barroso, J. (2003c). Toward a metasynthesis of qualitative findings on motherhood in HIV-positive women. *Research in Nursing & Health, 26,* 153–170.

*Sankar, A., Luborsky, I. M, Schuman, I. P., & Roberts, G. (2002). Adherence discourse among African-American women taking HAART. *AIDS Care, 14,* 203–218.

*Santacroce, S. J., Deatrick, J. A., & Ledlie, L. S. (2002). Redefining treatment: How biological mothers manage their children's treatment for perinatally acquired HIV. *AIDS Care, 14,* 247–260.

*Schrimshaw, E. W. & Siegel, K. (2002). HIV-infected mothers' disclosure to their uninfected children: Rates, reasons, and reactions. *Journal of Social and Personal Relationships, 19,* 19–43.

*Semple, S. J., Patterson, T. L., Temoshok, L. R., McCutchan, J. A., Straits-Troster, K. A., Chandler, J. L., et al. (1993). Identification of psychobiological stressors among HIV-positive women. *Women and Health, 20,* 15–36.

*Siegel, K., Kekas, H. M., Scrimshaw, E. W., & Johnson, J. K. (2001). Factors associated with HIV-infected women's use or intention to use AZT during pregnancy. *AIDS Education and Prevention, 13,* 189–206.[6]

*Siegel, K. & Scrimshaw, E. W. (2001). Reasons and justifications for considering pregnancy among women living with HIV/AIDS. *Psychology of Women Quarterly, 25,* 112–126.[6]

*Smith, K. V. & Russell, J. (1997). Ethical issues experienced by HIV-infected African-American women. *Nursing Ethics, 4,* 394–402.

*Sowell, R. L. & Misener, T. R. (1997). Decisions to have a baby by HIV-infected women. *Western Journal of Nursing Research, 19,* 56–70.[5]

*Tangenberg, K. M. (1998). *Marginalized epistemologies: Bodily and spiritual knowing among HIV-positive mothers.* Unpublished doctoral dissertation, University of Washington, Seattle, WA.[4]

Thorne, S. E. (1990). Mothers with chronic illness: A predicament of social construction. *Health Care for Women International, 11,* 209–221.

Thorne, S., Paterson, B., Acorn, A., Canam, C., Joachim, G., & Jillings, C. (2002). Chronic illness experience: Insights from a metastudy. *Qualitative Health Research, 12,* 437–452.

Thurer, S. (1994). *The myths of motherhood: How culture reinvents the good mother.* New York: Houghton Mifflin.

Treichler, P. A. & Warren, C. A. (1998). Maybe next year. Feminist silence and the AIDS epidemic. In P. A. Treichler, L. Cartwright, & C. Penley (Eds.). *The visible woman: Imagining technologies, gender, and science* (pp. 83–129). New York: New York University Press.

*Valdez, M. D. (1999). *La protectora (the protectress): A metaphor for HIV+ Hispanic women.* Unpublished doctoral dissertation, Texas Woman's University, Denton.

*Valdez, M. D. (2001). A metaphor for HIV positive Mexican and Puerto Rican women. *Western Journal of Nursing Research, 23,* 517–535.[7]

*Van Loon, R. A. (1996). *Coping and adaptation in women with AIDS.* Unpublished doctoral dissertation, University of Chicago, IL.

*Van Loon, R.A. (2000). Redefining motherhood: Adaptation to role change for women with AIDS. *Families in Society: The Journal of Contemporary Human Services, 31,* 152–161.[8]

*Van Servellen, G., Sarna, L., & Jablonski, K. J. (1998). Women with HIV: Living with symptoms. *Western Journal of Nursing Research, 20,* 448–464.

*Walker, S. E. (1996). *Vertically transmitted HIV+/AIDS: The impact on maternal attachment.* Unpublished doctoral dissertation, Antioch University, Keene, NH.[9]

*Walker, S. E. (1998). *Women with AIDS and their children.* New York: Garland Publishers.[9]

Weingarten, K, Surrey, J. L., Coll, C. G., & Watkins, M. (1998). Introduction. In C. G. Coll, J. L. Surrey, & K. Weingarten (Eds.), *Mothering against the odds: Diverse voices of contemporary mothers* (pp. 1–14). New York: Guilford Press.

*Wesley, Y., Smeltzer, S. C., Redeker, N., Walker, S., Palumbo, P., & Whipple, B. (2000). Reproductive decision making in mothers with HIV-1. *Health Care for Women International, 21,* 291–304.

West, P. (1990). The status and validity of accounts obtained at interview: A contrast between two studies of families with a disabled child. *Social Science & Medicine, 30,* 1229–1239.

*Winstead, B. A., Derlega, V. J., Burbee, A. P., Sachdev, M., Antle, B., & Greene, K. (2002). Close relationships as sources of strength or obstacles for mothers coping with HIV. *Journal of Loss & Trauma, 7,* 157–184.

*Wright, E. M. (1995). *Deep from within the well: African-American women living with AIDS.* Unpublished doctoral dissertation, Syracuse University, Syracuse, NY.

Complex Physical and Mental Health Needs of Rural Incarcerated Women

Mary Kane, MSN, CRNP, CS-P; Mary DiBartolo, PhD, RN, C

Despite the growing numbers of incarcerated women, there still remain few systematic analyses of their unique physical and mental health needs. A descriptive design was used in a convenience sample of 30 incarcerated female offenders in a rural detention center to investigate the complex health care needs of this population and formulate appropriate community-based nursing interventions. The participants received a detailed physical and mental health assessment as well as screening for alcohol and drug abuse. Sixty-three percent of the women reported drug problems and 80% reported alcohol problems, while 84% reported physical or sexual abuse. Serious health problems were identified, including AIDS, STDs, and delirium tremens. Scores on the Global Severity Index of the Brief Symptom Inventory showed that 70% of the women were in the clinical range for mental health problems. The scores on the Multidimensional Scale of Perceived Social Support were negatively correlated with the Global Severity Index on the BSI (r = −.377, p = .04), which may indicate some protective effect of social support with regards to psychiatric distress. The data demonstrate a need to develop a brief objective mental health-screening test for this specific population to identify psychiatric problems that require immediate attention during the incarceration period. The results also highlight incarcerations as an excellent opportunity for the advanced practice nurse to imitate focused health care interventions and other strategies, which can foster incarcerated women's reentry into the community. More research is needed in the underserved group, particularly concerning issues of maternal incarceration, STD prevention, detoxification, psychiatric treatment, and sources of social support.

More than 1.8 million people are currently in prisons or jails in the United States. At midyear 1999, 6.5% of these prisoners nationwide were women. City and county detention centers house approximately 67,000 women (Bureau of Justice Statistics, 2000). In jails and detention centers, the female population relative to male inmates is even higher than that in prisons, accounting for 11.2% of the total population (Bureau of Justice Statistics, 2000). In fact, the number of incarcerated women has nearly doubled since 1990 (Bureau of Justice Statistics, 2000). Although it is readily apparent that this proportion continues to increase at an alarming rate, very little attention has been given to imprisoned women (Fogel & Belyea, 1999; Keaveny & Zauszniewski,

Issues in Mental Health Nursing, 2002, Volume 23, pages 209–229

1999; Wilson & Leasure, 1991). Female offenders have historically gone unnoticed as a research concern because they constitute a comparatively minuscule percentage of the total prison population in a predominantly male system (Wilson & Leasure, 1991), and they are generally sentenced for nonviolent crimes punishable by shorter periods of imprisonment (Bureau of Justice Statistics, 2000).

It is also widely documented that incarcerated women are underserved when compared to jailed men (Teplin, Abram, & McClelland, 1996). The early research conducted in the female prison population focused primarily on the roles and function of women as inmates (Giallombardo, 1966), their adaptation to prison subculture (Ward & Kassebaum, 1965), the effects of imprisonment (Johnson & Toch, 1982), and the deprivations of confinement (Fogel & Martin, 1992; Fox, 1982). Mounting concerns regarding the prevalence of drug and alcohol abuse and sexually transmitted diseases in incarcerated women, along with other serious physical and mental health issues, have become the central focus in the literature more recently. The majority of incarcerated women are poorly educated, come from impoverished backgrounds, and have not been exposed to or been able to access routine health care (Brewer & Baldwin, 2000; Singer, Bussey, Song, & Lunghofer, 1995; Snell & Morton, 1994). Many have lives that are "steeped in physical sexual violence" (Maeve, 1997, p. 499). There is a high incidence of prostitution, as well as a burgeoning subpopulation of pregnant or postpartal inmates (Bureau of Justice Statistics, 2000; Wilson & Leasure, 1991) that presents its own special philosophical problems and challenges (Osborne, 1995). For these reasons, incarcerated women are not only one of the neediest populations, but also one that experiences the highest levels of social stigma and alienation from traditional service agencies.

Approximately 70% of female inmates are mothers of dependent children (Bureau of Justice Statistics, 2000). Maternal incarceration creates its own unique stresses (Fogel & Martin, 1992; Hairston, 1991) and places imprisoned mothers at high risk for mental distress resulting from the disruption in their family life (Bannach, 1985; LaPoint, Pickett, & Harris, 1985). Incarcerated women fear an erosion of the mother-child bond. They especially worry that their children are not being adequately cared for (Henriques, 1982; Stanton, 1980), and that they are missing the "growing-up" experiences of their children

and the developmental milestones that cannot be relived (Hairston, 1991).

Despite substantial gaps in knowledge regarding incarcerated women, even less is known about this population in a rural setting, where the numbers of incarcerated females is likely to be smaller relative to male inmates. Furthermore, health care resources are generally more limited in small rural jails than in large urban facilities. The mentally ill in a rural setting are more likely to be thought of as criminal and placed in jail for minor offenses or pending psychiatric hospitalization (Sullivan & Spritzer, 1997). Although female inmates in a rural area are similar in that their crimes are related to drugs and alcohol, they are different in their health and social linkages within the community. The rural population is likely to be more stable with large networks of people linked to each other and ongoing associations with service providers in the community. However, the services available in a jail are severely limited by local resources and funding. In small and poorer rural counties, the jail strongly reflects the local socioeconomic conditions. Although there may be greater concern from the more cohesive surrounding rural community, lack of access to health care in rural areas is magnified in the jail setting where part-time availability of health care providers is the norm. Thus, rural incarcerated women are less likely to benefit from what might be a rare opportunity for health care in the jail.

REVIEW OF THE LITERATURE

Incarcerated women often come from "deprived environments fraught with social problems" (Fogel & Martin, 1992), which are "significant for violence, drug abuse, and a kind of chronic chaos. Many enter the penal system with acute and chronic physical problems, along with mental health issues that have long gone unaddressed" (Maeve, 1997, p. 495). Imprisonment is a stressful life that necessitates drastic changes in one's life and is considered psychologically harmful (Berkman, 1995; Tanay, 1973). Furthermore, inmates are particularly vulnerable to the stress of incarceration because many enter the prison system in poor or compromised physical health from the outset (Fogel & Belyea, 1999). The most frequent medical problems among this group are drug and alcohol addiction and gynecological diseases, as well as exacerbation of chronic health conditions such as hypertension, epilepsy, and diabetes—not to mention undetected health problems. Incarceration itself has been found to exacerbate asthma, diabetes, peptic ulcers, and epilepsy (Wilson & Leasure, 1991). Weight gain is common due to limited dietary options combined with lack of exercise. The prevailing rate of prostitution, concomitant IV drug use, and sexually transmitted disease predisposes many inmates to AIDS. A Bureau of Justice report revealed that 44% of female inmates reported either physical or sexual abuse in the past (Bureau of Justice Statistics, 2000). Often, there are other preexisting mental health issues present, such as alcoholism or drug dependence as well as severe anxiety and depression, all of which are further magnified by the stresses of incarceration. Suicide persists as the second most common cause of death in jails (Bureau of Justice Statistics, 1995).

Only a few studies have explored the physical health issues in this group. Studies have focused on pregnancy, pregnancy outcome, and sexually transmitted diseases (Fogel & Belyea, 1999; Lindquist & Lindquist, 1999; Martin, Kim, Kupper, Meyer & Hays, 1997; Martin, Rieger, Kupper, Meyer, & Qaqish, 1997; Safyer & Richmond, 1995). In 1995, the incidence of HIV infection among women inmates was 4% compared to the 2.3% among male inmates (Gowdy et al., 1998). A study of county and city jails (Centers for Disease Control [CDC], 1998) showed that despite the recommendations of the National Commission on Correctional Health Care (1994), less than half of jails offered routine STD screening. While 6% of the women entering prison are pregnant, only 49% of facilities offered pregnancy testing and in those, only 4% of women actually received pregnancy testing (Snell & Morton, 1994; CDC, 1998).

Study findings also have supported high rates of mental health problems in populations of jailed women (Jordan, Schlenger, Fairbank, & Caddell, 1996; Novick, Della Penna, Schwartz, Remmlinger, & Lowenstein, 1977; Scott, Hannum, & Ghrist, 1982; Teplin et al., 1996). More than 40% of incarcerated women have some kind of DSM-III psychiatric diagnosis (Washington & Diamond, 1985). Turner and Tofler's (1986) study supported the premise that there are staggering numbers of women in prison with undetected and untreated mental illness. Of the 708 imprisoned women we studied, 30% reported drug use, 28% have a history of self-harm, and 18% have a history of psychiatric treatment. Fogel (1988) explored the mental health of female offenders ($N = 49$) at the time of incarceration and six months thereafter. Using Spielberger's (1983) State-Trait Anxiety Inventory [STAI] and the Center for Epidemiology Studies Depression Scale [CES-D] (Radloff, 1977), high levels of anxiety and depression were detected upon admission. In a subsequent study, Fogel and Martin (1992) investigated the mental health of incarcerated mothers versus nonmothers. Using the STAI and CES-D, they found that mothers and nonmothers evidenced somewhat differential patterns of emotional distress in prison. The mean depression level in this sample ($N = 46$) was more than twice that found in general population samples of women. Their anxiety levels declined significantly, while their depression scores continued to remain at clinically significant levels after six months. Fogel (1993) later conducted a descriptive, correlational study of female prisoners and selected health outcomes. Using standardized instruments (STAI-S and CES-D) and semi-structured interviews, data were collected from 35 incarcerated women during the first week of imprisonment and six months later. Specific stresses identified included separation from families, worry about their children, and loss of control over their own lives. Psychological stress was found to be positively related to depression and weight gain in jail. The initially high level of depression symptoms were possibly attributed to the separation from family and children. Hurley and Dunne (1991) screened 92 incarcerated women for psychological distress and identified high levels of depressive symptoms, the most frequent psychiatric diagnoses being adjustment disorder with depressed mood and personality disorder.

Using the National Institute of Mental Health Diagnostic Interview Schedule Version III-R (NIMH DIS-III-R) (Robins, Helzer, Croughan, & Ratcliff, 1981), Teplin et al. (1996) found that over 80% of a randomly selected, stratified sample of 1272 female pretrial detainees met the criteria for one or more lifetime psychiatric disorders; 70% had been symptomatic within six months prior to the initial interview. The most common disorders were drug and alcohol dependence and post-traumatic stress disorder, while the most common major mental disorder was depression. Jordan et al. (1996) focuses their investigation on incarcerated women entering prison as convicted felons. In a sample of 805 women, assessments were conducted for eight psychiatric disorders using the Composite International Diagnostic Interview (World Health Organization, 1990). Results indicated high rates of substance abuse and dependence, in addition to higher rates of antisocial and borderline personality disorders when compared to women in the community.

Singer et al. (1995) investigated psychosocial issues of ($N = 201$) jailed women. A majority (81%) reported some physical and sexual abuse and a lifestyle characterized by alcohol and illicit drug abuse (83%), as well as a social support system that is severely lacking or, for many, nonexistent (40%). Approximately 40% reported feelings of anxiety while 59% were depressed. Using the Global Severity Index of the Brief Symptom Inventory (BSI; Derogatis, 1992), 64% of the women were in the clinical range for mental health problems. In a larger scale effort, Teplin et al. (1996) identified women with significant mental illness awaiting trial. Over 75% of this group was classified as having a psychiatric diagnosis, most commonly drug abuse (52.4%), alcohol dependence (23.9%), major depressive disorder (13.7%), and dysthmia (6.7%). Furthermore, almost a quarter of the participants reported suffering from post-traumatic stress disorder as a past victim of rape or other violent assault. Using a descriptive, correlational design in a sample of 63 incarcerated female offenders, Keaveny and Zauszniewski (1999) systematically analyzed the factors that occurred in the 12 months preceding incarceration as possible precursors to the development of mental health problems. They found an average of 10 life events (e.g., jail term, change in living conditions, illness) during this period and a positive correlation between the number of life events and depression ($r = .24, p < .05$).

Despite the accumulating evidence of the physical and mental health care problems of incarcerated women, there still is insufficient empirical data regarding their complex needs and, more importantly, how to best address these issues during and after imprisonment. The purpose of this study is to identify the physical and mental health needs of incarcerated women so as to develop strategies and identify appropriate service that would be reasonable in light of the limited funds typically available in poor rural jails.

METHOD

Setting

The study was conducted at a county detention center located in rural Maryland. The county has a population of 24,235 with a population density of 74.1 persons per square mile, the lowest per capita income in the state, and over 21% of the population living below the poverty rate. Seventy-one percent of the population over age 25 graduated from high school (Bureau of the Census, 1999). The unemployment rate for 1999 was 7.7%, compared to a state average of 3.7% (Department of Labor, Licensing, and Regulation, 2000). Most of those arrested resided in two small cities located in the county. The detention center houses persons arrested in the county awaiting release on bond, awaiting trial, and persons sentenced to less than 18 months. Crimes generally ranged from petty theft to serious assaults. Some subjects in the study were released on bond within hours of their participation and others were eventually sentenced to many years in the state prison. During the fiscal year 1998, there was an average daily census of 84 inmates with an average daily census of seven women. The women's area was small, overcrowded, and at times, some women slept on makeshift cots on the floor. The health care was provided by contract with the County Health Department and health care personnel, including a nurse, nurse practitioner, and physician, who were available on a part-time basis.

Design and Sample

This descriptive study used a convenience sample consisting of 30 women. The data were collected by the principal investigator, a family nurse practitioner who was also providing primary care to all the inmates. During the study period (June 1987–July 1998) a total of 107 women were incarcerated. Permission was obtained from the Human Subjects Committee of the affiliated university and from the warden and the County Health Department. Women were asked if they wished to participate after they had received their initial health assessment. Each participant signed a written consent form and was informed of the right to participate in any or all components of the study or to withdraw completely at any time. Participants who declined to participate were not asked the reason why, as this was thought to be a form of coercion: moreover, it was feared that such questioning would interfere with requests for future health care. Two participants who initially refused later asked to participate and were included. Health care was provided in the same manner to all without regard to participation in the research. The only incentive for participation was the additional time spent in an air-conditioned office during data collection.

Interview Protocol

To obtain both the physical and mental health assessment data, each person was interviewed and received a physical examination by the nurse practitioner. A standard history form consisting of questions about physical health, mental health, addictions, and family history was used. When the responses were affirmative, follow-up questions were asked to clarify history of current symptoms. For example, if a participant identified that she had seizures, questions were asked about onset, most recent seizure, and current medications. Quantitative data were coded for analysis using SPSS. Qualitative comments were coded to preserve anonymity. Sixty percent of the study population participated during their first two weeks in jail. All interviews were held in private so that no one could overhear. After clients had completed their initial assessment, they were asked if they wished to participate in the study. If they agreed, they were asked additional questions about their social and family history and then administered the Brief Symptom Inventory (Derogatis, 1992) and the Multidimensional Scale of Perceived Social Support (Zimet, Dahlem, Zimet, & Farley, 1988). Where necessary, the questionnaires were verbally administered to those of low reading ability.

Instruments

Brief Symptom Inventory (BSI). The BSI (Derogatis, 1992) is a 53-item questionnaire design to reflect an individual's psychological symptom status. Participants are asked to identify how much distress they have experienced in the last seven days in relation to the 53 items. Items are rated on a five-point Likert-type scale; symptom distress ranged from 0 = "not at all" to 4 = "extremely." It yields nine primary symptom dimensions which include: Somatization, Obsessive-Compulsive, Interpersonal Sensitivity, Depression, Anxiety, Hostility, Phobic Anxiety, Paranoid Ideation, and Psychoticism. Additionally, a Global Severity Index (GSI) score, which is a general measure of psychological functioning, is also calculated. The internal consistency of the BSI has been well established with Cronbach's alpha coefficients ranging from .71 to .85. The test has been widely used, including with women with post-traumatic stress dis-

order (Allen, Huntoon, & Evans, 1999), incarcerated women (Singer et al., 1995), and pregnant and postpartal women (Otchert, Carey, & Adam, 1999).

The Multidimensional Scale of Perceived Social Support (MSPSS). The MSPSS (Zimet et al., 1988) is a 12-item scale with three subscales measuring perceived social support from three distinct groups: family, significant others, and friends. Norms for the general population have been published with higher scores indicating more social support (Dahlem, Zimet, & Walker, 1991). Social support is theorized to serve as a buffer in the experience of stress (Vaux, Burda, & Stewart, 1986; Vaux & Harrison, 1985). Diminished health in general was demonstrated among adolescents with fewer social supports (Resnick et al., 1997). This scale has shown that increased social support in neighborhood populations has been found to be significantly correlated with decreased incidence of childhood maltreatment (Coulton, Korbin, & Stu, 1999). For the incarcerated population, this support may prevent depression or other psychiatric illnesses and health problems. A seven-point Likert-type scale (very strongly disagree to very strongly agree) is used. The MSPSS has demonstrated good internal reliability (alpha coefficient of .88 for the total scale) and strong factorial validity (Zimet et al., 1988). Other studies using the instrument have reported excellent internal consistency (Cecil, Stanley, Carrion, & Swann, 1995; Dahlem et al., 1991). The MSPSS was modestly correlated with the Network Orientations Scale (Vaux et al., 1986), a measure of willingness to use available social supports (Cecil et al., 1995).

RESULTS

Data were analyzed using the Statistical Package for Social Sciences (SPSS) using descriptive statistics, including means and standard deviations.

Demographic Characteristics

Of the 30 women in the sample, the majority (13) was between 31–40 years of age, while nine were 21–30 years old, six were 41–50 years old, and two were less than 20 years old. Ten women were Caucasian, while 19 were African-American, and one was biracial. Twenty-one women had a high school education or GED, three reported some college, and six noted elementary school as their highest level of education.

Nineteen women stated that they were unemployed at the time of the arrest, compared to the remainder who reported either full-time or part-time employment. Nineteen women reported an annual income less than $5,000. Many of the women had multiple charges. Eight of the women were incarcerated for a violent crime; seventeen of the women were charged with a drug charge or a drug-related charge (e.g., stealing to support drug use). Fifteen were arrested for nonviolent crimes; and violation of probation charges were given to the 14 women who were on probation at the time of their arrest.

Physical Health

There were two confirmed cases of HIV infection. One woman who was severely immunocompromised was unable to comply with antiviral medication due to mental illness and limited intellectual capacity. Another woman was newly diagnosed in the jail and was offered antiviral medication because of a high viral load. She was found not guilty, however, was released, and resumed an alcoholic lifestyle. The other life-threatening problem requiring immediate treatment for two women was impending delirium tremens. In addition, other chronic illnesses were identified or reported by history; there were ten participants reporting asthma and two participants each reporting seizure disorder and diabetes. Two participants were on permanent disability (one from HIV infection and one due to a cerebrovascular accident [CVA] experienced while she was using crack cocaine). Two participants reported a history of hepatitis.

Reproductive Issues

Two of the women were pregnant at the time of interview, while all but one woman already had children. Thirty percent of the women reported that they previously had at least one sexually transmitted disease. While 16 participants reported they never used condoms, six reported they always used condoms. Of the 22 women who had gynecological examinations during incarceration, one third had abnormal examination with either an abnormal PAP or a current STD.

Mental Health

On initial interview nearly half of the women reported that they had been treated for psychiatric illness in the past. Six had a previous suicide attempt, six reported current depression beyond the depression associated with incarceration, two were overtly psychotic, and three were referred to a psychiatrist for immediate evaluation. Psychotropic medications prescribed during incarceration included anti-psychotics, anti-depressants, and anti-anxiety agents and medications used for alcohol and heroin withdrawal.

Seventy percent of the participants met the criteria on the BSI (Derogatis, 1992) to be defined as a psychiatric case. In two of the subscales, psychoticism and paranoia, 66% and 60% of the participants, respectively, had scores in the distress range. When these subscales were eliminated from the analysis, 50% of the women still were identified as in need of psychiatric care. Low scores were identified on the phobic anxiety and anxiety subscales. The study revealed high levels of general mistrust (90%) and high levels of expression of guilt (60%), low levels of blame (5%), and high levels of feeling taken advantage of (73%) (see Table 1).

Alcohol and Drug Use

Seventeen of the participants were in jail for drug offenses or drug-related offenses (stealing, violation of probation by using drugs, taking a possession charge for a friend, etc.). While only 13 openly admitted to a drug problem at the time of arrest, 16 noted that they had a current alcohol problem. As one might expect, a larger percentage reported a history of drug (63.3%) and alcohol problems (80%). Only 30% of the participants had ever been in an addictions treatment program.

Physical and Sexual Victimization and Abuse

Seventy percent of the women acknowledged physical abuse and half admitted to being the victim of sexual abuse. Only five of the participants said they had never been physically or sexually abused. Consistent with the general underreporting of abuse, several of the women had difficulty understanding the concept of sexual abuse and initially denied it until the question was rephrased. One participant clarified her response by saying, "Oh, yeah, I've been raped." One other woman asked, "Is it sexual abuse if a man broke your arm and leg and then had sex on you?"

Family Issues

Nineteen women in the sample were never married, one woman was currently married, and one third

TABLE A2-1

Comparison to Female Adult Nonpatient Norms

Scale	Norm *M*	Inmate *M*	Symptomatic
Somatization	0.35	0.95	37%
Obsessive-compulsive	0.48	1.13	33
Interpersonal sensitivity	0.40	1.0	43
Depression	0.36	1.06	37
Anxiety	0.44	1.01	33
Hostility	0.36	0.82	33
Phobic anxiety	0.22	0.59	23
Paranoid ideation	0.35	0.97	60
Psychoticism	0.17	0.5	66
Global indices			
GSI	0.35	0.76	47
PSDI	1.32	1.81	57
PST	12.86	27.00	37

Note: 70% of subjects met overall criteria for case definition.
GSI = Global Severity Index, PSDI = Positive Symptom Distress Index, PST = Positive Symptom Trial.

were either separated or divorced. All but one of the women identified themselves as mothers. Twenty-five of the women had preschool or school age children. There were a total of 47 children who were not being cared for by their mothers as a result of the current incarceration. Prior to incarceration, one third did not have legal custody, although some women voluntarily relinquished custody, while others lost custody through the courts. While their mothers were incarcerated, 40% of the children were cared for by grandparents, 20% by their fathers, and the remainder by other relatives, friends, or by the foster care system.

Social Support

The results of the MSPSS indicated that social support may have some protective effect in guarding against the experience of psychiatric distress. The total scores (mean = 4.71) on the MSPSS were significantly negatively correlated with the Global Severity Index on the BSI ($r = -.77$, $p = .04$). However, scores were markedly lower in two of the three subscales than any scores published in the literature. The mean score on the family subscale was 3.71, while the literature indicates a mean score of 54.5 among college students (Dahlem et al., 1991) and a lower mean (3.86) being

identified among depressed females (Cecil et al., 1995). The family subscale mean in this study was 4.51; compared to college student norm mean of 5.31 (Dahlem et al., 1991) and low mean score of 4.86 being identified among adolescents on an inpatient psychiatric unit (Kazarian & McCabe, 1991). The significant other subscale mean was 5.92. This approximates the mean (5.94) for college students and is higher than the mean published for other groups of students and patients (Dahlem et al., 1991).

DISCUSSION

As the data suggest, many incarcerated rural women have significant physical and mental health care problems. Physical health care needs were primarily focused on traditional women's health care needs. Routine gynecological examinations were the rare exception and yet their high risk behaviors predispose them to cancer, unplanned pregnancy, and sexually transmitted diseases. These findings reinforce the recommendation that gynecological examinations with routine screening for STDs and HIV should be an integral part of a jail admission physical. In this population, it is especially necessary to combine history with physical findings. Several of the women underestimated their alcohol intake and yet were found to be symptomatic for impending delirium tremens. It was fairly common to report asthma and obtain a bronchodilator inhaler, which was believed to make it easier to breathe in a stuffy cell. One woman was transferred from another jail with a supply of medications to treat HIV infection and sought leniency from the courts because of "end-stage AIDS," yet when repeat testing was done, she was found to be HIV negative. There were sexually transmitted diseases identified among women who reported always using a condom. The nurse practitioner providing screening and care must balance subjective and objective data in order to make appropriate diagnoses and avoid over-diagnosis. Health problems and pregnancy often foster leniency in the courts.

From a mental health standpoint, the results on the BSI support the notion that this group as a whole has high levels of psychiatric illness. The scores on the psychoticism and paranoid subscales had group means in a range that would place the entire group in a patient category. However, the validity of the scores is questionable as three of the five questions on the paranoid scale seemed to measure either precursors to incarceration, current living conditions, the extent that they were afraid of and avoided detection, or had developed relationships that fostered their addictions. This is evident by noting that 22 women endorsed (answered that they were distressed to some degree by the symptom) the item "Feeling that people will take advantage of you if you let them," 18 endorsed the item "Feeling that you are watched or talked about by others," and most strikingly, 27 endorsed the item "Feeling that most people cannot be trusted."

The questions on the psychoticism subscale yielded similar difficulties. Twenty-one subjects endorsed the item "Feeling lonely even when you are with people" and half endorsed the item "Never feeling close to anyone." These likely represent a longing for familiar people, and in the absence of other measures of psychotic behavior, they are not a reflection of psychotic thinking. Another item on the psychoticism subscale, "The idea that you should be punished for your sins" (endorsed by 18 women) and an item on the paranoid subscale, "Feeling that others are to blame for most of your trouble" (endorsed by 17 subjects), as well as the item "Feelings of guilt" (endorsed by 21 subjects, 70%) are more likely the

result of a sense of regret. These responses may potentially be interpreted as positive finding in that the women acknowledged responsibility and indicated amenability to change versus the "paranoia" they were intended to measure.

The questions on the anxiety subscale were endorsed by relatively few participants, and the group mean fell well within the nonpatient norm. The low levels of anxiety could imply that these women were not fearful, not easily scared, or were not willing to identify themselves as such in the presumably tense atmosphere of incarceration. The scores might also reflect that anxiety for them was at such a persistent level that they did not find it particularly distressing.

The results of MSPSS indicate that these women experienced low levels of emotional support from family and friends. While it is well known that incarcerated women do not have strong social support systems and that their habitual behavior and dysfunctional family and social networks make it difficult for others to be supportive, this issue requires more attention and specific interventions if women are to resume family roles in the community. If the behaviors that led to incarceration are to be changed and the cycle of addiction broken, friendships and families will need to be better maintained, and new social networks that exclude problematic friends and family members will need to be established. Furthermore, the trust that leads to supportive relationships will need to be earned and maintained by consistent behaviors on the part of the women.

The scores on the significant other subscale of the MSPSS, while within the range of the norms, may be equally troubling. All other indicators demonstrated that these women are typically involved in a series of dysfunctional relationships with men who have abused them and share their problems with addictions. Anecdotal evidence also attests to the involvement of incarcerated women with men who have destructive influence on them. These include achieving social status and favors in the jail by association with men—some of whom they may have never met but with whom they correspond on an intimate level and claim as a significant other or fiancé. Men easily step into the role of significant other by simply providing small tokens or gifts like commissary money or underwear. Incarcerated women repeatedly demonstrated loyalty to drug dealers or pimps. Very often, women pled guilty to a charge and accepted jail time in order to spare their man. At one point in the study, there were three incarcerated women who had intense relationships with one incarcerated man. One woman was married to him, another had a child with him, and the third had a long-standing intimate relationship with him. These codependent behaviors were not studied directly here, but are certainly issues that need to be examined further so that interventions can be focused on helping these women to develop self-reliance and overcome their involvement with the criminal life.

As a whole, this group also demonstrated tremendous needs in terms of psychiatric illness, addictions, and difficulty with maintaining family and maternal roles, and yet the nature of these problems calls for action beyond mere identification. Practitioners have a unique opportunity to improve the health care provided to incarcerated women, a segment of the population that has more health concerns statistically than the rest of society, yet the fewest available medical resources to address these problems (Wilson & Leasure, 1991). Nursing intervention to reduce psychological distress at the time of admission to the detention center may reduce levels of depression and mistrust. While the problems are complex and interrelated, and trust in the nurse is not to be assumed, the nursing interventions must begin with specific actions that will bring immediate benefit. Obtaining a detailed health history can in itself provide support and a firm basis for individualized care. A complete physical with appropriate interventions in the treatment of depression, psychoses, and addictions is critical. For women who have been abused or involved in exploitive relationships and are severely lacking social support, delivering concrete benefits is key to assisting the women in addressing current problems and engaging in self-help activities. The incarcerated mother, in particular, requires special attention, as she is part of a family that is at risk. While care during incarceration focuses on the inmate, the issues of addiction and abuse are known to be repeated in families and must be addressed. This is an appropriate time to ask women about their children, to identify their health risks, and make referrals for them. The incarcerated woman most often will not have any visits with her children under age 12 and yet she needs support that her role as a mother is valued.

The admission assessment represents a crucial point of intervention and referral (Teplin et al., 1996)

although for short-term incarceration, the services must be delivered with a focus on prompt intervention and fairly rapid discharge. Maintaining positive health behaviors and outcomes for the long term will only be achieved if preventive strategies are implemented to keep these women safe and well. The model used in this detention center where health care is provided by the county health department does provide for continuity of care because clients are linked with appropriate community resources while in jail. The period of incarceration can provide an excellent opportunity for linking these women and their children with appropriate services that were generally lacking preincarceration.

Cost issues, however, both in terms of staff time and availability of medications and referrals, are real barriers to achieving positive health outcome in a rural jail. Many citizens are opposed to allocating funds for the health care of the imprisoned, yet dollars spent up-front for prompt treatment and preventive care and counseling may by money well spent and prevent more costly treatments in the future. For example, while the cost of a gynecological examination and single-dose treatment for STDs is high, this may be the only opportunity to help these vulnerable women, and these measures do prevent the spread of disease and more costly sequelae. Furthermore, prescribing the newer but more costly psychotropic medications has a higher degree of compliance because of the side-effect profile.

Although the data obtained from this population of rural incarcerated women overwhelmingly supports findings of previous studies, it must be interpreted with caution. There are obvious limitations both in terms of sample size and the lack of generalizability from this convenience sample in one rural detention center. Another limitation to be considered is the reliability of retrospective self-report data, especially in this population. While the majority of the women appeared to be truthful and openly admitted to a variety of socially undesirable behaviors, problems related to recall, exaggeration, and potentially dishonest responses must be recognized. Although a strength of the study was its consistency in data collection methods via the use of one individual performing assessments and administering the instruments to all participants, one could suspect that there was some potential bias in that the primary investigator was also the same individual providing health care. All steps were taken to ensure that women could freely choose whether to participate or not without fear of reprisal. However, the verbal administration of tests for women who have difficulties with reading comprehension, as well as the overall lack of familiarity with Likert-type scale testing, may have influenced responses.

Another concern is that of instrumentation. At present, there are very few tools that have been adequately tested in this specialized population. The BSI is certainly a well-established and psychometrically stable instrument. Although it has been widely used in the general adult population, as well as adolescent and adult psychiatric outpatients, it has been used minimally with incarcerated women who have a different set of norms and life circumstances. There were obvious problems with some of the questions when administered to those living in a jail. Four of the five questions on the phobic anxiety subscale were questions, which did not apply to those who have been incarcerated during the last week. The items were: "Feeling afraid in open spaces and on the street," "Feeling afraid to travel on buses, subways, or trains," "Feeling uneasy in crowds, such as shopping or at the movies," and "Feeling nervous when you are left alone." Thus, the phobic anxiety could not be accurately measured by this scale. However, one should note that even if the problematic psychoticism, paranoid, and phobic anxiety subscales were eliminated, 50% of the women met the criteria to be defined as a psychiatric case. Nonetheless, there is a need to accurately assess these subscales with items that would reveal valid paranoia, psychoticism, and phobic anxiety. As a practical alternative to the 53-item BSI, a brief objective mental health screening tool could be administered upon admission to jail, where the incidence of mental illness is high, the risk of suicide is real, and the cancer for undertreatment of psychiatric disorders is great. This could provide a vital means to accurate diagnosis, which would guide more immediate interventions, as well as a discharge map with appropriate providers in the community.

CONCLUSION

The issues surrounding the care of incarcerated women pose great challenges to nursing and warrant continued investigation (Fogel & Martin, 1992). Despite the aforementioned methodological constraints, the results of this study do add to the current research base and shed some light on important

issues present in a rural detention center. First, the results identified a variety of complex physical and mental health care needs of incarcerated women, which provide a compelling rationale for nursing involvement. One such intervention would be the development of a brief mental health screening tool specifically geared to this population. Through prompt identification of problems and subsequent implementation of therapeutic interventions, the nurse can use the incarceration episode as an entry point for continuing care. The physical assessment can serve as a vehicle to address new or ongoing physical concerns via specific interventions or education to prevent more costly expenditures down the line. The care must include an orientation toward the future, as these problems are long term and not resolved during incarceration. Education and appropriate referrals for counseling regarding problems with addictions, abuse, and other health care or family issues are central to comprehensive care.

Mental health nurse practitioners and other advanced practice nurses are well-suited to work in this setting. The life-threatening issues of detoxification and suicide require the skills of someone who can make immediate assessments and interventions in this area. Nurses are in an optimal position to collaborate with community health departments in providing ongoing services essential to enhancing the health of women in rural areas post incarceration.

More research is justified in this neglected area of inquiry. Correctional facilities remain "a fertile field for doing research and are virtually untapped by nurse researchers" (Drake, 1998, p. 52). Not only will this vital information add to the existing knowledge base, but also it will provide insight into the special health care needs and problems inherent to this group. The aforementioned health care delivery suggestions are proposed with the belief that correctional health care is not a site-specific service but rather part of a continuum of community health care for this vulnerable group. Addressing these specialized needs at the point of contact enables incarcerated women to receive immediate and necessary interventions with referrals for appropriate continuing care when reentering the rural-based community.

References

Allen, J. G., Huntoon, J., & Evans, R. (1999). Complexities in complex posttraumatic stress disorder in inpatient women: Evidence from cluster analysis of MCMI-III personality disorder scales. *Journal of Personality Assessment, 73,* 449–471.

Bannach, P. J. (1985). *Mothers in prison.* New Brunswick, NJ: Transaction Books.

Brewer, M. K. & Baldwin, D. (2000). The relationship between self-esteem, health, habits, and knowledge of BSE in female inmates. *Public Health Nursing, 17*(1), 16–24.

Bureau of the Census. (1999). *Somerset County Quickfacts from the U.S. Census Bureau* (Online). Available: http://quickfacts.census.gov/cgi-bin/cnty_quicklinks?24039

Bureau of Justice Statistics. (2000). *Prison and jail inmates at midyear 1998.* Washington, DC: NCI-173414.

Cecil, H., Stanley, M., Carrion, P., & Swann, A. (1995). Psychometric properties of the MSPSS and NOS in psychiatric outpatients. *Journal of Clinical Psychology, 51,* 593–602.

Centers for Disease Control. (1998). Assessment of sexually transmitted diseases service in city and county jails—United States, 1997. *Morbidity and Mortality Weekly Report, 47*(21), 429–431.

Coulton, C., Korbin, J., & Stu, M. (1999). Neighborhoods and child maltreatment: A multi-level study. *Child Abuse & Neglect, 23*(11), 1019–1040.

Dahlem, N. W., Zimet, G. D., & Walker, R. R. (1991). The Multidimensional Scale of Perceived Social Support: A confirmatory study. *Journal of Clinical Psychology, 47,* 756–761.

Department of Labor, Licensing, and Regulation. (2000). *Civilian Labor Force, Employment, and Unemployment by Place of Residence. 1999.* (Online). Available: www.dllr.state.md.US/mi/981aus.htm

Derogatis, L. (1992). *BSI administration, scoring and procedures manual—II.* Baltimore: Clinical Psychometric Research.

Drake, V. K. (1998). Process, perils and pitfalls of research in prison. *Issues in Mental Health Nursing, 19,* 41–52.

Fogel, C. I. (1993). Hard time: The stressful nature of incarceration for women. *Issues in Mental Health Nursing, 14,* 366–377.

Fogel, C. I. (1988). Health status of incarcerated women. *Dissertation Abstracts International, 49,* 1582.

Fogel, C. I. & Belyea, M. (1999). The lives of incarcerated women: Violence, substance abuse and at risk for HIV. *Journal of the Association of Nurses in AIDS Care, 19*(6), 66–74.

Fogel, C. I. & Martin, S. L. (1992). The mental health of incarcerated women. *Western Journal of Nursing Research, 14,* 30–47.

Fox, J. (1982). Women in prison: A case study in the social reality of stress. In R. Johnson & H. Toch (Eds.), *The pains of imprisonment* (pp. 205–220). Beverly Hills, CA: Sage.

Gaillombardo, R. (1966). *Society of women: A study of women's prisons.* New York: Wiley.

Gowdy, V. B., Cain, T., Corrothers, H., Katsel, T. H., Parmley, A. M., & Schmidt, A. (1998). *Women in the criminal justice system—A twenty-year update.* Washington, DC: National Institute of Justice.

Hairston, C. F. (1991). Mothers in jail: Parent-child separation and jail visitation. *Affilia, 6,* 9–27.

Henriques, Z. W. (1982). *Imprisoned mothers and their children.* Washington, DC: University Press of America.

Hurley, W. & Dunne, M. (1991). Psychological distress and psychiatric morbidity in women prisoners. *Australian/New Zealand Journal of Psychiatry, 25,* 461–470.

Johnson, R. & Toch, H. (1982). *The pains of imprisonment.* Beverly Hills, CA: Sage.

Jordan, B. K., Schlenger, W. E., Fairbank, J. A., & Caddell, J. M. (1996). Prevalence of psychiatric disorders among incarcerated women. II: Convicted felons entering prison. *Archives of General Psychiatry, 53,* 513–519.

Kazarian, S. S. & McCabe, S. B. (1991). Dimensions of social support in the MSPSS: Factorial structure, reliability, and theoretical implications. *Journal of Community Psychology, 19,* 150–160.

Keaveny, M. D. & Zauszniewski, J. A. (1999). Life events and psychological well-being in women sentenced to prison. *Issues in Mental Health Nursing, 20,* 73–89.

LaPoint, V., Pickett, M. O., & Harris, B. F. (1985). Enforced family separation: A descriptive analysis of some experiences of children of black imprisoned mothers. In M. B. Spencer, G. K. Brookins, & W. R. Allen (Eds.), *Beginnings: The social and affective development of black children* (pp. 143–183). Hillsdale, NJ: Firlbaum.

Lindquist, C. H. & Lindquist, C. A. (1990). Health behind bars: Utilization and evaluation of medical care among jail inmates. *Journal of Community Health, 24*(4), 285–303.

Maeve, M. K. (1997). Nursing practice with incarcerated women: Caring within mandated (sic) alienation. *Issues in Mental Health Nursing, 18,* 495–510.

Martin, S. L., Kim, J. Kupper, L. L., Meyer, R. E., & Hays, M. (1997). Is incarceration during pregnancy associated with infant birthweight? *American Journal of Public Health, 87*(9), 1526–1531.

Martin, S. L., Rieger, R. H., Kupper, L. L., Meyer, R. E., & Qaqish, B. F. (1997). The effect of incarceration during pregnancy on birth outcomes. *Public Health Report, 112*(4), 340–346.

National Commission on Correctional Health Care. (1994). *Position statement: Women's health care in correctional settings.* (Online). Available: www.corrections.comneche/statements.html

Novick, L. F., Della Penna, R., Schwartz, F. S., Remmlinger, F. E., & Lowenstein, B. (1977). Health status of the New York City prison population. *Medical Care, 11,* 210–216.

Osborne, O. H. (1995). Jailed mothers: Further explorations in public sector nursing. *Journal of Psychosocial Nursing, 33,* 23–28.

Radloff, L. (1977). The CES-D Scale: A self-report depression scale for research in the general population. *Applied Psychological Measurement, 3,* 385–401.

Resnick, M. D., Bearman, P. S., Blum, R. W., Badman, K. E., Harris, R. M. Jones, J., Tabor, J., Beahing, T., Sieving, R. E., Shaw, M., Ireland, M, Bearnger, L. H., & Udry, J. R. (1997). Protecting adolescents from harm. Findings from the national longitudinal study on adolescent health. *Journal of the American Medical Association, 278,* 823–832.

Robins, L.N. Helzer, J. E., Croughan, J., & Ratcliff, K. (1981). National Institute of Mental Health Diagnostic Interview Schedule: Its history, characteristics and validity. *Archives of General Psychiatry, 38,* 381–389.

Safyer, S. M. & Richmond, L. (1995). Pregnancy behind bars. *Seminars in Perinatology, 19*(4), 314–322.

Scott, N., Hannum, T., & Ghrist, S. (1982). Assessment of depression among incarcerated females. *Journal of Personality Assessment, 46,* 372–379.

Singer, M. I., Bussey, J., Song, L., & Lunghofer, L. (1995). The psychosocial issues of women serving time in jail. *Social Work, 40,* 103–112.

Snell, T. & Morton, D. (1994). *Women in prison* (NJ-145321). Washington, DC: US Department of Justice: Office of Justice Programs, Bureau of Justice Statistics.

Spielberger, C. D. (1983). *Manual for the State-Trait Anxiety Inventory.* Palo Alto, CA: Counseling Psychologists Press.

Stanton, A. M. (1980). *When mothers go to jail.* Lexington, MA: Lexington.

Sullivan, G. & Spritzer, K. (1997). The criminalization of persons with serious mental illness living in rural areas. *The Journal of Rural Health, 13,* 6–13.

Tanay, E. (1973). Psychiatric morbidity and treatment of prison inmates. *Journal of Forensic Sciences, J8,* 53–59.

Teplin, L. A., Abram, K. M., & McClelland, G. M. (1996). Prevalence of psychiatric disorders among incarcerated women. I: Pretrial jail detainees. *Archives of General Psychiatry, 53,* 505–512.

Turner, T. & Tofler, D. (1986). Indicators of psychiatric disorder in women admitted to prison. *British Journal of Medicine, 292,* 651–653.

Vaux, A., Burda, P., & Stewart, D. (1986). Orientation toward utilization of support resources. *Journal of Community Psychology, 14,* 159–170.

Ward, D. & Kassebaum, G. (1965). *Women's prison: Sex and social structure.* Chicago: Aldine.

Washington, P. & Diamond, R. J. (1985). Prevalence of mental illness among women incarcerated in five California county jails. *Research in Community and Mental Health, 5,* 33–41.

Wilson, J. S. & Leasure, R. (1991). Cruel and unusual punishment: The health care of women in prison. *Nurse Practitioner, 16,* 33–39.

World Health Organization. (1990). *Composite International Diagnostic Interview (CIDI).* Version 1.0. Geneva, Switzerland: World Health Organization.

Zimet, G., Dahlem, N., Zimet, S., & Farley, G. (1988). The Multidimensional Scale of Perceived Social Support. *Journal of Personality Assessment, 52,* 30–41.

Correlates of Recovery Among Older Adults After Major Abdominal Surgery

Margarete Lieb Zalon

Background: *Little research has examined the recovery patterns of older adults who have had major abdominal surgery.*

Objective: *To determine whether pain, depression, and fatigue are significant factors in the return of older adults who had major abdominal surgery to functional status and self-perception of recovery in the first 3 months after discharge from the hospital.*

Methods: *A correlational predictive study involved adults 60 years of age or older who had undergone major abdominal surgery. Data were collected during hospitalization (n = 192), then 3 to 5 days (n = 141), 1 month (n = 132), and 3 months after discharge to home (n = 126) using the Brief Pain Inventory, the Geriatric Depression Scale–Short Form, the Modified Fatigue Symptom Checklist, the Enforced Social Dependency Scale, and the Self-Perception of Recovery Scale.*

Results: *Multiple regression analysis indicated that pain, depression, and fatigue are significantly related to patients' self-perception of recovery and functional status. Pain, depression, and fatigue explain 13.4% of the variation in functional status at 3 to 5 days, 30.8% at 1 month, and 29.1% at 3 months after discharge. These three factors also explain 5.6% of the variation*

in self-perception of recovery during hospitalization, 12.3% at 3 to 5 days, 33.2% at 1 month, and 16.1% at 3 months after discharge.

Conclusions: *Pain, depression, and fatigue are important factors to consider in the provision of care to abdominal surgery patients with a relatively uncomplicated postoperative course. Specific interventions to reduce pain, depression, and fatigue need to be evaluated for their impact on the postoperative recovery of older adults.*

Key Words: *depression, fatigue, function recovery, pain, surgery.*

The leading complication of hospitalization for older patients is functional decline, which is associated with longer hospital stays, increased mortality, higher rates of institutionalization, greater need for rehabilitation and home care services, and higher costs (Inouye, Bogardus, Baker, Leo-Summers, & Cooney, 2000). Yet lengths of hospital stay for individuals 65 years of age or older decreased from 10 days in 1980 to 6 days in 2000 (National Center for Health Statistics, 2002, p. 253). Thus, nurses are responsible for facilitating patients' recovery in less time for an increasingly older population at greater risk for functional decline.

Nursing Research, 2004, Volume 53, Number 2, pages 99–106.

Considering nurses' greater accountability for nursing care, the nature of recovery from surgery needs to be examined. Research has demonstrated that pain, depression, and fatigue occur after joint arthroplasty and coronary artery bypass graft (CABG), and that they occur in relation to the functional status of older adults in residential care (Gallagher, Verma, & Mossey, 2000; Liao & Ferrell, 2000; Redeker, 1993). However, few studies have specifically examined pain, depression, and fatigue in relation to the recovery of older adults after their discharge to community after major abdominal surgery. The extent of inadequate postoperative pain relief after discharge is not known. Patients may limit activities because of pain, fatigue, and functional status. Depression may make the resumption of activities difficult after surgery, contributing to poorer outcomes. It is important to examine pain, depression, and fatigue together in relation to postoperative recovery because of their complex interrelations. Therefore, this study, using Levine's (1991) Conservation Model as a framework, aimed to describe the relation of pain, depression, and fatigue to recovery in older adults during the first 3 months after abdominal surgery.

Recovery from surgery is defined as improvement in functional status and the perception that one is recovering. In the context of Levine's (1991) Conservation Model, recovery is a return to wholeness that occurs by conservation of energy and restoration of integrity. Four conservation principles guide nursing practice: energy, structural integrity, personal integrity, and social integrity. Thus, when pain and depressive symptoms are decreased, energy is conserved, and when fatigue is decreased, more energy is available to the individual.

Acute pain depletes energy and generally indicates impaired structural integrity after surgery. Unrelieved pain is a persistent problem during hospitalization for surgery and after discharge (Devine et al., 1999; Moore, 1994; Redeker, 1993; Warfield & Kahn, 1995). Older patients are more likely to have persistent pain, to experience less relief from analgesics, and to use fewer analgesics (Lay, Puntillo, Miaskowski, & Wallhagen, 1996; MacIntyre & Jarvis, 1996). Pain is a concern for patients with abdominal aortic aneurysm and older surgical patients after discharge (Galloway, Rebeyka, Saxe-Braithwaite, Bubela, & McKibbon, 1997; McDonald, 1999). Elderly women restrict their movement to deal with postoperative pain (Zalon, 1997). Decreasing

movement places patients at risk for functional decline during hospitalization and after their return home.

None of the aforementioned studies examined the relation of pain to functional status in the first few months after discharge. Retirement center residents whose pain interfered with their lives rated their health as worse, were more likely to be depressed, and had lower physical functioning (Gallagher et al., 2000). Older adults discharged to community after surgery may be different because of their capabilities, and may have fewer formal services available to them. However, the research suggests that older adults, because they are more likely to have unrelieved or persistent pain after surgery, are at greater risk for its interference with function and thus delaying recovery.

Depression depletes the conservation of personal integrity. The prevalence of depression in late life is reported to be 15% (Mulsant & Ganguli, 1999). Its prevalence in older hospitalized patients ranges from 5% to 50% (Koenig, 1997; Pouget, Yersin, Wietlisbach, Bumand, & Bula, 2000). Surgery is an additional burden for older adults already at increased risk for depression, and may exacerbate the symptoms of those with some level of depression. Depression has been associated with lower functional status after colorectal cancer surgery, medical-surgical illness, and hip fracture repair (Barsevick, Pasacreta, & Orsi, 1995; Johnson, Kramer, Lin, Kowalsky, & Steiner, 2000; Mossey, Knott, & Craik, 1990), and with late mortality after CABG (Baker, Andrew, Schrader, & Knight, 2001). The relation between depression and functional status after major abdominal surgery may be similar to that associated with the other surgeries because of the surgery itself, or it may be different because of the meaning attributed to the underlying illness and expectations about recovery. Therefore, it is important to examine depression in relation to functional status in a broader population of older surgical patients.

Fatigue is a manifestation of limited energy resources (Levine, 1991, p. 7). Postoperative fatigue has been examined in the context of a stress response model and correlated with the degree of trauma, heart rate, and deteriorating nutritional status (Christensen & Kehlet, 1993). Physiologic studies of postoperative fatigue have used small samples, have measured different variables, and generally have not examined age or functional status. A meta-analysis of postoperative fatigue intervention studies indicates that increased analgesia is effective in reducing fatigue during the immediate postoperative period after abdominal surgery (Rubin

& Hotopf, 2002). However, 23 of 66 studies used fatigue measures untested for reliability and validity, and few examined functional status. Fatigue is prevalent after CABG and minimally invasive direct coronary artery bypass (Redeker, 1993; Zimmerman, Barnason, Brey, Catlin, & Nieveen, 2002). It has its most significant impact after hysterectomy during the first few months after surgery (DeCherney, Bachmann, Isaacson, & Gall, 2002). However, the cited study was a retrospective investigation of premenopausal women whose hormonal changes also may have contributed to their fatigue.

The most distressing symptoms after the discharge of patients who underwent abdominal aortic aneurysm repair are fatigue and sleep loss (Galloway et al., 1997). Abdominal surgery generally requires more time for return of bowel function, which may in turn have an impact on nutritional status and fatigue. It is not known to what extent postoperative fatigue is related to functional status or for how long. In analyzing physiologic studies, Westerblad and Allen (2002) concluded that central fatigue, referring to decreased central nervous system activation, may be more pronounced in the elderly. Liao and Ferrell (2000) found that depression, pain, number of medications, and a 3-minute walk predicted fatigue intensity among older adults in residential care, concluding that fatigue is poorly recognized and probably undertreated. Thus, older adults may be more vulnerable to the effects of postoperative fatigue on functional status. Therefore, the following research question was addressed: What is the relation of pain, depression, and fatigue to recovery, as measured by functional status and self-perception of recovery in older adults who have had major abdominal surgery?

RESEARCH DESIGN AND METHODS

Design

This study used a correlational, predictive design to measure the relation of pain, depression, and fatigue to functional status and self-perception of recovery during the first 3 months after discharge among abdominal surgery patients 60 years of age or older.

Sample

Patients 60 years of age or older who had undergone abdominal surgery were recruited from three community hospitals. The criteria for inclusion in the study required that the subjects be alert and ori-

ented, able to speak and read English, and accessible by telephone. Those who had laparoscopic surgery, neurologic dysfunction, a psychotic disorder, or surgery specifically for cancer were excluded.

Instruments

Pain. Pain was measured with the Brief Pain Inventory (BPI), which was developed originally to obtain data about the prevalence and severity of pain in the general population (Daut, Cleeland, & Flanery, 1983). The BPI uses numeric scales ranging from 0 (no pain) to 10 (pain as bad as you can imagine) to measure the severity of pain (worst, least, average, right now) and pain's interference with daily life (general activity, mood, walking, work, relationships with others, sleep, and enjoyment of life). Two items related to pain relief measures were not included in the regression analysis.

The BPI has been used widely in studies involving patients with cancer. Zalon (1999) demonstrated the reliability and validity of the BPI for use with surgical patients. The Cronbach alpha reliability coefficient for the current sample ranged from .90 to .95.

Depression. Depression was measured with the short form of the Geriatric Depression Scale (GDS-SF) (Sheikh & Yesavage, 1986). This 15-item yes/no checklist contains questions specifically related to geriatric depression. The GDS has been used widely with both community-dwelling elders and elderly people hospitalized for depression. The short form is correlated significantly with the long form ($r = .84; p \leq .001$) (Sheikh & Yesavage, 1986). The Cronbach alpha reliability coefficient for the current sample ranged from .61 to .77.

Fatigue. Fatigue was measured with the Modified Fatigue Symptom Checklist (MFSC) (Yoshitake, 1971) as modified by Pugh (1993). The MFSC has 30 items (e.g., "I feel my head is heavy;" "I feel tired in my legs") measuring fatigue from a multidimensional perspective in three subscales: drowsiness, concentration, and physical symptoms measured on a 4-point Likert scale. The reliability and validity of the MFSC has been established in different clinical populations including the elderly. In the current sample, the Cronbach alpha reliability coefficient ranged from .87 to .92.

Functional Status. Functional status was measured with the Enforced Social Dependency Scale (ESDS), which indicates how disease and its treatment influence patient responses by measuring the degree of assistance required to perform ordinary activities of daily living from the patient's perspective (Benoliel, McCorkle, & Young, 1980).

The ESDS consists of 10 items in two subscales: personal and social competence. The personal competence subscale evaluates dependence on others for eating, walking, dressing, traveling, bathing, and toileting on a 6-point scale. The social competence subscale consists of activities at home, work, and recreation evaluated on a 4-point scale, and communication evaluated on a 3-point scale.

The ESDS is administered as a semi-structured interview. Scores range from 10 to 51, with the higher scores indicating greater dependency. The ESDS has been used with elderly postoperative patients with cancer. The Cronbach alpha reliability coefficient for the current sample ranged from .69 to .80.

Self-Perception of Recovery after Surgery. Self-perception of recovery after surgery was measured by asking participants to indicate on a 0 to 100 numeric rating scale how much they had recovered from their surgery. A single-item scale rating health in general has been used widely by the National Center for Health Statistics (Ware, Nelson, Sherbourne, & Stewart, 1992). If a participant indicated that the answer was less than 10%, clarification was sought to make sure the scale was not being confused with a 0 to 10 rating scale.

Cognitive Status. The Mini-Mental State Examination (MMSE) (Folstein, Folstein, & McHugh, 1975) was used as a screening tool to assess cognitive status. The MMSE consists of 11 items assessing orientation, recall, registration, attention, calculation, language, and praxis. Scores range from 0 to 30, with a score less than 24 indicating cognitive impairment. Those with a score less than 24 were excluded from the study.

DEMOGRAPHIC AND MEDICAL RECORD DATA

Background data included age, gender, education, marital status, religion, race, ethnocultural identification, previous pain, previous pain medication experience, depression treatment, occupation, living arrangements, and household income. Related medical data included type of surgery, American Society of Anesthesiologists (ASA) score, type and length of anesthesia, pain ratings and analgesics ordered and administered for the 24 hours before the interview,

hematocrit, albumin, total protein, height, weight, length of stay, diagnostic related group, discharge medication, and activity restrictions.

Procedures

Institutional review board approval was obtained at each site. Data were collected in an initial face-to-face interview during hospitalization, and via telephone 3 to 5 days, 1 month, and 3 months after hospital discharge directly to a home setting.

Consents were obtained postoperatively, allowing for the inclusion of participants who had undergone emergency surgery. Potential participants were identified from surgical records. Nurses then were interviewed to determine whether the patients were medically unstable or whether they had experienced episodes of delirium in the preceding 24 hours.

Patients were approached about participation while resting comfortably. If patients consented, the BPI, GDS-SF, MFSC, and evaluation for self-perception of recovery were completed then or at another mutually agreeable time. Demographic and related chart data also were obtained at that time. Participants were given a copy of the consent form, tentative interview schedule, and contact information. A copy of the instruments was provided to decrease respondent burden. Reminders were sent before the 1- and 3-month interviews. Rehospitalized patients were not included in subsequent interviews. The following were administered during each telephone interview: BPI-SF, MFSC, GDS-SF, ESDS, and evaluation for self-perception of recovery after surgery. Research assistants received a standard orientation. The same data collector was used for the participants whenever possible.

Results

The sample consisted of 192 male and female patients 60 years of age or older recovering from abdominal surgery, who were then followed 3 months after discharge directly to a home setting. Initially, 295 persons met the criteria. Of these, 192 consented, 84 refused, and 19 were missed. Those who refused to participate were significantly older than those who consented (mean, 75 vs. 71.2 years; $t = 4.28$). The most common reasons for refusal were related to the person's perception of well-being (too sick, too depressed, not up to it, too weak) ($n = 15$) followed by a desire not to be bothered ($n = 6$). Two persons withdrew consent during the initial interview; 13 subsequently had a change

TABLE A3-1

Descriptive Data for Pain, Depression, Fatigue, Functional Status, and Self-Perception of Recovery

Scale	Initial Mean (SD)	3–5 Days Mean (SD)	1 Month Mean (SD)	3 Months Mean (SD)
Pain	39.93 (24.43)	20.86 (20.50)	11.79 (16.44)	8.76 (16.23)
Depression	2.97 (2.19)	3.27 (1.88)	2.17 (2.20)	1.79 (2.28)
Fatigue	47.58 (13.83)	41.45 (9.49)	39.18 (9.42)	38.42 (9.13)
Functional Status	—	30.82 (5.07)	20.17 (5.63)	13.84 (3.88)
Self-Perception of Recovery	57.03 (23.30)	65.60 (19.69)	81.45 (18.63)	92.30 (12.57)

in discharge plans from home to another type of healthcare facility; 10 did not want to be bothered after discharge; 4 stated that they were "too sick"; 1 could not be reached; and 1 died. The remainder did not provide a reason. Eleven of the individuals were rehospitalized.

The age of participants ranged from 60 to 87 years ($SD = 6.8$). The sample was 46.9% male and 99.5% non-Hispanic White. The majority had at least a high school education. Specifically, 32.6% had one or more years of post-secondary education; 48.1% had completed high school; and 19.3% had not finished high school.

The most common type of surgery was abdominal aortic aneurysm repair (26.6%), followed by colon resection (22.4%), cholecystectomy (18.2%), appendectomy (5.7%), and abdominal hysterectomy (3.6%), with the remaining 20.3% categorized as "other." The average length of hospital stay was 9.6 days for the patients who initially enrolled in the study and 8.3 days for those who completed the 3-month interview. On the average, the initial interview was conducted on postoperative day 5 ($SD = 2.2$ days). The patients were categorized as retirees (79.5%), employed workers (16.8%), homemakers (2.6%), or unemployed individuals (1.1%). The majority of the participants were married (59.4%), followed by those who were widowed (24.1%), then by those who were single, divorced, or separated (16.3%). Those living alone comprised 29.5% of the sample.

The presence of a chronic painful condition was reported by more than half of the participants (59.2%), and this was most commonly arthritis.

Home care services were received by 32.9% of the participants.

The means for the BPI and MFSC decreased over time, and there was a concomitant decrease in the standard deviations, indicating that pain and fatigue decreased over time, and that there was less variance in the sample at 3 months after discharge (Table 1). Depression scores were increased at the 3- to 5-day interval, and subsequently decreased. The ESDS scores declined, indicating an improvement in functional status.

The participants' perception of how much they recovered increased over time from a mean of 57% recovered from surgery while in the hospital to a mean of 92.3% recovered from surgery at 3 months after discharge. The correlation between pain and depression was significant at each time point, ranging from .26 to .37, with the highest correlation for the initial measurement (Table 2). Pain and fatigue were significantly correlated at each time interval, ranging from 0.22 to 0.52. Fatigue and depression were highly correlated at each time interval, with the correlations ranging from 0.51 to 0.60. Functional status and self-perception of recovery were significantly correlated at 1 and 3 months.

The results of the multiple regression analysis with the variables entered at once indicate that pain, depression, and fatigue significantly accounted for 13.4% of the variation in functional status during the immediate postoperative period (3–5 days after discharge) (Table 3). The primary contribution to the variation in functional status during this period was depression. At 1 month after discharge, pain, depression, and

TABLE A3-2

Correlation Matrix for Study Variables at Each Time Interval

	1	2	3	4	5
Initial (Hospitalization)	—	.37**	.52**	—	−.20**
1. Pain		—	.53**	—	−.09
2. Depression			—	—	—
3. Fatigue				—	—
4. Functional Status					—
5. Self-Perception of Recovery					
3–5 Days Post-Discharge					
1. Pain	—	.27**	.39**	.12	−.25**
2. Depression		—	.60**	.36**	−.28**
3. Fatigue			—	.26**	−.13
4. Functional Status				—	−.09
5. Self-Perception of Recovery					—
One Month Post-Discharge					
1. Pain	—	.33**	.22**	.33**	−.44**
2. Depression		—	.51**	.50**	−.50**
3. Fatigue			—	.42**	−.32**
4. Functional Status				—	−.50**
5. Self-Perception of Recovery					—
Three Months Post-Discharge					
1. Pain	—	.26**	.50**	.39**	−.24**
2. Depression		—	.54**	.43**	−.35**
3. Fatigue			—	.46**	−.34**
4. Functional Status				—	−.53**
5. Self-Perception of Recovery					—

$**p < .01$

fatigue accounted for 30.8% of the variation in functional status. Pain, depression, and fatigue were significant contributors to the variation in functional status at 1 month. At 3 months after discharge, pain, depression, and fatigue significantly accounted for 29.1% of the variation in functional status. Pain, depression, and fatigue each made significant contributions to the variation in functional status at 3 months after discharge.

The results of the multiple regression analysis with the variables entered at once indicate that pain, depression, and fatigue significantly accounted for 5.6% of the variation in self-perception of recovery at the initial measurement during hospitalization (Table 3). None of the variables (pain, depression, or fatigue) alone contributed significantly to self-perception of recovery initially. At 3 to 5 days after discharge, pain, depression, and fatigue significantly accounted for 12.3% of the

variation in self-perception of recovery (Table 3). Pain and depression made significant contributions to the variation in self-perception of recovery 3 to 5 days after discharge. At 1 month after discharge, pain, depression, and fatigue significantly accounted for 33.2% of the variation in self-perception of recovery. Depression and pain made significant contributions to the variation in self-perception of recovery at 1 month. At 3 months after discharge, pain, depression, and fatigue significantly accounted for 16.1% of the variation in self-perception of recovery (Table 3). Depression alone made a significant contribution to the variation in self-perception of recovery at 3 months after discharge. Diagnostics conducted for each of the multiple regression analyses indicated that multicollinearity was not a problem.

Pain medication was taken by 76.9% of the participants in the 24 hours before the hospital interview,

TABLE A3-3

Regressions of Pain, Fatigue, and Depression in Functional Status and Self-Perception of Recovery

n Dependent Variables	Independent Variables	169 Initial B	137 3–5 Days B	131 1 Month B	126 3 Month B
Functional Status					
	Pain		.001	.06*	.05*
	Depression		.85**	.84***	.44**
	Fatigue		.04	.13*	.09*
F			6.94***	18.82***	16.69***
R²			.134	.308	.291
Self-Perception of Recovery					
	Pain	−.15	−.22*	−.35***	−.08
	Depression	.79	−3.23**	−3.01***	−1.31*
	Fatigue	−.25	.31	−.13	−.22
F		3.28*	6.24**	21.06***	7.83***
R²		.056	.123	.332	.161

*$p < .05$, **$p < .01$, ***$p < .0001$

by 53.2% before the 3- to 5-day interview, by 28% 24 hours before the 1-month interview, and by 22% 24 hours before the 3-month interview. Fatigue in the hospital was not significantly correlated with hematocrit, albumin, or total protein.

Discussion

The results of this study demonstrate that pain, depression, and fatigue are significantly related to functional status as well as self-perception of recovery in older postoperative abdominal surgery patients. The findings are consistent with the Conservation of Energy Model (Levine, 1991, p. 7), in which it is hypothesized that pain and depression have effects on energy and on structural, personal and social integrity; that fatigue is a manifestation of energy depletion; and that together they are related to a return to wholeness or functional status.

The results of this investigation are consistent with those of others addressing functional status and illness from a more global perspective as well as findings of studies focusing on patients undergoing specific surgical procedures in that pain, depression, and fatigue were related to functional status at all three data collection times: 3 to 5 days, 1 month, and 3 months after

discharge. This indicates that interventions to address pain, depression, and fatigue are important regardless of the reason for hospitalization.

The lower contribution of pain, depression, and fatigue to the variation in functional status 3 to 5 days after discharge may reflect homogeneity of patients during the first few days after discharge. Surgical patients in general may experience a lower functional status regardless whether they have pain, fatigue, or depressive symptoms.

The proportion of variation explained by pain, depression, and fatigue 1 and 3 months after discharge highlights the importance of factors that have the potential for effective treatment during the postoperative period. Although pain contributed to the variation in functional status at 1 and 3 months, it should be noted that a number of participants reported that their pain at 3 months was not related to the incision or surgery, but rather to a chronic painful condition. Thus, patients with chronic painful conditions need to have their pain managed well to maximize their recovery from surgery. Individuals with chronic pain are more likely to have a subthreshold or major depression (Gallagher et al., 2000). The findings highlight the need to address not only the management of acute postoperative pain, but also chronic painful conditions to enhance the return of postoperative patients to their previous functional status.

Home care reimbursement has been limited in recent years. This is evident in that only one third of the study participants received home care services. Therefore, strategies to facilitate effective pain management after discharge, including the management of chronic pain, need to be addressed in the acute care setting.

The sample in this study consisted of patients discharged directly to their home, indicating either a higher level of functioning at discharge or a stronger support system than abdominal surgery patients as a whole enjoy. Despite this, depression made a significant contribution to functional status at each time point, indicating that the emotional component of postoperative recovery may be critical to the successful return of patients to their previous functional status.

Although fatigue contributed to the variation in both regression models, the t for fatigue was significant only in the functional status model 1 and 3 months after discharge. This may be related to the measurement of fatigue. Inclusion of ratings for the degree of fatigue and the degree of fatigue's interference with daily activities would provide more information and more direction for nursing interventions.

Pain and depression contribute to functional loss in older persons, which may be exacerbated when surgery is needed. Postoperative interventions have been standardized for patients undergoing certain types of surgeries with high volumes such as CABG or joint replacement. They are less likely to be standardized for low-volume surgeries. As such, there may not be the same impetus for attention to specific outcomes for these patients. It has been demonstrated that nursing interventions can make a difference in physical functioning and distress after CABG and ambulatory surgery (Ai, Dunkle, Peterson, Saunders, & Bolling, 1998; Moore & Dolansky, 2001; Swan, 1998).

The significant relation of pain, depression, and fatigue to self-perception of recovery in older adults indicates that healthcare providers need to consider their patients' perspective and their involvement in specific postoperative care regimens. Self-perception of recovery may be closely related to self-rated health, although research is needed to determine whether they are the same or conceptually distinct phenomena.

Pain contributed to the variance in self-perception of recovery. Therefore, institution of appropriate pain relief measures in the postoperative period, particularly in the first month after discharge, is important. Correcting misconceptions about pain medication and teaching patients about the importance of taking medication would facilitate the resumption of daily activities. Only 53.2% of the participants took pain medication in the 24 hours before the 3- to 5-day postdischarge interview. Efforts to improve pain management for patients who have chronic pain by incorporating an existing pain management regimen into the postoperative pain management protocol are suggested.

The group investigated in this study was not a random sample of abdominal surgery patients. Patients not discharged directly to a home setting were excluded. Some patients who declined participation or dropped out of the study indicated that they were "too sick" to participate. It is possible in the investigation of unpleasant symptoms that a greater number of individuals experiencing extreme distress are not included. Thus, the participants in this study may have been relatively well as compared with abdominal surgery patients in general. Increasingly, patients are being transferred to rehabilitation facilities, skilled nursing facilities, and personal care homes before they return home. It is likely, but not known, that these particular subsets of patients have more extended postoperative recoveries.

A limitation of this study is that baseline data were not available because the participants did not complete the instruments preoperatively. Therefore, additional research including baseline data is recommended to describe the impact of surgery on recovery. The close relation of pain, depression, and fatigue to functional status indicates that a multifaceted approach including psychosocial interventions has the potential to enhance the recovery of older patients after major surgery.

References

Ai, A. L., Dunkle, R. E., Peterson, C., Saunders, D. G., Bolling, A. F. (1998). Self-care and psychosocial adjustment of patients following cardiac surgery. *Social Work in Health Care, 27,* 75–95.

Baker, R. A., Andrew, M. J., Schrader, G., & Knight, L. (2001). Preoperative depression and mortality in coronary artery bypass surgery: Preliminary findings. *Australia New Zealand Journal of Surgery, 71,* 139–142.

Barsevick, A. M., Pasacreta, J., & Orsi, A. (1995). Psychological distress and functional dependency in colorectal cancer patients. *Cancer Practice, 3,* 105–110.

Benoliel, J. Q., McCorkle, R., & Young, K. (1980). Development of a social dependency scale. *Research in Nursing and Health, 3,* 3–10.

Christensen, T. & Kehlet, H. (1993). Postoperative fatigue. *World Journal of Surgery, 17,* 220–225.

Daut, R. L., Cleeland, C. S., & Flanery, R. C. (1983). Development of the Wisconsin Brief Pain Questionnaire to assess pain in cancer and other diseases. *Pain, 17,* 197–210.

DeCherney, A. H., Bachmann, G., Isaacson, K., & Gall, S. (2002). Postoperative fatigue negatively impacts the daily lives of those recovering from hysterectomy. *Obstetrics and Gynecology, 99,* 51–57.

Devine, E. C., Bevsek, S. A., Brubakken, K., Johnson, B. P., Ryan, P., Sliefert, M. K., et al. (1999). AHCPR clinical practice guideline on surgical pain management: Adoption and outcomes. *Research in Nursing & Health, 22,* 119–130.

Folstein, M. F., Folstein, S. E., & McHugh, P. R. (1975). "Mini-Mental State": A practical method for grading the cognitive state for the clinician. *Journal of Psychiatric Research, 12,* 189–198.

Gallagher, R. M., Verma, S., & Mossey, J. (2000). Chronic pain: Sources of late-life pain and risk factors for disability. *Geriatrics, 55*(9), 40–44, 47.

Galloway, S. C., Rebeyka, D., Saxe-Braithwaite, M., Bubela, N., & McKibbon, A. (1997). Discharge information needs and symptom distress after abdominal aortic surgery. *Canadian Journal of Cardiovascular Nursing, 8*(3), 9–15.

Inouye, S. K., Bogardus, S. T., Baker, D. I., Leo-Summers, L., & Cooney, L. M. (2000). The Hospital Elder Life Program: A model of care to prevent cognitive and functional decline in older hospitalized patients. *Journal of the American Geriatrics Society, 48,* 1697–1706.

Johnson, M. F., Kramer, A. M., Lin, M. K., Kowalsky, J. C., & Steiner, J. F. (2000). Outcomes of older persons receiving rehabilitation for medical and surgical conditions compared with hip fracture and stroke. *Journal of the American Geriatrics Society, 48,* 1389–1397.

Koenig, H. G. (1997). Differences in psychosocial and health correlates of major and minor depression in medically ill older adults. *Journal of the American Geriatrics Society, 45,* 1487–1495.

Lay, T. D., Puntillo, K. A., Miaskowski, C. A., & Wallhagen, M. I. (1996). Analgesics prescribed and administered to intensive care cardiac surgery patients: Does patient age make a difference? *Progress in Cardiovascular Nursing, 11*(4), 17–24.

Levine, M. E. (1991). The conservation principles: A model for health. In K. M. Shaefer & J. B. Pond (Eds.), *Levine's conservation model: A framework for practice* (pp. 1–11). Philadelphia: F. A. Davis.

Liao, S. & Ferrell, B. A. (2000). Fatigue in an older population. *Journal of the American Geriatrics Society, 48,* 426–430.

MacIntyre, P. E. & Jarvis, D. A. (1996). Age is the best predictor of postoperative morphine requirements. *Pain, 64,* 357–364.

McDonald, D. D. (1999). Postoperative pain after discharge. *Clinical Nursing Research, 8,* 355–367.

Moore, S. M. (1994). Development of discharge information for recovery after coronary artery bypass surgery. *Applied Nursing Research, 7,* 170–177.

Moore, S. M. & Dolansky, M. A. (2001). Randomized trial of a home recovery intervention following coronary artery bypass surgery. *Research in Nursing & Health, 24,* 93–104.

Mossey, J. M., Knott, K., & Craik, R. (1990). The effects of persistent depressive symptoms on hip fracture recovery. *Journal of Gerontology, 45,* M163–M168.

Mulsant, B. H. & Ganguli, M. (1999). Epidemiology and diagnosis of depression in late life. *Journal of Clinical Psychiatry, 60*(Suppl 20), 9–15.

National Center for Health Statistics. (2002). *Health, United States, 2002 with chartbook on trends in the health of Americans.* Hyattsville, MD: Author.

Pouget, R., Yersin, B., Wietlisbach, V., Bumand, B., & Bula, C. J. (2000). Depressed mood in a cohort of elderly medical inpatients: Prevalence, clinical correlates, and recognition rate. *Aging (Milano), 12,* 301–307.

Pugh, L. C. (1993). Childbirth and the measurement of fatigue. *Journal of Nursing Measurement, 1,* 57–66.

Redeker, N. S. (1993). Symptoms reported by older and middle-aged adults after coronary bypass surgery. *Clinical Nursing Research, 2,* 148–159.

Rubin, G. J. & Hotopf, M. (2002). Systematic review and meta-analysis of interventions for postoperative fatigue. *British Journal of Surgery, 89,* 971–984.

Sheikh, J. I. & Yesavage, J. A. (1986). Geriatric Depression Scale (GDS): Recent evidence and development of a shorter version. *Clinical Gerontologist, 5,* 166–173.

Swan, B. A. (1998). Postoperative nursing care contributions to symptom distress and functional status after ambulatory surgery. *Medsurg Nursing, 7,* 148–151, 154–158.

Ware, J. E., Nelson, E. C., Sherbourne, C. D., & Stewart, A. L. (1992). Preliminary tests of a 6-item general health survey: A patient application. In A. L. Stewart & J. E. Ware (Eds.), *Measuring functioning and well-being: The medical outcomes study approach* (pp. 291–303). Durham, NC: Duke University.

Warfield, C. A. & Kahn, C. H. (1995). Acute pain management: Programs in U.S. hospitals and experiences and attitudes among U.S. adults. *Anesthesiology, 83,* 1090–1094.

Westerblad, H. & Allen, D. G. (2002). Recent advances in the understanding of skeletal muscle fatigue. *Current Opinion in Rheumatology, 14,* 648–652.

Yoshitake, H. (1971). Relations between the symptoms and the feeling of fatigue. *Ergonomics, 14,* 175–186.

Zalon, M. L. (1997). Pain in frail, elderly women after surgery. *Image: Journal of Nursing Scholarship, 29,* 21–26.

Zalon, M. L. (1999). Comparison of pain measures in surgical patients. *Journal of Nursing Measurement, 7,* 135–152.

Zimmerman, L., Barnason, S., Brey, B. A., Catlin, S. S., & Nieveen, J. (2002). Comparison of recovery patterns for patients undergoing coronary artery bypass grafting and minimally invasive direct coronary artery bypass in the early discharge period. *Progress in Cardiovascular Nursing, 17,* 132–141.

Evolution of the Caregiving Experience in the Initial 2 Years Following Stroke

Carole L. White, Nancy Mayo, James A. Hanley, Sharon Wood-Dauphinee

Abstract: *Relationships between stroke survivor and family caregiver factors and the caregiver's health-related quality of life (HRQL) and overall quality of life (QoL) were examined in 97 dyads during the first and second years after stroke. Compared to age- and sex-matched population norms, caregivers scored significantly lower on the mental subscales of HRQL, and differences were greater for women than for men. Caregiver characteristics (older age, less burden, and fewer physical symptoms) were associated with better HRQL (mental summary scale) in the first year, with similar findings in the second year. Moderate stroke survivor physical impairment and caregiver characteristics (younger age and better HRQL) were associated with better QoL in the first year. During the second year poorer caregiver physical and mental health and caring for a stroke survivor with communication difficulties were associated with diminished QoL.*

Key Words: family caregiver, quality of life, health-related quality of life, stroke.

At least 50% of stroke survivors have some degree of disability or other sequelae of stroke. Even so, the majority will return to live in the community (Hochstenbach, Donders, Mulder, Van Limbeek, & Schoonderwaldt, 1996; Mayo, Wood-Dauphinee, Côté, Durcan, & Carlton, 2002). This positive outcome is achieved largely through the assistance provided by informal care providers, most of whom are family members (R. Anderson, 1992). Previous researchers have demonstrated, however, that the provision of this care is not without negative consequences for the caregiver (Han & Haley, 1999; Low, Payne, & Roderick, 1999). The prevalence of emotional disorders among caregivers, including depression and anxiety, has been studied most frequently and has been estimated to range from 20% to 55% (C. S. Anderson, Linto, & Stewart-Wynne, 1995; Carnwath & Johnson, 1987; Dennis, O'Rourke, Lewis, Sharpe, & Warlow, 1998; Wade, Legh-Smith, & Hewer, 1986). Fewer researchers have examined the impact on the caregiver's physical health. In these studies caregivers have reported a decline in physical health and an increase in physical strain and fatigue since undertaking the caregiving role (Greveson, Gray, French, & James 1991; Silliman, Fletcher, Earp, & Wagner, 1986).

Research in Nursing & Health, 2003, Volume 26, pages 177–189

The almost exclusive focus on the emotional consequences has limited the understanding of family caregiving for stroke survivors. Increased attention to other effects, including social, physical, and overall quality of life (QoL), will contribute to a more comprehensive representation of the caregiving role (Low et al., 1999). Furthermore, the majority of studies have been cross-sectional, thereby limiting the understanding of the evolution of the caregiving role. The functional recovery of the stroke survivor that takes place over time and the caregiver's responses over time suggest that time is an important variable that must be considered in the design, analysis, and interpretation of the results of caregiving studies. The purpose of this study, therefore, was to describe the health-related quality of life (HRQL) and overall QoL of family caregivers in the initial 2 years following stroke and to examine the impact of stroke survivor and caregiver characteristics on HRQL and QoL. Clarification of the dynamic relationship between the caregiver and the stroke survivor and of the impact of the caregiving experience on the caregiver's HRQL and QoL may provide researchers with needed information for the design and testing of interventions for family caregivers (Han & Haley, 1999).

HRQL encompasses the physical, emotional, and social domains. This construct has been defined as "the value assigned to duration of life as modified by the impairment, functional states, perceptions, and social opportunities that are influenced by disease, injury, treatment or policy" (Patrick & Erickson, 1993; page 22). Although there is growing recognition among health care researchers of the importance of measuring HRQL, this perspective has been addressed in few studies of family caregiving. Even in those studies that examined aspects of physical or social health, nonstandardized measures were often used (Low et al., 1999). More comprehensive than HRQL is the concept of overall QoL, defined as "individuals' perception of their position in life in the context of the culture and value systems in which they live and in relation to their goals, expectations, standards, and concerns" (The WHOQOL Group, 1995, page 1405). Although HRQL and QoL have often been used interchangeably, they are two distinct constructs (Smith, Avis, & Assmann, 1999). Health, as defined by the individual, has been recognized as an important component of overall QoL (Flanagan, 1978; Smith et al., 1999). QoL in some cases may refer to the notion of health, but it encompasses much more than health, particularly because individuals consider other aspects of their lives when assessing their overall QoL. QoL is subjective, reflects the balance of positive and negative effects, and is multidimensional. These characteristics make QoL a particularly relevant outcome for the study of family caregiving.

Few longitudinal studies of stroke caregiving have been done, thereby limiting the understanding of the evolution of the caregiving experience (Han & Haley, 1999). A period of high initial stress followed by a reduction in stress over time has been hypothesized as a likely pattern for caregivers of those sustaining a disease with a sudden onset, such as a stroke (Biegel, Sales, & Schulz, 1991; Seltzer & Li, 1996). However, findings from the available longitudinal research suggest several contrasting patterns.

Brocklehurst, Morris, Andrews, Richards, and Laycock (1981) interviewed 97 caregivers from 4 to 6 weeks after the patient's stroke and at regular intervals thereafter for 1 year. During this time there was a considerable increase in the proportion of caregivers who reported their health as poor (10% to 28%). Without a comparison group, however, it is impossible to determine in a group of caregivers most of whom are more than 60 years old, how much of this change could be attributed to caregiving and how much to the normal aging process.

Wade et al. (1986) assessed psychiatric morbidity in caregivers at 3 weeks, 6 months, and 1 and 2 years after the patient's stroke. Two different trajectories were reported: little change over time; and initial high distress decreasing and thereafter remaining stable. The pattern varied according to the outcome measure used. Stability over time was the pattern suggested by the scores on the Wakefield Depression Inventory (Snaith, Ahmed, Mehta, & Hamilton, 1971) with about 20% scoring depressed or probably depressed at each interview. In contrast, the percentage of caregivers with abnormal scores on the second measure of psychiatric morbidity, the General Health Questionnaire (Goldberg & Hillier, 1979), decreased from 21% at 3 weeks to 12% at 6 months and thereafter remained at this level. Although the Wakefield Depression Inventory focuses on depression, the General Health Questionnaire covers four elements of distress including anxiety. Understandably, anxiety may be more prevalent in the early weeks following the stroke.

Finally, the data from several other studies of caregivers of stroke survivors suggest a pattern of stability for the group over time, with little change in health outcomes, including psychological morbidity and HRQL, over the first 6 months (Bugge, Alexander, & Hagen, 1999; Schulz, Tompkins, & Rau, 1988; Teel, Duncan, & Lai, 2001) and the first year (Hodgson, Wood, & Langton-Hewer, 1996) of caregiving. Although Hodgson et al. reported little change in mean well-being for the group, examination of individual scores revealed that about half the caregivers experienced a decrease in well-being between 3 and 12 months of caregiving. This suggests that examination of subgroups, such as those stratified by gender, may reveal important information. Although gender discrepancies in caregiver psychological outcomes have been noted previously (Yee & Schulz, 2000), most studies have been cross-sectional, and the scores have not been compared to a noncaregiving group or to population norms. As a result, the differential effects of caregiving over time are not clear.

To summarize, although the results from these studies suggest a pattern of stability over time for the group, several researchers reported considerable within-person variability, with some individuals improving over time and others reporting decreased health. It is important to examine subgroups and to identify those individuals who may be at risk for negative consequences, such as diminished HRQL and overall QoL. To further advance our understanding of family caregiving for stroke survivors, it is also important to examine the impact of caregiving over a longer period of time. With one exception (Wade et al., 1986), the follow-up in these studies has been limited to the first year or less following stroke. Given the incomplete recovery from stroke for at least 50% of stroke survivors (Thorngren, Westling, & Norrving, 1990), caregiving will likely continue indefinitely, and it may take longer for a chronic stressor such as caregiving to declare itself.

To characterize the evolution of the caregiving experience over the initial 2 years of caregiving, the following specific objectives were addressed: (a) to describe caregiver characteristics (physical health symptoms, burden, HRQL, and overall QoL) in the first and second years of caregiving; (b) to compare the caregiver's HRQL in the first and second years of caregiving to age- and sex-adjusted population norms; (c) to examine the impact of stroke survivor characteristics (physical and communication disabilities) and caregiver characteristics (age, gender, kin relationship to stroke survivor, physical health symptoms, and burden) on HRQL; and (d) to examine the impact of stroke survivor characteristics (physical and communication disabilities) and caregiver characteristics (age, gender, kin relationship to stroke survivor, physical health symptoms, burden, and HRQL) on overall QoL.

METHODS

Sample

The study reported here is derived from the Montreal Cohort Study (Mayo et al., 2002). The focus of the parent study was to examine the long-term impact of stroke on individuals experiencing stroke. This study examines the evolution of the stroke caregiving experience over a 2-year period on a subset of data generated by the caregivers. Caregivers were recruited into the parent study only if stroke survivors were unable to provide study data independently. Caregivers then provided the requested information regarding the stroke survivor and also were asked to provide important information about themselves as caregivers.

To be concordant with the objectives of the present study, only those caregivers interviewed in both the first and second years of their caregiving role, a subset of the total sample of 181 caregivers, were eligible for participation. There were 75 caregivers who underwent only one interview and were not included in these analyses. Reasons for undergoing only one interview were: caregiver recruited only in the second year following stroke ($n = 5$), stroke survivor admitted to a long-term care institution prior to a second interview ($n = 8$), individual with stroke died prior to a second interview ($n = 10$), and caregiver refused follow-up after the initial interview ($n = 52$). Reasons for refusing further follow-up were: (a) near-normal to normal recovery of stroke survivor, and caregiver stated that she/he was no longer in a caregiving role ($n = 34$), and (b) caregiver reported being too busy in the role to respond to the interview ($n = 3$). Reasons were unknown for 15 caregivers. From this group of 106 caregivers who underwent two interviews, caregivers were further excluded from these analyses for the following reasons: paid for being a caregiver ($n = 5$), and two caregivers for the same stroke survivor completed the interviews

($n = 4$). This left 97 caregiver/stroke survivor dyads, who comprised the sample for this study.

To assess the potential bias in excluding those who underwent one interview only, this group was compared to the study sample. There were no significant differences on baseline characteristics (age, gender, living arrangements, education, kin relationship to person with stroke) between the group of caregivers who completed 2 years of follow-up and those who underwent only one interview ($p > .05$).

As seen in Table 1, most caregivers in this sample were women. They were more likely to be spouses than adult children or other relatives. The majority lived with the care recipient. About one-third of caregivers were currently employed. The most frequently reported prevalent health conditions were arthritis and hypertension. In comparison with the general Canadian population, however, the rates among this group of caregivers were lower for arthritis (34% versus 30%) and hypertension (35% versus 25%; Statistics Canada, 1999).

Stroke survivors were older on average than the caregivers. As indicated by the scores on the Barthel Index (Granger, Dewis, Peters, Sherwood, & Barrett, 1979), which measures physical function, the majority of stroke survivors required assistance with activities of daily living in the first year following stroke. The prevalence of comorbid conditions was high in these stroke survivors.

Procedures

The study was approved by the research ethics committees of the participating hospitals. Informed consent was provided by all caregivers.

TABLE A4-1

Baseline Characteristics of Participants ($n = 97$)

Characteristic	Caregivers	Stroke Survivors
Age: *M (SD)*	56.8 (15.3)	73.6 (11.2)
Female (%)	77.3	42.3
Barthel index (%)		
≤60		30.4
>60 and ≤90		31.5
>90 to 100		38.0
Communication problems (%)		38.1
Destination from acute care (%)		
Directly home		34.0
Rehabilitation and home		63.9
Transfer and home		2.1
Relationship to stroke survivor (%)		
Spouse	60.0	
Adult child	38.0	
Other	2.0	
Live in same house with stroke survivor (%)	86.6	
Employed (%)	31.0	
Prevalent health problems (%)		
Hypertension	24.7	53.7
Arthritis	30.0	46.3
Cataracts	7.2	29.3
Bronchitis	17.5	24.4
Angina	9.3	22.0
History of myocardial infarction	4.1	20.7
Diabetes	10.3	20.7
Asthma	3.1	14.6
Ulcer disease	4.1	11.0

During their hospitalization for stroke, patients and their caregivers were provided with information about the study. Informed consent was obtained while in the hospital or shortly after discharge. All consenting stroke survivors and their caregivers were contacted by telephone following discharge, either straight from the acute care hospital or following inpatient rehabilitation, to arrange for the follow-up interviews. All follow-up interviews were conducted by telephone at a time convenient for the stroke survivor or caregiver. The initial interview was planned for 6 months following stroke; however, because of difficulty scheduling interviews, the average time between the stroke and the first interview was 7 months. Caregivers also were interviewed in the second year following stroke, on average, 23 months after the stroke.

The feasibility of telephone interviews was demonstrated in a recent study designed to obtain information about stroke survivors and their caregivers (Christopher, 1999). Telephone interviews were found to provide information comparable to that received from face-to-face interviews (Korner-Bitensky, 1994). The interviews were completed by health professionals who underwent specific training to improve the reliability of the interviewing process. Interviews averaged 30–45 min.

All information that was reported for the present study was provided by the caregivers. The stroke survivors were unable to respond, necessitating the recruitment of the caregivers to provide the information, for several reasons: communication problems related to aphasia or dysarthria, cognitive impairment, being too frail to complete interviews, and inability to communicate in English or French. In addition to information that the caregivers provided about themselves and their caregiving role, they provided the information about the stroke survivors. Several researchers have examined patient-proxy responses related to health and functional status and have consistently demonstrated that proxies tend to underestimate health status (Knapp & Hewison, 1999). Proxy ratings appear to be more accurate, however, when the information sought is concrete and observable (Knapp & Hewison, 1999; Pierre, Wood-Dauphinee, Korner-Bitensky, Gayton, & Hanley, 1998). Because of the discrepancies involved in using proxy responses, particularly with measures assessing emotional responses, each caregiver provided information only on demographic characteristics, the presence of comorbid conditions, and the functional status of the stroke survivor.

Measures

Stroke Survivors. The caregivers provided information on whether the persons with stroke had sustained a communication disability (yes/no). To assess a stroke survivor's functional status, a caregiver completed the Barthel Index (Granger et al., 1979), a measure of basic activities of daily living. This scale measures three categories of function: self-care, continence of bowel and bladder, and mobility. It comprises 10 items, and the score can range from 0 to 100. Internal consistency reliability in a sample of 258 stroke patients ranged from 0.87 to 0.92 (Shah, Vanclay, & Cooper, 1989), and in this study Cronbach's alpha was 0.93. Predictive validity has been reported for survival, functional recovery, and discharge disposition (Roy, Togneri, Hay, & Pentland, 1988). Guidelines have been proposed for interpreting the scores. A score of 60 or less suggests severe dependency; 61–90, moderate dependence; and above 90, slight dependence to independence (Shah et al., 1989). A proxy respondent can provide the information.

Caregivers. To measure the presence of physical symptoms, caregivers completed a checklist (yes/no) of 24 physical symptoms that they might have experienced over the past 30 days (Aday & Andersen, 1975). The checklist has been used in several studies assessing access to health care (Shapiro, Ware, & Sherbourne, 1986) and includes physical symptoms that account for a large proportion of self-initiated medical ambulatory visits in the United States. Items include those that assess "minor" symptoms, such as coughing, fatigue, and headache, and "serious" symptoms, such as weight loss, diarrhea, and chest pain (Shapiro et al., 1986). The unweighted number of symptoms has been found to correlate highly ($r = .95$) with the weighted version (Baumgarten et al., 1992), so the unweighted number of symptoms present was used in this study.

To estimate the stress associated with caregiving, caregivers completed the Burden Index (Zarit, Reever, & Bach-Peterson, 1980; Zarit, Todd, & Zarit, 1986). This 22-item measure, designed to assess feelings of anger, frustration, and stress as well as the burden of being a caregiver, has been used frequently with caregivers of persons who are mentally or physically impaired. Caregivers are asked to rate how often they feel the way described in each question, from 0 *(never)* to 4 *(nearly always)*. A total burden score is calculated, with higher scores indicating more burden. The Burden Index has high internal consistency ($\alpha = .91$) and fair test-retest reliability ($r = .71$; Vitaliano, Young, & Russo, 1991). Support for its construct validity has been suggested by its negative association with morale and its positive association with hours spent caregiving (Pratt, Schmall, & Wright, 1986). Although the Burden Index was originally developed for caregivers of the demented elderly, and it has been used with caregivers of the demented elderly, it has been used with caregivers of those with stroke (Christopher, 1999; Reese, Gross, Smalley, & Messer, 1994), and in the present study internal consistency was high ($\alpha = .89$).

HRQL was measured using the Medical Outcome Study 36-Item Short Form Health Survey (SF-36) (Ware & Sherbourne, 1992). The well-known SF-36 is a generic scale of perceived health status that includes eight multi-item scales measuring physical functioning, role limitations because of physical health problems, bodily pain, general health perceptions, vitality, social functioning, role limitations resulting from emotional problems, and mental health. The items on the SF-36 subscales do not provide a total score but can be aggregated into a mental component summary (MCS) scale and a physical component summary (PCS) scale (Ware, Kosinski, & Keller, 1994). These summary scales are standardized to have a mean of 50 and a standard deviation (*SD*) of 10. To decrease the number of outcomes, the two summary scales were used as dependent variables in this study. The SF-36 has been used with a variety of populations, including family caregivers of stroke survivors (Bugge et al., 1999). Internal consistency reliability has been extensively demonstrated ($\alpha = $ .73–.96; Brazier et al., 1992; McHorney, Ware, Lu, & Sherbourne, 1994) as has test-retest reliability (ICC = .76–.93; Ruta, Hurst, Kind, & Stubbings, 1998). In the current study, internal consistency of the subscales ranged between 0.78 and 0.94. Construct validity has been tested in a number of studies using convergent/discriminant and known-groups approaches, and the hypotheses have been supported (Ware, 2000).

Finally, overall QoL was measured using a 0–10 numerical rating scale. Single-item measures of this type ask respondents for a global rating of a construct. The single global item may be the most valid measure in that it most closely represents the subjective nature of QoL (Cohen, Mount, & MacDonald, 1996). Caregivers were asked to rate their QoL for that day, where 0 was the worst it could be and 10 the best. A measure of overall QoL for family caregivers of stroke survivors was not available. Although there are published scales for caregivers persons with cancer (Weitzner, Jacobsen, Wagner, Friedland, & Cox, 1999) and for spouses of persons with cardiac disease (Ebbesen, Guyatt, McCartney, & Oldridge, 1990), many items in these scales are not relevant to caregivers of persons with chronic neurological diseases. Therefore, the numerical rating scale was chosen to assess overall QoL.

Data Analysis

To address the first objective—a description of caregiver characteristics in the first and second years after stroke—*t* tests were used to compare the computed mean scores of these variables in the first and second interviews. For the second objective—the impact of caregiving in HRQL—*t* tests were used to compare caregiver scores with published age- and sex-matched norms (Hopman et al., 2000). These comparisons to the population norms were undertaken for both the first and second years after the stroke.

To address the third and fourth objectives—the impact of patient characteristics and caregiver characteristics on caregiver HRQL (MCS and PCS) and overall QoL—a series of linear regression models was used. Models were developed for both the first and second years of caregiving. The impact of stroke-related variables (patient physical function and communication disability) and their relationship to caregiver outcomes have been examined most frequently in the literature, and these were entered first in all analyses, followed by caregiver characteristics. In the models with overall QoL as the dependent variable, HRQL was considered as an explanatory variable and was entered into these models. Effect modifiers were assessed using interaction terms in the models. Because the explanatory variables were measured on different scales, standardized regression coefficients were used and β weights reported. Only those variables that were statistically significant ($p < .05$) were included in the final models.

RESULTS

Caregiver Characteristics in First and Second Years Following Stroke

To address the first objective, scores on the measures of caregiver characteristics were compared between the initial and the final interviews. As shown in Table 2, mean scores changed little between the two interviews. From the list of 24 physical symptoms, caregivers reported an average of 4 to 5 symptoms in the past 30 days in both the first and second years of caregiving. The most frequently reported symptoms at both times, reported by 30% to 50% of the caregivers, were feeling tired, headaches, stiff joints, and trouble falling asleep (not shown in table).

The total burden score did not change between the first and second years. To understand the aspects of the caregiving role that may be burden-some to caregivers, the distribution of the individual items on the Burden Index was examined. For five items at least 50% of caregivers at both interviews responded that they felt *sometimes* to *nearly always* about the item described. These items were: having enough time for themselves, stressed trying to meet all responsibilities, afraid of what the future holds for family member with stroke, feeling that family members are dependent on them, and feeling that family members expect caregivers to take care of them as if they are the only one on which they can depend.

The mean scores on the subscales of the measure of HRQL did not change with the exception of the "social function" subscale of the SF-36, which increased significantly between the first and second years of caregiving ($p < .01$). Finally, overall QoL, as measured by the numerical rating scale, did not change between the first and second years.

TABLE A4-2

Caregiver Characteristics in Years 1 and 2 Following Stroke and Comparison of HRQL Scores to Age-Matched Norms

Construct (Measure)	First Interview ($n = 97$) M (SD)	Last Interview ($n = 97$) M (SD)	Age-Matched Norms M (SD)
Months since stroke	7.3 (5.4)	22.7 (9.2)	
Physical symptom checklist (24–0)	4.2 (3.5)	4.5 (4.0)	
Burden (Burden Index: 88–0)	24.0 (16.1)	26.1 (19.9)	
HRQL (SF-36)			
Physical function (0–100)	85.5 (23.9)	85.9 (23.1)	82.3 (19.3)
Role—physical (0–100)	80.9 (35.5)	76.8 (40.2)	81.3 (33.1)
Bodily pain (0–100)	76.0 (31.0)	74.7 (32.6)	74.9 (23.7)
General health (0–100)	76.8 (24.6)	79.7 (22.2)	74.8 (19.4)
Vitality (0–100)	57.4 (25.2)[1**]	56.7 (25.4)[1**]	68.3 (17.7)[1**]
Social function (0–100)	70.6 (27.6)[2**]	82.0 (24.1)[2**]	88.1 (18.8)
Role—emotional (0–100)	80.1 (37.2)	78.0 (38.2)[1*]	87.8 (28.3)[1*]
Mental health (0–100)	64.2 (24.4)[1**]	63.6 (23.9)[1*]	79.5 (14.7)[1**]
PCS[†]	52.1 (10.1)[1*]	52.1 (10.5)[1*]	49.0 (9.2)[1*]
MCS[†]	44.9 (12.4)[1**]	45.9 (11.0)[1**]	53.7 (8.2)[1**]
Quality of life (NRS: 0–10)	6.8 (2.2)	6.7 (2.1)	

HRQL, health-related quality of life; NRS, numerical rating scale.
[*]$p < .05$, [**]$p < .01$.
[1]Interview scores significantly different from population means.
[2]First interview and second interview scores significantly different.
[†]Physical (PCS) and mental (MCS) component summary scores from the SF-36, standardized to have a mean of 50 and a SD of 10.

Caregiver HRQL Compared to Population Norms

To address the second question, caregiver scores on the SF-36 were compared to the age- and sex-matched Canadian norms (Hopman et al., 2000). The availability of population norms allowed an examination of the impact of caregiving beyond that related to normal stress and aging. These comparisons showed two remarkable differences. As can be seen in Table 2, caregivers scored significantly higher on the PCS and significantly lower on the mental subscales and the MCS. Further examination of the MCS and PCS score distributions compared to the age-matched norms showed that about 30% of the caregivers scored at least 1 SD below the population norms on the MCS at both interviews, whereas only 7% scored at least 1 SD below on the PCS. Those caregivers who consistently scored low on the MCS were significantly more likely to be female, be unemployed, and report higher burden scores and lower overall QoL ($p < .01$). There were no significant differences in stroke survivor disability, kin relationship to the recipient of care, and caregiver age.

Comparing caregiver scores to age- and sex-matched norms showed that the magnitude of the differences on the mental subscales and the MCS was greater for women (9%–21% below the norms) than for men (9%–13% below the norms). As can be seen

in Figure 1, female caregivers scored significantly lower ($p < .06$) at both interviews than the age-matched female norms on three of the four mental subscales ("vitality," "social functioning," and "mental health") and on the MCS. In contrast, they scored significantly higher on the PCS. Although male caregivers scored lower on the mental subscales and the MCS than the age-matched male norms, these differences were not statistically significant (see Fig. 2). This may be a function of power, however, given the small sample of male caregivers. Examination of HRQL over time showed that whereas men improved on all mental subscales and the MCS, women showed little change over time. This differential change over time further increased the gap between male and female caregivers.

The comparisons to the age- and sex-matched population norms suggested that the impact of caregiving was different for men and women. To understand what could be driving these differences in outcomes, patient and caregiver characteristics were examined by gender. Male and female caregivers cared for stroke survivors with similar physical disability. Despite similar overall burden scores and few mean changes over time, the more burdensome aspects of the role were different by gender. The most notable difference between the first and last interviews was that for more than half of the items,

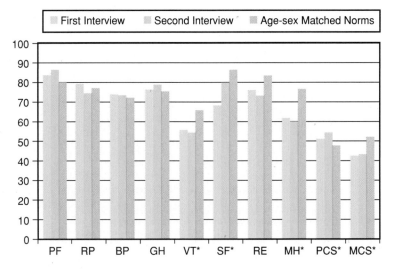

FIGURE A4-1 • Female caregiver SF-36 scores compared to Canadian age-adjusted norms. PF, physical functioning; RP, role—physical; BP, bodily pain; GH, general health; VT, vitality; SF, social functioning; RE, role—emotional; MH, mental health; PCS, physical component summary; MCS, mental component summary. *$p < 0.05$ (caregiver scores at both interviews different from norms).

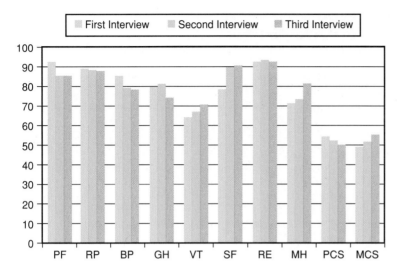

FIGURE A4-2 • Male caregiver SF-36 scores compared to Canadian age-adjusted norms. PH, physical functioning; RE, role—emotional; MH, mental health; PCS, physical component summary; MCS, mental component summary.

men reported little change or improvement, whereas women reported more burden over time. In particular, an increased proportion of women reported burden on items related to managing the caregiving role and the other aspects of their lives (not enough time for self, time for other responsibilities, caregiving impact on family relationships).

Factors Affecting HRQL and Overall QoL

To address the third and fourth research objectives, the impact of patient characteristics and caregiver characteristics on HRQL (MCS and PCS) and overall QoL was estimated using a series of linear regression models. The final models are shown in Table 3.

Approximately 42% of the variation in MCS, measured within the first 6 months of caregiving, was explained by caregiver age, physical symptoms reported by the caregiver, and caregiver burden. Older age, less burden, and fewer physical health symptoms were associated with increased mental health as measured by the MCS. Some 41% of the variation in MCS after approximately 2 years of caregiving was again explained by both caregiver physical symptoms and caregiver burden, except that rather than age, caregiver gender was associated with MCS. Interestingly, patient characteristics were not associated with MCS at either the first or second interviews.

Relationships for PCS were similar at both interviews. Caregiver age and physical health symptoms explained 22% and 26% of the variation in PCS at the initial interview and the final interview, respectively. Increasing age and increasing reports of physical symptoms were associated with decreased PCS. There was no association between patient characteristics or reports of burden and the caregiver's physical health.

Finally, QoL was regressed on patient characteristics and caregiver characteristics, including HRQL. At the first interview caring for a stroke survivor with moderate impairment, being younger, reporting a higher PCS, having a higher vitality, and an interaction between caregiver gender and MCS explained 56% of the variability in caregiver QoL. Using standardized beta coefficients, the interaction term can be interpreted as follows. Adjusting for all other variables in the model, groups of men who are 1 *SD* higher on the MCS would be 0.44 units lower on overall QoL. For groups of women, however, a 1 *SD* increase in MCS would be associated with a 0.88 unit increase in a self-reported QoL, adjusting for all other variables in the model. At the final interview, both higher PCS and higher MCS were associated with higher QoL, and the effect with MCS was not modified by sex. Although functional status of the stroke survivor was no longer associated with QoL, caring for a stroke survivor with aphasia was associ-

TABLE A4-3

Regression Models for Health-Related Quality of Life and Overall Quality of Life

	First Interview			Last Interview		
	sβ	*SE*	*R²*	*sβ*	*SE*	*R²*
			95% CI			*95% CI*
HRQL: MCS			0.42			0.41
Caregiver age	1.90	0.98	(−0.02, 3.82)			
Caregiver gender				−2.11	0.87	(−3.82, −0.40)
Symptoms	−5.99	1.05	(−8.05, −3.93)	−5.05	0.92	(−6.85, −3.25)
Burden	−3.86	1.03	(−5.88, −1.84)	−2.58	0.91	(−4.36, −0.80)
HRQL: PCS			0.22			0.26
Caregiver age	−2.14	0.92	(−3.94, 0.34)	−2.75	0.92	(−4.55, 0.95)
Symptoms	−4.34	0.91	(−6.12, −2.56)	−4.37	0.92	(−6.17, −2.57)
Quality of life (NRS)			0.56			0.35
Moderate impairment[1]	0.46	0.16	(0.15, 0.77)			
Aphasia[1]				−0.57	0.18	(−0.92, −0.22)
Caregiver age	−0.43	0.18	(−0.78, −0.08)			
Caregiver gender	−2.09	0.88	(−3.81, −0.37)			
Vitality	0.73	0.30	(0.14, 1.32)			
PCS	0.57	0.22	(0.14, 1.00)	0.55	0.18	(0.20, 0.90)
MCS	−0.53	0.57	(−1.65, 0.59)	0.88	0.18	(0.53, 1.23)
MCS*caregiver gender						
Men	−0.44	0.51	(−1.44, 0.56)			
Women	0.88	0.27	(0.35, 1.41)			

HRQL, health-related quality of life; MCS, mental component summary; PCS, physical component summary; NRS, numerical rating scale.
sE is the standard error (β/ sE is equivalent to a *t* test value); 95% confidence interval; sβ= standardized regression coefficient = β χ standard deviation (*SDs* are taken from Tables 1 and 2).
[1] Patient deficits.
The interpretation of this interaction required examining the effect of MCS separately in men and in women. To find the variance for the estimated effect for women (included variance for MCS and the interaction term), the following formula was used: $V_1 + V_2 + 2Cov_{12}$. The variance for men was just the variance for MCS. These variances were taken from a variance-covariance matrix of the parameter estimates. These betas were subsequently standardized.

ated with a diminished QoL. Together these variables explained 35% of the variance in QoL.

DISCUSSION

We have described the evolution of the caregiving experience over the first 2 years following stroke. Although there is general agreement that HRQL is an important outcome, it has been measured infrequently in studies of family caregivers. Several findings about HRQL measurement in this study are noteworthy. The first relates to the impact of caregiving on the mental health of these caregivers. The group on average scored about 10 points lower than their age-matched Canadian counterparts on the mental dimensions. A 5-point difference on the subscales has been considered clinically and socially meaningful (Ware, Snow, Kosinski, & Gandek, 1993). Secondly, this effect was different for men and women. Whereas men scored on average about 10% below the population norms, women scored approximately 20% below. Further, although men showed improvement over time, women reported very little improvement, except for the social dimension, thus widening gender differences.

There were also dissimilarities between women and men in the elements of the role that were perceived as more stressful, as measured by the Burden Interview, and this may suggest differences in how men and women cope with stressful events and in their subsequent responses (Rose-Rego, Strauss, & Smyth, 1998). There are several theoretical perspectives on gender effects in caregiving that suggest that gender influences the amount and type of care provided and access to social resources that may alleviate the burden associated with caregiving (Miller & Cafasso, 1992). Women spend more time on caregiving activities and are more likely to perform personal care activities than are men. Instrumental tasks that are time-limited and may be performed at the caregiver's discretion, such as money management, are more likely to be congruent with the roles of male caregivers (Ford, Goode, Barrett, Harrell, & Haley, 1997). Further, women are less likely to obtain informal support for caregiving and consequently to report higher levels of burden. It may also be that men are more likely to receive home care services. Information on the home care services used by caregivers in this study was not available. However, services are usually available to those who require assistance with bathing. In this sample more than 60% of the care recipients were unable to bathe independently, yet the percentage of those caring for a stroke survivor requiring assistance with bathing was slightly higher for female caregivers (69%) than for male caregivers (60%).

Although there was little change in the mental health of the caregiver group over the 2 years, there was considerable change at the individual level. Comparing the group of caregivers to population norms showed that almost one third of the caregivers scored at least one *SD* lower than the population norms on the MCS. In the Medical Outcomes Study the mean score on the MCS of those participants with clinical depression was 34.8, with an SD of 12.2 (Ware et al., 1994). It is notable that scores reported by at least 40% of the caregivers were consistent with depression at either or both interviews. This is almost double the prevalence reported for age-matched norms (Bellerose, Lavallée, & Camirand, 1994) and at least as high as that reported for stroke survivors (Hermann, Black, Lawrence, Szekely, & Szalai, 1998).

Interestingly, despite lower scores on the mental subscales, scores on the physical subscales of the SF-36 were marginally higher than the Canadian age-sex matched norms (Hopman et al., 2000). There is evidence supporting the existence of a hierarchy of caregiving, with spouses the first to take on the role, and adult children, most frequently daughters, taking over when the spouse is deceased or unable to function as a caregiver (Dwyer & Coward, 1992). This would suggest that caregivers are selected into this role because of their good physical health, a "healthy caregiver effect." Over time caregivers reported little change in their physical health. In a review of the dementia caregiving literature, Schulz, O'Brien, Bookwala, and Fleissner (1995) reported that although caregivers reported their health to be worse than noncaregivers, the evidence concerning physical morbidity was weak and inconsistent.

Global QoL, as measured by the numerical rating scale, seemed to reflect more fully the complexity of the caregiving role, including the aspects of the caregiving situation and caregiver characteristics. HRQL was not associated with stroke survivor characteristics, which may suggest a limitation in measuring only HRQL in studies of family caregiving. A large component of the measure is made up of physical domains, and there was no noticeable effect on the physical health of caregivers. The importance of QoL as an outcome has been widely recognized in the health care literature; specifically, the need to study the QoL for family caregivers was expressed more than a decade ago (Anderson, 1987). The use of the numerical rating scale allowed the caregiver to subjectively determine the important content when reporting on QoL. However, a global summary score does not identify the specific aspects of the caregiving role that affect QoL. Furthermore, the use of a summary measure does not provide the specific information needed to guide the development of appropriate interventions (Cohen et al., 1996). Therefore, based on these results, to more fully capture the impact on the caregiver's QoL, a measure of outcome developed from caregiver-generated content is recommended.

Almost half the participants at the time of both interviews reported worrying about the future of the care recipients, which was unrelated to the functional status of the patients. Even in the context of a mild stroke with minimal residual neurological deficit, caregivers have reported increased emotional distress related to the fear of a second stroke (Hanger, Walker, Paterson, McBride, & Sainsbury, 1998; van Veenendaal, Grinspun, & Adriaanse, 1996). This finding suggests an important avenue for intervention. Providing information to a caregiver about secondary prevention will not only benefit the care recipient but also may help to reduce the caregiver's fear about potential future events.

This study is limited in several aspects. There are many challenges in conducting longitudinal studies including attrition and difficulty obtaining interviews at the scheduled times. The challenge is particularly high in caregiving as well as other roles of spouse, parent, and employee contribute to this problem. Caregivers often were too busy in their caregiving role to be interviewed, and interviews were rescheduled several times before completion, leading to variability in the interview times. Data from the few longitudinal studies of informal caregiving for stroke survivors suggest similar difficulties. In those studies in which this information was reported, the proportion completing all scheduled follow-up interviews ranged from 56% to 79% (Hodgson et al., 1996; Teel et al., 2001; Tompkins, Schulz, & Rau, 1988).

A further limitation relates to the sample selection. Because the primary objective of the main study was to describe the long-term outcomes of persons with stroke, caregivers of only those stroke survivors unable to respond for themselves were included in this study. This most likely reflects those patients with the greatest needs (i.e., physical frailty, cognitive and communication impairments), and therefore this caregiver sample may be biased toward those caring for more functionally disabled patients.

Despite these limitations, this study makes important contributions to increasing the understanding of family caregiving in stroke. Many researchers have measured only burden, and few researchers have examined both HRQL and QoL. Information on HRQL compared to population norms supported the impact of the caregiving role in addition to normal aging. Although there have been several longitudinal studies, in most cases follow-up was limited to the initial 6 months following stroke. This time frame limits the understanding of long-term caregiving that is required for many stroke survivors. As reported here, even at 2 years following stroke, there was a significantly high proportion of caregivers who reported scores on the MCS consistent with depression. Because care by families to functionally dependent members is the most effective means of maintaining them in the community, these results therefore highlight the importance of preventing and treating health problems among caregivers. Further, depression in the caregiver has been associated with depression in the stroke survivor (Carnwath & Johnson, 1987). This suggests that interventions aimed at treating emotional disturbances in the family caregiver will benefit not only the caregiver but may also benefit the person with stroke.

References

Aday, L. A. & Andersen, R. (1975). *Development of indices of access to medical care*. Ann Arbor, MI: Health Administration Press.

Anderson, C. S., Linto, J., & Stewart-Wynne, E. G. (1995). A population-based assessment of the impact and burden of caregiving for long-term stroke survivors. *Stroke, 26,* 843–849.

Anderson, R. (1987). The unremitting burden on carers. *British Medical Journal, 294,* 73–74.

Anderson, R. (1992). *The aftermath of stroke*. Cambridge, UK: Cambridge University Press.

Baumgarten, M., Battista, R., Infante-Riverd, C., Hanley, J., Becker, R., & Gauthier, S. (1992). The psychological and physical health of family members caring for an elderly person with dementia. *Journal of Clinical Epidemiology, 45,* 61–70.

Bellerose, C., Lavallée, C., & Camirand, J. (1994). *1992–1993 Health and Social Survey: Highlights*. Québec, Qc, Gouvernement du Québec, Santé Québec.

Biegel, D. E., Sales, E., & Schulz, R. (1991). *Family caregiving in chronic illness*. London: Sage.

Brazier, J. E., Harper, R., Jones, N. M., O'Cathain, A., Thomas, K. J., Usherwood, T., et al. (1992). Validating the SF-36 health survey questionnaire: A new outcome measure for primary care. *British Medical Journal, 305,* 160–164.

Brocklehurst, J. C., Morris, P., Andrews, K., Richards, B., & Laycock, P. (1981). Social effects of stroke. *Social Science & Medicine, 15,* 35–39.

Bugge, C., Alexander, H., & Hagen, S. (1999). Stroke patients' informal caregivers. Patient, caregiver, and service factors that affect caregiver strain. *Stroke, 30,* 1517–1523.

Carnwath, T. C. M. & Johnson, D. A. W. (1987). Psychiatric morbidity among spouses of patients with stroke. *British Medical Journal, 294,* 409–411.

Christopher, A. B. (1999). *The caregivers of stroke patients: The evolution of health status over the first three months after the patient returns home*. McGill University, Montreal, Quebec.

Cohen, S. R., Mount, B. M., & MacDonald, N. (1996). Defining quality of life. *European Journal of Cancer, 32A,* 753–754.

Dennis, M., O'Rourke, S., Lewis, S., Sharpe, M., & Warlow, C. (1998). A quantitative study of the emotional outcome of people caring for stroke survivors. *Stroke, 29,* 1867–1872.

Dwyer, J. W. & Coward, R. T. (1992). Gender, family, and long-term care of the elderly. In J. W. Dwyer & R. T. Coward (Eds.), *Gender, families, and eldercare* (pp. 3–17). London: Sage.

Ebbesen, L. S., Guyatt, G. H., McCartney, N., & Oldridge, N. B. (1990). Measuring quality of life in cardiac spouses. *Journal of Clinical Epidemiology, 43,* 481–487.

Flanagan, J. C. (1978). A research approach to improving our quality of life. *American Psychologist, 33,* 138–147.

Ford, G. R., Goode, K. T., Barrett, J. J., Harrell, L. E., & Haley, W. E. (1997). Gender roles and caregiving stress: An examination of subjective appraisals of specific primary stressors in Alzheimer's caregivers. *Aging & Mental Health, 1,* 158–165.

Goldberg, D. P. & Hillier, V. F. (1979). A scaled version of the General Health Questionnaire. *Psychological Medicine, 9,* 139–145.

Granger, C. V., Dewis, L. S., Peters, N. C., Sherwood, C. C., & Barrett, J. E. (1979). Stroke rehabilitation: Analysis of repeated Barthel Index measures. *Archives of Physical Medicine and Rehabilitation, 60,* 14–17.

Greveson, G. C., Gray, C. S., French, J. M., & James, O. F. W. (1991). Long-term outcome for patients and carers following hospital admission for stroke. *Age and Ageing, 20,* 337–344.

Han, B. & Haley, W. E. (1999). Family caregiving for patients with stroke. Review and analysis. *Stroke, 30,* 1478–1485.

Hanger, H. C., Walker, G., Paterson, L. A., McBride, S., & Sainsbury, R. (1998). What do patients and their carers want to know about stroke? A two-year follow-up study. *Clinical Rehabilitation, 12,* 45–52.

Hermann, N., Black, S. E., Lawrence, J., Szekely, C., & Szalai, J. P. (1998). The Sunnybrook Stroke Study: A prospective study of depressive symptoms and functional outcome. *Stroke, 29,* 618–624.

Hochstenbach, J., Donders, R., Mulder, T., Van Limbeek, J., & Schoonderwaldt, H. (1996). Long-term outcome after stroke: A disability-orientated approach. *International Journal of Rehabilitation Research, 19,* 189–200.

Hodgson, S. P., Wood, V. A., & Langton-Hewer, R. (1996). Identification of stroke carers 'at risk': A preliminary study of the predictors of carers' psychological well-being at one year post stroke. *Clinical Rehabilitation, 10,* 337–346.

Hopman, W. M., Towheed, T., Anastassiades, T., Tenenhouse, A., Poliquin, S., Berger, C., et al. (2000). Canadian normative data for the SF-36 health survey. *Canadian Medical Association Journal, 163,* 265–271.

Knapp, P. & Hewison, J. (1999). Disagreement in patient and carer assessment of functional abilities after stroke. *Stroke, 30,* 934–938.

Korner-Bitensky, N. (1994). Eliciting health status information by telephone after discharge from hospital: Health professionals versus trained lay persons. *Canadian Journal of Rehabilitation, 8,* 23–34.

Low, T. S., Payne, S., & Roderick, P. (1999). The impact of stroke on informal carers: A literature review. *Social Science & Medicine, 49,* 711–725.

Mayo, N. E., Wood-Dauphinee, S., Côté, R., Durcan, L., & Carlton, J. (2002). Activity, participation, and quality of life 6 months poststroke. *Archives of Physical Medicine and Rehabilitation, 83,* 1035–1042.

McHorney, C. A., Ware, J. E., Jr., Lu, J. F., & Sherbourne, C. D. (1994). The MOS 36-Item Short-Form Health Survey (SF-36): II. Tests of data quality, scaling assumptions, and reliability across diverse patient groups. *Medical Care, 32,* 40–66.

Miller, B. & Cafasso, L. (1992). Gender differences in caregiving: Fact or artifact? *The Gerontologist, 32,* 498–507.

Patrick, D. L. & Erickson, P. (1993). *Health status and health policy: Quality of life in health care evaluation and resource allocation* (p. 22). New York: Oxford University Press.

Pierre, U., Wood-Dauphinee, S., Korner-Bitensky, N., Gayton, D., & Hanley, J. (1998). Proxy use of the Canadian SF-36 in rating health status of the disabled elderly. *Journal of Clinical Epidemiology, 51,* 983–990.

Pratt, C. C., Schmall, V., & Wright, S. (1986). Family caregivers and dementia. *Social Casework, 67,* 119–124.

Reese, D. R., Gross, A. M., Smalley, D. L., & Messer, S. C. (1994). Caregivers of Alzheimer's disease and stroke patients: Immunological and psychological considerations. *The Gerontologist, 34,* 534–540.

Rose-Rego, S. K., Strauss, M. E., & Smyth, K. A. (1998). Differences in the perceived well-being of wives and husbands caring for persons with Alzheimer's disease. *The Gerontologist, 38,* 224–230.

Roy, C. W., Togneri, J., Hay, E., & Pentland, B. (1988). An inter-rater reliability study of the Barthel Index. *International Journal of Rehabilitation Research, 11,* 67–70.

Ruta, D. A., Hurst, N. P., Kind, P., & Stubbings, A. (1998). Measuring health status in British patients with rheumatoid arthritis: Reliability, validity and responsiveness of the Short Form 36-Item Health Survey (SF-36). *British Journal of Rheumatology, 37,* 425–436.

Schulz, R., O'Brien, A. T., Bookwala, J., & Fleissner, K. (1995). Psychiatric and physical morbidity effects of dementia caregiving: Prevalence, correlated, and causes. *The Gerontologist, 35,* 771–791.

Schulz, R., Tompkins, C. A., & Rau, M. T. (1988). A longitudinal study of the psychosocial impact of stroke on primary support persons. *Psychology and Aging, 3,* 131–141.

Seltzer, M. M. & Li, L. W. (1996). The transitions of caregiving: Subjective and objective definitions. *The Gerontologist, 36,* 614–626.

Shah, S., Vanclay, F., & Cooper, B. (1989). Improving the sensitivity of the Barthel Index for stroke rehabilitation. *Journal of Clinical Epidemiology, 42,* 703–709.

Shapiro, M. F., Ware, J. E., Jr., & Sherbourne, D. D. (1986). Effects of cost sharing on seeking care for serious and minor symptoms: Results of a randomized controlled trial. *Annals of Internal Medicine, 104,* 246–251.

Silliman, R. A., Fletcher, R. H., Earp, J. L., & Wagner, E. H. (1986). Families of elderly stroke patients. Effects of home care. *Journal of the American Geriatrics Society, 34,* 643–648.

Smith, K. W., Avis, N. E., & Assmann, S. F. (1999). Distinguishing between quality of life and health status in quality of life research: A meta-analysis. *Quality of Life Research, 8,* 447–459.

Snaith, R. P., Ahmed, S. N., Mehta, S., & Hamilton, M. (1971). Assessment of the severity of primary depressive illness. Wakefield Self-Assessment Depression Inventory. *Psychological Medicine, 1,* 143–149.

Statistics Canada. (1999). *How healthy are Canadians?* Ottawa, Ontario: Government of Canada.

Teel, C. S., Duncan, P., & Lai, S. M. (2001). Caregiving experiences after stroke. *Nursing Research, 50,* 53–60.

The WHOQOL Group. (1995). The World Health Organization Quality of Life Assessment (WHOQOL): Position Paper from the World Health Organization. *Social Science & Medicine, 41,* 1403–1409.

Thorngren, M., Westling, B., & Norrving, B. (1990). Outcome after stroke in patients discharged to independent living. *Stroke, 21,* 236–240.

Tompkins, C. A., Schulz, R., & Rau, M. T. (1988). Post-stroke depression in primary support persons: Predicting those at risk. *Journal of Consulting and Clinical Psychology, 56,* 502–508.

Van Veenendaal, H., Grinspun, D. R., & Adriaanse, H. P. (1996). Educational needs of stroke survivors and their family members, as perceived by themselves and by health professionals. *Patient Education and Counseling, 28,* 265–276.

Vitaliano, P. P., Young, H. M., & Russo, J. (1991). Burden: A review of measures used among caregivers of individuals with dementia. *The Gerontologist, 31,* 67–75.

Wade, D. T., Legh-Smith, J., & Hewer, R. L. (1986). Effects of living with and looking after survivors of a stroke. *British Medical Journal, 293,* 418–420.

Ware, J. E., Jr. (2000). SF-36 Health Survey update. *Spine, 25,* 3130–3139.

Ware, J. E., Jr., Kosinski, M., & Keller, S. D. (1994). *SF-36 Physical and Mental Health Summary Scales: A user's manual.* Boston: The Health Institute, New England Medical Center.

Ware, J. E., Jr. & Sherbourne, D. D. (1992). The MOS 36-item Short-Form Health Survey (SF-36). I. Conceptual framework and item selection. *Medical Care, 30,* 473–483.

Ware, J. E., Jr., Snow, K. K., Kosinski, M., & Gandek, B. (1993). *SF-36 Health Survey: Manual and interpretation guide.* Boston: The Health Institute, New England Medical Centre.

Weitzner, M. A., Jacobsen, P. B., Wagner, H., Jr., Friedland, J., & Cox, C. (1999). The Caregiver Quality of Life Index–Cancer (CQOLC) scale: Development and validation of an instrument to measure quality of life of the family caregiver of patients with cancer. *Quality of Life Research, 8,* 55–63.

Yee, J. L. & Schulz, R. (2000). Gender differences in psychiatric morbidity among family caregivers: A review and analysis. *The Gerontologist, 40,* 147–164.

Zarit, S. H., Reever, K. E., & Bach-Peterson, J. (1980). Relatives of the impaired elderly: Correlates of feelings of burden. *The Gerontologist, 20,* 649–655.

Zarit, S. H., Todd, P. A., & Zarit, J. M. (1986). Subjective burden of husbands and wives as caregivers: A longitudinal study. *The Gerontologist, 26,* 260–266.

APPENDIX
A-5

Needs of Family Members of Patients with Severe Traumatic Brain Injury: Implications for Evidence-Based Practice

A. Elaine Bond, DNSc, APRN, CCRN; Christy Rae Lee Draeger, RN, BSN; Barbara Mandleco, RN, PhD; Michael Donnelly, RN, BSN, CCRN

Traumatic brain injury occurs in 500,000 persons each year in the United States; approximately 50,000 of these die before they reach a hospital. Of those who do reach a hospital, approximately 80% have mild traumatic injuries (Glasgow Coma Scale [GSC] score 14–15) and require little, if any, care in an intensive care unit (ICU). About 10% have moderate traumatic brain injuries (GCS score 9–13) and may be admitted to an ICU simply for observation. For the remaining 10% (approximately 45,000 patients) who have severe traumatic brain injury (GCS score 3-8), rapid intervention and stabilization in an ICU can improve morbidity and mortality.[1]

Initially, patients with severe traumatic brain injury are in an extremely unstable condition and may require surgery for removal of epidural and/or subdural hematomas and repeated computed tomography scans. They may need intracranial pressure monitoring, hyperosmolar agents to control increasing pressures, and ventilator support.[1,2] Although ICU nurses become accustomed to working in such crisis situations, the families of patients with

severe traumatic brain injury may be overwhelmed by the patients' critical, constantly changing status. While the families experience the whirlwind of care, often without understanding what is happening, they must also address the possibility of their relatives' future dysfunction or untimely death.[3] This time can be extremely stressful for these families.

Indeed, all admissions to an ICU are stressful for patients' families, but the sudden unexpected onset of severe traumatic brain injury, coupled with its unstable nature and strong probability of death, makes the families of patients with such injuries especially vulnerable. As Landsman et al[4] reported, the severity of the injury may place demands on patients' families beyond the families' ability to cope. By following the vision of the American Association of Critical Care Nurses (AACN) of advocacy for patients and patients' families (see Table A5-1), compassionate ICU nurses can alleviate the anxiety and concern of these families. Even though research findings indicate that staffing and time restrictions impinge on the care nurses give to patients' family

Critical Care Nurse, 2003, Volume 23, Number 4, pages 63–72

Box A5-1 Qualitative Research

Qualitative research involves broadly stated questions about human experiences and realities, and is conducted by using sustained contact with persons in their natural environments. The information gathered is rich and descriptive and helps in understanding the participant's experiences. Researchers search for patterns and theories in the data rather than focus on testing hypotheses. An inductive rather than a deductive approach is used, leading to a narrative summary of the information, then synthesizing the experiences of participants.

Purposes of Qualitative Research

- Explore and describe topics that little is known about or gain insight about a particular group of patients or health condition.
- Account for and illustrate quantitative findings to answer "why" and "how" questions.
- Discover and explain phenomena.
- Extend knowledge about a theory.

Principles of Qualitative Research

- The focus is broad and holistic.
- Data are usually oral or written responses to open-ended questions.
- The wholeness of human experiences in naturalistic settings is studied.
- Comment analysis of the data involves examining the information and creating categories of data that are similar; analysis and collection of data occurs simultaneously.
- Data collection continues until no new information is learned (saturation).
- The number of participants (sample size) varies and usually is small; researchers continue to interview participants until no new information is obtained.
- The term "rigor" is used instead of reliability and validity. Rigor is judged in 3 ways: credibility, auditability, and fittingness.

  Credibility means faithful description or interpretations of a human experience that the persons having that experience would immediately recognize from those descriptions or interpretations as their own.

  Auditability means leaving a clear decision trail concerning the study from the beginning to the end, so other researchers can follow the progression of events in the study and understand the logic of the researcher.

  Fittingness occurs when the audience views the study findings as meaningful and applicable in terms of the audience's own experience.

Phenomenology

Phenomenology (also called hermeneutics) is rooted in a philosophical tradition developed by Husseri and Heidegger. It is an approach to think about what the experiences of persons are like and the process of learning and constructing the meaning of human experience through intensive dialogue with persons who are living the experience. Often the researcher will ask what it is like to live or experience something. Participants are purposively chosen because they are experiencing whatever the researcher is studying. Data are presented by using direct quotes that relate to a particular theme the researcher has identified.

members[11] and some nurses consider interaction with patients' family members a low-order priority,[7] appropriate interactions with the families are essential if nurses are to remain advocates for these patients and families and provide holistic nursing care.

Determining better ways to empower patients' families and meet their needs requires learning what they perceive their needs to be. The purpose of this qualitative descriptive study was to discover the needs of families of patients with severe traumatic brain injury during the families' experience in a neurosurgical ICU.

REVIEW OF THE LITERATURE

Providing care for patients' families arises from crisis theory, which states that the whole is greater than the sum of the parts: family adaptation or resiliency can affect patients' outcomes, both short- and long-term, either positively or negatively.[8,12] In the late 1970s, Dracup and Breu[13] urged nurses to use Hampe's research findings,[14] which identified the importance of meeting the needs of families of acutely or terminally ill patients. Soon thereafter, Molter published her study[11] of the needs of families of critically ill patients (Table 1). Molter and Leske refined Molter's randomized list of 45 family needs into the Critical Care Family Needs Inventory.[17] The inventory clustered Molter's original 45 items into 5 categories:

1. support
2. comfort
3. information
4. proximity, and
5. assurance.

The inventory was used throughout the 1980s and 1990s to quantitatively identify family needs.[10,15-23] In the AACN protocols for practice series on creating a healing environment, the booklet on the needs of patients' families[8] has an annotated bibliography of 24 studies and a reference list of 122 other studies, all of which address the needs of, assessment of, interventions for, or satisfaction of patients' families. Clearly, the needs of families who have a family member in an ICU have been examined in many studies.

On the basis of the results of these earlier investigations, numerous researchers have attempted to address the needs of patients' families, with mixed results. For example, Appleyard et al[24] evaluated the effectiveness of a "nurse-coached" volunteer program to meet the needs of patients' families in an ICU. Volunteers provided information, comfort, and support to the families and notified the staff nurses of any family's concerns. At the conclusion of the study, according to families' ratings, comfort was the only category with statistically significant improvement. The scores for support improved slightly, the scores for proximity remained the same, and the scores for assurance and information actually decreased. Even so, the families who received the intervention reported less anxiety and stated that they received better information than the families that did not receive the intervention reported.

In contrast, in a study on the effectiveness of a structured communication program, Medland and Ferrans[25] found that having families meet with a nurse about 24 hours after admission to discuss the patient's condition, giving them an information booklet, and then following up with a daily telephone call significantly decreased the number of telephone calls into the ICU, without affecting the families' perception of how well information was provided ($P < .05$).

Other studies indicated that assistive personnel can facilitate nurses' work with families. In one study,[28] family advocates, who worked directly with the families of trauma patients, helped the families throughout the hospital stay, as the families dealt with severe injury and death. The advocates received training in crisis intervention, grief counseling, and customer service, which helped them address families' concerns. Surveys of patients' families after the inception of the program indicated that the families felt greater satisfaction than families had indicated before the program began.

In recent years, investigators have broadened the search to retrospectively identify needs of patients' families. In several studies,[27,28] family members of patients who died were interviewed or filled out questionnaires. In the study by Malacrida et al,[29] 17% of 123 respondents thought that the information they received about the condition of their family member was neither clear nor adequate. In addition, 30% of the respondents were not satisfied with the information they received about the cause of the patient's death. Similarly, Abbott et al[27] found that 46% of respondents thought a conflict existed between healthcare professionals and the respondents. The respondents stated that healthcare professionals disregarded or ignored

TABLE A5-1

Comparison of Molter's Original Findings of Needs of Families of Critically Ill Patients With the Needs of Families of Patients With Severe Traumatic Brain Injury

Molter[11]: Family needs of relatives of critically ill patients
1. To feel there is hope
2. To feel that hospital personnel care about the patient
3. To have the waiting area near the patient
4. *To be called at home about changes in the condition of the patient*
5. *To know the prognosis*
6. *To have questions answered honestly*
7. *To know specific facts concerning the patient's progress*
8. *To receive information about the patient at least once a day*
9. *To have explanations given in terms that are understandable*
10. To see the patient frequently

Mathis[15]: Personal needs of family members of critically ill patients with and without acute brain injury
1. To feel that hospital personnel care about my relative
2. *To be called at home about changes in the condition of the patient*
3. *To know exactly what is being done for my relative*
4. To be reassured that the best care possible was being given to my relative
5. *To have my questions answered honestly*
6. *To be told about how my relative was going to be treated medically*
7. *To receive information about my relative's condition at least once a day*
8. To feel accepted by hospital personnel
9. To feel there was hope
10. *To have specific facts concerning my relative's progress*

Engli and Kirsivali-Farmer[16]: Needs of family members of critically ill patients with and without acute brain injury
1. *To know the prognosis*
2. *To have questions answered honestly*
3. *To be assured that the best possible care is being given to the patient*
4. *To be called at home about changes in the patient's condition*
5. *To feel that the hospital personnel care about the patient*
6. *To have a specific person to call at the hospital when unable to visit*
7. *To know how the patient is being treated medically*
8. *To have explanations that are understandable*
9. *To know specific facts concerning the patient's progress*
10. To see the patient frequently

*Items italicized are need-to-know needs.
Reprinted from Molter,[11] copyright 1979, with permission from Elsevier Science; Mathis,[15] copyright 1984, with permission from the American Association of Neuroscience Nurses; and Engli and Kirsivali-Farmer,[16] copyright 1984, with permission from the American Association of Neuroscience Nurses.

their input into treatment plans. Curtis et al[28] strongly recommended that family conferences be used more effectively to improve "physician-family" and "nurse-family" communication in instances of impending death.

Families of patients with severe traumatic brain injury may be in a state of distress as they face the possibility of impending death for their loved one. In early studies of brain injury,[15,16] the needs of families of patients with traumatic brain injury differed significantly from those of families of patients without such injuries (Table 1). The No. 1 need for the families of patients with brain injury was information about the patients' condition and what to expect. The families reported they needed to have questions answered honestly and realistically. Other researchers[10,32] also found that the No.1 need of families of patients with severe traumatic brain injury was information.

However, some investigators have recognized that some needs are still unmet, that the result of intervention studies and recommendations might not be universally applied, and that deeper, as yet unrecognized, needs may exist. For instance, Dyer[33] noted that many studies are merely repetitions of the work of Molter and Leske and urged researchers to engage in new research. Burr maintained that use of a single measure alone does not provide an adequate assessment of all needs of families of brain-injured patients. She suggested that qualitative information could strengthen quantitative findings and determine if any needs existed that were not easily ascertained by quantitative means.[31] Our qualitative study was designed to explore the needs of patients' families through individual interviews during the course of the patients' stay in the ICU.

METHODS

Setting and Participants

We used an exploratory qualitative descriptive design and a convenience sample of family members of patients admitted to an 11-bed neurological ICU in a level 1 trauma center. After approval was obtained from the appropriate institutional review boards, family members who met the criteria were contacted by one of us (C.R.I.D.; see box A5-1 for an explanation of qualitative research). Consent forms signed by the participants provided an explanation of the project, the risks, the benefits, the time commitment, the measures taken to ensure anonymity and confidentiality, and the voluntary nature of the study.

Inclusion criteria were: (1) 1 family member of a patient with a diagnosis of severe traumatic brain injury who was at least 18 years or older; (2) the patient had a GCS score of 8 or less upon hospitalization; and (3) the patient was hospitalized in the neurological ICU for at least 24 hours.

Procedure

Initial data collection occurred in the privacy of a nearby waiting room. The same researcher (C.R.I.D.) interviewed all the participants to ensure consistency in the interviewing. On each of the remaining days of a patient's ICU stay, the patient's family member was asked to describe the family's needs and concerns and also was asked if any new needs had arisen. Subsequent interviews were conducted either at the hospital or by telephone, at the participants' convenience, building upon the trust developed during the first in-person interviews.

Recruitment of participants continued until saturation of the initial data occurred, with additional daily interviews of the original participants until their relative who was the patient died or was discharged from the ICU. Appropriate follow-up and probing questions were included as required. Interviews were recorded on audiotape and were transcribed verbatim; all identifying information was removed.

DATA ANALYSIS AND RESULTS

Seven family members of patients with severe traumatic brain injury (GCS score <8) participated in the study. Two mothers, a daughter, a father, a grandmother, a sister, and an uncle were interviewed during a 4-month period from January to April 2001. Their ages ranged from 41 to 61 years.

Although each participant had individual and unique situations and needs, content analysis indicated 4 common themes (Table 2):

1. need to know
2. need for consistent information
3. need for involvement in care
4. need to make sense of the experience

(In the following sections, the grammar of the material from the interviews was corrected slightly for readability.)

Need to Know

The most common phrase, heard from every participant on day 1 was "I just need to know." One participant stated that "a better relay system between physician and family would be much more helpful." Of the 7 participants, 4 had not been able to talk with the doctor yet when they were interviewed initially, a situation that partially contributed to their lack of and need for information. Family members preferred to be told the truth about the patient's conditions, even if the information conflicted with or compromised their need for hope. As one participant emphatically stated, "Don't sugarcoat! I can take it. Please give me some reality. If there is no hope, tell me there is no hope!"

Need for Consistent Information

Each participant spontaneously reported inconsistencies in information given to them by doctors, nurses,

TABLE A5-2

Overview of the Needs of Families of Patients With Severe Traumatic Brain Injury

Day of Hospitalization	Need
1	*To know* "Don't sugarcoat." "If there is no hope, tell me there is no hope."
2	*For consistent information* "Each doctor said something different. And since not all of us were together, each person heard something different." ". . . is it going to help or not?"
3–6	*For involvement in care* "I want to help, to be involved in [the patient's] care." "If there is anything we can do physically, tell us. The nurses haven't volunteered that." "Now I could have easily and gladly done that [the patient's bath]. But she [the nurse] told us to wait outside."
7–22	*To make sense of the experience* "It was a roller coaster. At first we didn't know how to handle it. One day were told we needed to start thinking about donating [the patient's organs], and the next were told to wait it out for 2 more weeks. Do you know what that does to you? It's like watching ER and hearing Dr. Green tell Dr. Carter to call it [the code], but he won't." Dealing with the death of the patient: "We don't want her to be dragged on. We don't want to prolong [the patient's] life for the sake of her being a learning instrument."

technicians, and other hospital staff by the second day in the hospital. One family member reported, "You get so much personality from them that you are unable to know what is real and what is just opinion." Of the 7 participants, 5 expressed wishes that some kind of uniform, condensed information could be given by a single doctor to all of the family members, although the entire family was usually not present at one time:

Each doctor said something different. And since not all of us were there together, each person heard something different. When we came together as a family, it was very confusing and very problematic, and we almost started fighting. We had conflicting information. More harm was done that should have been.

Another participant recounted the frustration of receiving different information from physicians:

One doctor said that [the patient] "absolutely could not hear anything." But then I go in there, and I notice that as I touch her arm and tell her who I am, the top line on the screen [heart rate] started to go up. I think she knew it was me; she recognized me and she was reacting to that. But that [the first] doctor said it wasn't possible. Then another doctor and I were talking and I told him about it and he suggested playing her favorite music for her on a little stereo. Now, is it going to help or not? Can she hear it or not? I want to do it if it is going to help her. This does not help me. I can take the bad news. Just don't tell us things that are not true and think that we need to hear happy things.

Need for Involvement in Care

On days 3 through 6 of the ICU stay, family members began to discuss their wish to participate in the care of their family member. Several participants expressed frustration at being restricted from the patient at times and why they could not help with the care the patient required. As one participant stated, "It doesn't matter whether or not I can be in there, so much as it does [matter] why I can't be in there." Another family member remarked on this situation: "We just sit around, waiting. And we don't want to get in the way, but we want to be with our loved one as much as possible. If there is anything we can do physically, tell us. The nurses haven't volunteered that. I want to help, to be involved in [the patient's] care." Two other participants also clarified the need related to what they could do for the patient. The first one stated:

> If I had more instruction as to what to do by the bedside, I would do it. I am not afraid of that stuff [monitors, catheters, tubes]. But when I am told that nothing I do will make a difference, I just sit there and exist with [the patient]. And that is not what I am here to do. I am here to help [the patient].

Another participant remarked on this lack of information about patients' care by family members and recalled the nurse giving a bath to the participant's relative:

> Now I could have easily and gladly done that [the patient's bath]. But she [the nurse] told us to wait outside. So I asked her if she would come tell us when she was done, so that I could come right back into the room. But she forgot and we sat and sat and sat. I know that the nurses are busy, but we were just sitting there. I guess we have nothing better to do, but we want to spend as much time with her as we can. But even when we are in the room, we don't know what to do and what not to do. We just sit and stare at her [the patient] and each other. And what good is that doing [the patient]?

Need to Make Sense of the Experience

As new needs arose on subsequent days of hospitalization, previous needs for consistent and honest information remained unmet for the family members, compounding their emotional distress. They attempted to make sense of or to understand what they and their loved one had experienced. Some family members

relied on their faith as they learned to accept that their loved one might not recover at all.

Three patients with severe traumatic brain injury had stays in the neurological ICU ranging from 11 to 22 days. One participant approached the doctors on day 8, stating, "We don't want her to be dragged on. We don't want to prolong [the patient's] life for the sake of her being a learning instrument." The participant's assertiveness, coupled with the patient's deterioration, resulted in family conference on day 9. After the conference, mechanical ventilation was stopped, and the patient died 2 days later. The participant stated:

> The biggest thing is the miscommunication. . . . But it would have helped if they could have talked through the procedures as they did them, instead of our having to ask. We would like to know why certain things are being done, what they hope to find out, what certain results mean. But when I have to ask, I feel intrusive. And then sometimes I get an answer that isn't English. I need an analogy, something to relate it to for normal [nonmedical] people.

Another family member with a long-staying relative recounted what the experience had been like on day 12:

> It was a roller coaster. At first we didn't know how to handle it. One day we were told we needed to start thinking about donating [the patient's organs], and the next we were told to wait it out for 2 more weeks. Do you know what that does to you? It's like watching *ER* and hearing Dr. Green tell Dr. Carter to call it [the code], but he won't. The family gets frightened, because it is too intricate for us to understand. I don't know if there is a right or wrong anymore, but I do know that God is the one in charge.

On day 22, the same participant spoke about the death of the patient:

> It's just a terrible thing and you hope no one ever has to go through this. It is scary, but you rely on your faith and on your family. . . . You know, everybody has to walk through this some way and we are trying to do that.

Discussion and Application for Nurses

Interviewing each participant each day of the patient's hospitalization entailed more than 60 interviews and provided a rich understanding of the stress of that family's experience. Additionally, when 4 of the 7 participants' relatives died, the data reinforced the seriousness of severe traumatic brain injury and the extreme need to support families of such patients during the patients' ICU stay.

The most pressing initial family need was the need to know, a finding that suggests family members want information about the diagnosis, the treatments, and the rationale for those treatments. This finding is similar to the results of earlier studies.[12,16,21,31,41] Although families expect factual information from a single source, nurses and physicians know that all facts are not readily available during the early part of hospitalization of patients with severe traumatic brain injury and that there will not be just one person who can address all issues. Initial brain edema can mask diffuse axonal injury that will not become apparent until the swelling subsides. The patients may also have multiple other injuries that require additional time for identification. However, having healthcare providers meet with the patients' family members early on and communicate what is known and what additional information is being explored would enable family members to begin processing the enormity of the injury and its continuing challenges.

As the patients' families began to receive inconsistent information during the second and third days of the hospitalization, the family members discussed the need for consistent information. Other researchers[27,28,31,32] have addressed the need of patients' families for consistent information, the conflicting information the families receive, and the families' dissatisfaction with the information given. In Burr's triangulated study,[31] she used the Critical Care Family Needs Inventory and qualitative interviews to examine the extreme distress of family members of patients with brain injury. She found that the unmet need of knowing was a main contributor to the family's intense feeling of anxiety and distress and that it remained a main contributor until the families obtained sufficient information to help with their understanding. Johnson et al[35] discovered that discussions and interactions with multiple attending physicians and different nurses every day resulted in inconsistencies and increased families' stress.

Having a designated healthcare provider meet daily with patient's family members to provide updated information can lessen this stress. Continuity in nursing assignments could also decrease the families' anx-

iety. In addition, ICU nurses know that patient's family members may not assimilate all information at once but will need continual reinforcement over time. Families also need to have information presented in terms they can understand. As changes in the condition of a patient with severe traumatic brain injury are identified, with accompanying changes in procedures, the patient's family members need additional explanations and information. A comparison of the needs of families of critically ill patients originally described by Molter[11] with the needs of families of patients with severe traumatic brain injury[15,16] indicates some form of the need to know as mentioned 6 or 7 times in each study (Table 1). Two of AACN's Values specifically support meeting these informational needs (see box A5-2).[38] Clearly, information is important to alleviate families' distress.

After the first few days, the family members in our study voiced their need for involvement in the patient's care and were prepared to spend long hours at the hospital to support their relatives. The family members felt frustrated when they were not allowed to help with the patients' ordinary care. As Leske[17] pointed out, families can be beneficial to help alleviate patients' stress and improve patients' outcomes.

Certainly, nurses can include patients' families in basic care. Assisting with a patient's bath (if the relationship is appropriate) or other basic care would provide a sense of inclusion and increase the family member's understanding of the gravity of the patient's situation. It would also help prepare family members for their upcoming caregiving role or help them realize that they may need to think about an extended-care facility when the patient is discharged from the ICU. Such an experience would benefit both patients and family members.

A close look at the needs identified in our study indicates that the families' initial needs for information

---

Box A5-2 Items 1 and 2 from AACN's Values[36]

Advocate for organizational decisions that are driven by the needs of patients and families.
Act with integrity by communicating openly and honestly, keeping promises, honoring commitments, and promoting loyalty in all relationships.

continued over time. Although the families reported that their needs for information remained unmet, they asserted themselves. First they tried to obtain information, and then when they realized that the information was not consistent, they tried to move into an adaptive behavior: providing care for their family member to validate the information they had and seeking additional information. When patients remained unconscious for a long period, and had an extremely poor prognosis, the patient's family members attempted to put the experience in perspective and to reach closure. (Current family members of patients with severe traumatic brain injury have reviewed the experiences and interpretations reported here and have agreed with our findings.)

As the family members in our study reviewed their stay in the ICU, they reflected on the overall experiences, trying to make sense of it all, reaching for closure. On the basis of information and suggestions they provided, the recommendations of earlier intervention studies[14,22–35] and the work of Leske,[11] we recommend simple interventions to empower patients' families and meet these needs (Table 3). Nurses also need to remember that individual family needs are subjective and require individualized attention and support. Harvey,[38] recommended a "strong multidisciplinary approach and a unit culture that encourages keeping the family informed." Johnson[39] agreed and also recommended that nursing and medical students be acculturated into the notion of family-centered care and practice.

IMPLICATIONS FOR EVIDENCE-BASED PRACTICE

Since Molter's seminal work[11] on the needs of families of critically ill patients, ICUs have undergone many changes. New diagnostic procedures and technology enable staff to treat patients more aggressively with improved outcomes; most hospitals now have one-patient rooms to provide more privacy; many hospitals have lenient visiting hours for patient's immediate family members; and waiting rooms are more convenient in size, décor, and proximity to patients. In order to further improve ICU experiences for patients' families, the AACN protocols for practice series includes the booklet *Family Needs and Interventions in the Acute Care Environment.*[19] Additional articles have reinforced the value of the AACN series.[9] Yet, with all these improve-

ments and materials, nurses continue to recognize that needs of patients' family members are not being met, as evidenced by numerous new studies that continue to describe these needs.

A closer scrutiny of the results of studies on the needs of families of patients with traumatic brain injury may indicate nurses have overlooked an important concept, namely, empowerment of patients and patients' families, and have continued to follow an older, paternalistic model in which healthcare professionals take charge. Nurses may pay lip service to patient-centered care and think their studies and interventions have been carried out to support patient's families but may not recognize why the top needs of patients' families consistently include the need for information (Table 2). Healthcare issues of today, such as informed consent, do not resuscitate orders, and managed care, require including patient's families in decision making for the care of the patients. Without adequate information, families cannot determine the correct care of their family member and consequently feel powerless and out of control. Williams[40] defined empowerment as "the creation of an environment in which individuals can behave as responsible adults, and where decision making is made at the point where the knowledge is greatest." Empowered families of patients with severe traumatic brain injury, armed with information, can work with healthcare providers to achieve quality care.

LIMITATIONS

The focus of our study was strictly the needs of families of patients with severe traumatic brain injury during the patients' ICU stay. We did not evaluate the families' home dynamics or the stresses that accompany disruption of regular routines, financial disruption, or other lifestyle changes. Qualitative research, with small sample size, can provide insights about a particular group of patients or health condition and can illustrate quantitative finding, but is limited in its generalizability.

RECOMMENDATIONS FOR FURTHER RESEARCH

Using the concept of empowerment of patients and their families[41] and Leske's contribution[9] in the AACN protocols for practice series, researchers should focus on ways to meet the needs of patients'

TABLE A5-3

Collaborative Intervention Plan for Families of Patients With Severe Traumatic Brain Injury*

Intervention	Steps in the Intervention
Initiate information protocol.	• Meet with the patient's family when the patient is admitted to the hospital. • Provide current information about the extent of the patient's injury and prognosis. • Arrange to meet the family again immediately after the patient's condition is initially stabilized. • Allow the family to see the patient immediately, regardless of the patient's condition. • Arrange support through social worker or pastoral leader. • Provide a beeper or telephone number for necessary updates. • Provide booklet with information on severe traumatic brain injury.
Arrange daily time for family briefing.	• Have the family designate a spokesperson to receive information and to relay that information to other family members. • Reinforce understanding and clarify misconceptions. • Review the information in the booklet on severe traumatic brain injury. • Be professional in discussions with the family: provide accurate information, suppress personal bias, and support the family in their decisions.
Be sensitive to the families' individual characteristics.	• Be sensitive to family issues, feelings, and religious considerations; differences in educational and cultural backgrounds; and the dynamics of divorced or estranged families.
Validate the family's feelings throughout the patient's stay in the Intensive Care Unit.	• Help family members draw upon their personal beliefs and practices. • Recognize that the major source of frustration is the patient's unstable conditions and uncertain outcome.
Encourage continuity of information support for patients' family members.	• Provide in-service training for staff members of the neurological intensive care unit.
Provide comfort to patients'[1] family members.	• Use hospital volunteers, social workers, or family advocates to provide comfort measures.
Meet the families' need to be involved in the patients' care.	• Allow the family to assist with the patients' basic care.

*Based on suggestions from patients' families, recommendations of earlier studies, and Lesko.[9]

families for information and ways to incorporate the families' input in decision making about the patients' care. Investigators should evaluate the effectiveness of the interactions, by working with families, rather than merely examining family interventions.[41] Evidence-based practice requires healthcare providers to identify interventions that lead to the intentional, systematic improvements in informed decision making by patients' families, decrease the families' stress, and improve the patients' outcomes.

CONCLUSIONS

We identified specific needs of families of patients with severe traumatic brain injury during the patients' stay in the neurological ICU: the need to know, the need for consistent information, the need for involvement, and the need to make sense of the experience. On the basis of the results of earlier intervention studies,[24,25,34] suggestions from the families in our study, Leske's contribution[9] to the AACN protocols for practice series, and AACN's Values,[36] nurses can alleviate the stress of patients' families by providing information and way for the families to be involved in the patients' care. Such a model of holistic care, based on evidence, will validate the role of patients' families during patients' hospitalization and improve outcomes for families and, possibly, for patients.

Acknowledgments

This study was funded in part by the Office of Research and Creative Activities at Brigham Young University, Provo, Utah.

References

1. American College of Surgeons. (1907). *Advance trauma life support for doctors* (6th ed., pp. 181–201). Chicago, Ill: Author.

2. Littlejohns, L. R. & Bader, M. K. (2001). Guidelines for the management of severe head injury: Clinical application and changes in practice. *Critical Care Nurse, 21,* 48–98.

3. Hall, K. M., Karzmark, P., Stevens, M., Englander, J., O'Hare, P., & Wright, J. (1994). Family stressors in traumatic brain injury: A two year follow-up. *Archives of Physical Medicine and Rehabilitation, 75,* 876–884.

4. Landsman, I. S., Baum, C. G., Arnkoff, D. R., Craig, M. J., Lynch, I., Copes, W. S., & Champion, H. R. (1990). The psychosocial consequences of traumatic injury. *Journal of Behavioral Medicine, 13,* 561–581.

5. American Association of Critical-Care Nurses. *Vision, 2002.* Retrieved June 2, 2003 from http://www.aacn.org

6. Curry, S. (1995). Identifying family needs and stresses in the intensive care unit. *British Journal of Nursing, 4,* 15–19.

7. Scullion, P. (1994). Personal cost, caring and communication: An analysis of communication between relatives and intensive care nurses. *Intensive Critical Care Nurse, 10,* 64–70.

8. Agulera, D. C. & Messick, J. M. (1985). *Crisis intervention theory and methodology.* (5th ed.). St. Louis, MO: CV Mosby.

9. Leske, J. S. (1997). *Family needs and interventions in the acute care environment.* Aliso Viejo, CA: American Association of Critical-Care Nurses.

10. Lopex-Puglin, I. (1995). Critical Care Family Needs Inventory: A cognitive research utilization approach. *Critical Care Nurse, 15*(21), 23–26.

11. Molter, N. C. (1979). Needs of relatives of critically ill patients: A descriptive study. *Heart and Lung, 8,* 332–339.

12. Woolley, N. O. (1990). Crisis theory: A paradigm of effective intervention with families of critically ill people. *Journal of Advanced Nursing, 15,* 1402–1408.

13. Dracup, K. A. & Breu, C. S. (1978). Using nursing research findings to meet the needs of grieving spouses. *Nursing Research, 27,* 212–216.

14. Hampe, S. O. (1975). Needs of the grieving spouse in a hospital setting. *Nursing Research, 24,* 113–120.

15. Mathis, M. (1984). Personal needs of family members of critically ill patients with and without acute brain injury. *Journal of Neuroscience Nursing, 16,* 36–44.

16. Engli M. & Kirsivali-Farmer K. (1993). Needs of family members of critically ill patients with and without acute brain injury. *Journal of Neuroscience Nursing, 25,* 78–85.

17. Leske J. (1986). The needs of relatives of critically ill patients a follow-up. *Heart and Lung, 15,* 189–193.

18. Bernstein L. P. (1990). Family-centered care of the critically ill neurologic patient. *Critical Care Nursing Clinics of North America, 2,* 42–50.

19. Bauman, C. C. (1984). Identifying priority concerns of families of ICU patients. *Dimensions of Critical Care Nursing, 3,* 313–319.

20. Daley, I. (1984). The perceived immediate needs of families with relatives in the intensive care setting. *Heart and Lung, 13,* 231–237.

21. Melvor, D. & Thompson, F. J. (1988). The self-perceived needs of family members with a relative in the intensive care unit (ICU). *Intensive Care Nurse, 4,* 139–145.

22. Mendonca, D. & Warren, N. A. (1998). Perceived and unmet needs of critical care family members. *Critical Care Nursing Quarterly, 21,* 58–67.

23. Miracle, V. A. & Hovekamp, G. (1994). Needs of families of patients undergoing invasive cardiac procedures. *American Journal of Critical Care, 3,* 155–157.

24. Appleyard, M. E., Gavnghan, S. R., Gonzalez, C., Annian, I., Tyrell, R., & Carroll, D. I. (2000). Nurse-coached intervention for the families of patients in critical care units. *Critical Care Nurse, 20,* 40–48.

25. Medland, J. J. & Ferrans, C. E. (1998). Effectiveness of a structured communication program for family members of patients in an ICU. *American Journal of Critical Care, 7,* 24–29.

26. Washington, G. T. (2001). Family advocates; caring for families in crisis. *Dimensions of Critical Care Nursing, 20,* 36–40.

27. Abbott K. H., Sage, J. G., Breen, C. M., Abernathy, A. P., & Tulsky, J. A. (2001). Families looking back: One year after discussion of withdrawal or withholding of life sustaining support. *Critical Care Medicine, 29,* 197–201.

28. Curtis, J. R., Patrick, D. L., Shannon, S. L., Treece, P. D., Engelberg, R. A., & Rubernfield, G. D. (2001). The family conference as a focus to improve communication about end-of-life care in the intensive care unit: Opportunities for improvement. *Critical Care Medicine, 29*(Suppl. 2), N26–N33.

29. Malacrida R., Bettelini, C. M., Degrate A., Martinez, M., Badia, F., Piazza J., Vizzardi N., Wullschleger, R., & Rapin C. H. (1998). Reasons for dissatisfaction: A survey of relatives of intensive care patients who died. *Critical Care Medicine, 26(7),* 1187–1193.

30. Serin, C. D., Kreutzer, J. S., & Witel, A. D. (1997). Family needs after traumatic bran injury: A factor analytic study of the Family Needs Questionnaire. *Brain Injury, 11,* 1–9.

31. Burr, G. (1998). Contextualizing critical care family needs through triangulation; an Australian study. *Intensive Critical Care Nurse, 14,* 161–169.

32. Testani-Dufour, L., Chappel-Aiken, L., & Gueldner, S. (1992). Traumatic brain injury: A family experience. *Journal of Neuroscience Nursing, 24,* 317–323.

33. Dyer, I. Research into visitor needs using Molter's tool: Time to move on. *Critical Care Nurse, 2,* 285–290.

34. Gavaghan, S. R. & Carroll, D. L. (2002). Families of critically ill patients and the effect of nursing interventions. *Dimensions of Critical Care Nursing, 21,* 64–71.

35. Johnson, D., Wilson, M., Cavanaugh, B., Bryden, C., Gudmundson, D., & Moodley, O. (1998). Measuring the ability to meet family needs in an intensive care unit. *Critical Care Medicine, 26,* 268–271.

36. American Association of Critical-Care Nurses. *Values. 2002.* Retrieved June 2, 2003 from http://www.aacn.org

37. Leske, J. S. (1998). Interventions to decrease family anxiety. *Critical Care Nurse, 18,* 92–95.

38. Harvey, M. (1998). Evolving toward—but not to—meeting family needs. *Critical Care Medicine, 26,* 206–207.

39. Johnson, B. H. (2000). Family-centered care; facing the new millennium. Interview by Elizabeth Ahmann. *Pediatric Nursing, 21,* 100–104.

40. Williams, T. Patient empowerment and ethical decision-making: The patient/partner and the right to act. *Dimensions of Critical Care Nursing, 21,* 100–104.

41. Andrew, C. M. (1998). Optimizing the human experience: Nursing the families of people who die in intensive care. *Intensive Critical Care Nursing, 14,* 59–65.

Efficacy of an In-Home Nursing Intervention Following Short-Stay Breast Cancer Surgery

Gwen K. Wyatt, Laurie Friedman Donze, Kathryn Christensen Beckrow

Abstract: *This randomized controlled trial (n = 240) was designed to test the efficacy of sub-acute home nursing intervention participants following short-stay surgery for breast cancer. Intervention participants received the in-home nursing protocol, whereas non-intervention participants received agency nursing care or no nursing care. Data, collected via questionnaire, telephone interview, and chart audit, included surgical recovery/self-care knowledge, functional status, anxiety, quality of life (QOL), and health service utilization. There were no significant group differences on postoperative functional status, anxiety, QOL, further surgeries, or complications. Intervention participants were more likely to receive instruction on surgical self-care (p ≤ .001) and report improved social/family QOL (p ≤ .05), with fewer home visits (p ≤ .001). These findings suggest that a target nursing protocol may, at reasonable cost, improve QOL and enhance health-related knowledge.*

Keywords: *breast cancer, quality of life, short-stay surgery, nursing care.*

Over the past decade in the United States, the length of hospital stay following breast cancer surgery has changed dramatically. Patients undergoing a mastectomy used to be hospitalized for 10 to 14 days until their surgical drains were removed (Gross, 1998). Currently, a long stay is considered to be anything over 48 hours (Krug, 1997). This evolving change in the standard for hospital stay, coupled with the inherent decrease in nursing care, has created much controversy and debate over acceptable standards of care for women following surgery for breast cancer.

There are clearly proponents on each side of the long- versus short-stay debate, and clinical practice continues to evolve with or without an evidence-base. Therefore, the purpose of this study was to report on the impact of a short-term (14 days post-surgery), sub-acute care intervention for women who underwent short-stay surgery (48 hours or less) for breast cancer.

A commonly cited advantage of short-stay surgery involves the minimization of nosocomial infection and allowing patients to return home to their normal routines (Oncology Nursing Society, 1998). In addition, health maintenance organizations (third party insurers) have argued against lengthy hospitalization for breast surgeries such as axillary node dissection,

Research in Nursing & Health, 2004 Volume 27, Number 5, pages 322–331

lumpectomy, and mastectomy, stating that physical recovery can occur at home, and that extended hospital stays contribute little to addressing self-image, pain, and disfigurement that patients experience (Kambouris, 1995). As a result, surgeons are required to document that an overnight stay is "medically necessary" in order for patients to obtain insurance coverage for an overnight stay. Short-stay and outpatient surgery provides economic savings to health plans, estimated at $1,200 saved per patient if the patient is not hospitalized (Pederson, Douville, & Eberlein, 1994). Kambouris estimated that for each day the length of hospital stay is shortened for breast cancer patients in the United States, approximately $92 million could be saved nationally. Pedersen et al. determined that short hospital stays following breast cancer surgery reduced medical costs without compromising the quality of care that patients receive. It also has been argued that family members can be taught how to care for the surgical site and surgical drain for patients once they return home (Kambouris) and that patients are happier when they are able to be at home and provide their own care (Pederson et al.).

Representing the other side of this argument, many patients and members of the health care community have voiced concern, asserting that money, rather than clinical judgment, is controlling too much of the health care system in the United States today (Canavan, 1997). These critics contend that many disadvantages to short-stay surgery exist, including delays in identifying complications, lack of care in the home for patients who live alone, and the risk that post-operative care instructions will not be followed properly. In addition, it has been argued that the cost of re-admitting a surgical outpatient to the hospital because of post-surgical infection could potentially more than triple the original cost of a longer initial recovery in the hospital without complications (Oncology Nursing Society, 1998).

The research to date regarding short-stay surgery for breast cancer is limited, with most studies focusing on feasibility. In a study by Bundred et al. (1998), a sample of 100 women undergoing mastectomy with axillary dissection or breast conserving surgery was assessed for the presence of physical and psychological sequelae resulting from early discharge (2 days after surgery). Increased rates of complications were not found in this sample, leading the researchers to conclude that the short-stay surgery policy can be recommended if patients have sufficient support at home. Bonnema et al. (1998) also assessed the psychosocial and medical effects of early discharge after surgery in a sample of 125 women with breast cancer, comparing patients discharged 4 days after surgery (with the surgical drain still in place) with patients discharged after the drain was removed ($M = 9$) days post-surgery, with a range of 2–14 days. The investigators found no difference in duration of drainage or incidence of wound complications among groups, with high satisfaction among those who had the shorter stay. This research team also found that opportunities for social support within the family were enhanced by early discharge.

In a study of 52 women undergoing modified radical mastectomy, simple mastectomy, lumpectomy with axillary dissection, or other breast procedures, Burke, Zabka, McCarver, and Singletary (1997) found that most patients had no problems with drain or incision care and were prepared to leave the hospital on the first post-operative day. These investigators concluded that short-stay surgery was feasible for post-operative patients who receive appropriate educational support in preparation for their return to the home. Finally, in his study of 133 breast cancer patients, Seltzer (1995) found that limited axillary node dissection and partial mastectomy can be performed safely as a same-day procedure. Advantages to this approach are that patients do not have to be hospitalized, the surgeon's in-hospital responsibilities and paperwork are reduced, and third-party insurers have reduced costs. From these studies, short-stay surgery appears to be feasible. The question remains, however: what are the physical and psychological costs of short-stay surgery for the patient and her family, which are no longer addressed by the health care system?

Although the majority of the research has focused on the length of hospital stay, little has been done to assess or address the needs of the patients once they return home. Warren et al. (1998) conducted a study of elderly women to determine outcomes for outpatient mastectomies. They found that few data were available on patient satisfaction following surgery, and they concluded that larger studies were needed to provide information on the patient experience following short-stay breast cancer procedures. In a 4-week in-home intervention study, Hughes, Hodgson, Muller, Robinson, and McCorkle (2000) found that extensive information needs existed for elderly cancer patients as they transitioned from the hospital to home following surgery. Several experts have made the point that women's needs may vary greatly, especially in relationship to available family and social support (Canavan, 1997; Wyatt & Friedman, 1998).

Wang, Cosby, Harris, and Liu (1999) found that the major concerns and needs experienced by breast cancer patients were related to health, family, self-esteem, work, finances, future, and counseling and support for the family and themselves. Although some women received agency in-home nursing care to address physical health concerns (such as dressing changes and surgical drain care), many received no follow-up care to manage their numerous other needs, such as protection against the development of lymphedema, anxiety, quality of life (QOL) problems, and obtaining access to necessary community resources. As a result, these women were left to care for themselves or depend on family members to provide physical and emotional support.

Although having family or friends at home may be a great comfort to women, there are still several factors that each individual faces after surgery that may be outside the realm of family or friendship support. Such factors include: psychosocial issues related to the change in body image and anxiety about follow-up adjuvant therapy; physical issues related to post-surgical self-care (e.g., dressing changes and drain care) and prevention of complications (such as lymphedema or diminished surgical arm range-of-motion); and cost-related issues involving use of health services, purchase of supplies, and other costs not covered by insurance but essential to post-surgical recovery. Therefore, based on these issues, a nursing intervention was developed and piloted to address the following research question: can a focused nursing intervention that targets the needs of women following short-stay breast cancer surgery improve the outcomes of physical functioning, QOL, and anxiety in a cost-effective manner, and ultimately, empower women to care for themselves?

The nursing intervention of this study was based on the holistic framework for QOL developed by Wyatt & Friedman (1996). This model includes four life domains: biological, social, psychological, and spiritual/existential. The intervention tapped the biological component via addressing surgical recovery, self-care knowledge, and physical functioning. The social domain was included by involving the patient's

family or other members of her support system, when available, in the intervention. The psychological domain was addressed by the nurse attending to the patient's reported anxiety and emotional QOL. The spiritual domain was not an element of this particular intervention.

The study's specific research questions were as follows: (a) were there any differences among three groups in the post-surgery outcomes of functional status or activities of daily living (ADLs), QOL, and anxiety; (b) were there any differences in self-care education received among the groups; (c) were there differences in health service utilization among groups in changes over time on the outcome variables?

METHOD

Sample

This study provides data on 240 women, with 121 participants in the intervention (Group A), 64 in agency-based home nursing care (Group B), and 55 in no home nursing care (Group C). Women in the intervention (Group A) did not receive agency-ordered home care. The participating surgeons agreed that if women were assigned to the intervention group (Group A), they would not order additional agency-based home care. There were no exceptions to this agreement.

All women were aged 21 and above, able to speak and write the English language, with a positive diagnosis of breast cancer, and undergoing short-stay surgery (anticipated hospital stay of 48 hours or less). The majority were Caucasian (91.7%), married (62.5%), had at least some college education (68.3%), and were employed prior to surgery (56.7%). The mean age of the sample was 56 years ($SD = 11.6$). The average annual household income was $55,164 ($SD = $37,117$). The majority of the women were diagnosed with stage 1 or 2 tumors (94.2%) and had a lumpectomy with axillary node dissection (76.7%) for their surgical treatment (see Table 1). Exclusion criteria included pregnancy, in situ tumors, immediate reconstructive surgery, pre-surgical chemotherapy, or an acute episode of medically diagnosed mental illness at the time of cancer diagnosis.

There were no significant differences among the three groups (A, B, and C) at baseline on demographic variables, functional status, QOL, or anxiety. Therefore, demographics are shown for the total sample (Table 1). In addition, there were no significant differences in demographic or baseline variables across data collection sites.

Measures

In addition to the items assessing demographic information, measures of surgical recovery/self-care knowledge and health service utilization were designed or adapted especially for this study (Given & Given, 1993), and were included in the telephone interview conducted 4 weeks after surgery. Other instruments included standardized tools measuring functional status, anxiety, and QOL.

The items assessing surgical recovery and self-care knowledge were "yes/no" questions to obtain self-reported information on four areas: (a) infection status

TABLE A6-1

Demographics for Total Sample

	Study Total ($n = 240$)	
	n	**Percent**
Ethnicity		
Caucasian	220	91.7
Other	20	8.3
Marital Status		
Married	150	62.5
Divorced/separated	43	17.9
Widowed	29	12.1
Never married	18	7.5
Employment Status		
Employed before surgery	136	56.7
Returned to work after surgery	72	52.9
Did not return to work after surgery	64	47.1
Not employed before surgery	87	36.3
Missing	17	7.1
Education		
Completed graduate school	44	18.3
Completed college	32	13.3
Completed some college	88	36.7
Completed high school	58	24.2
Completed some high school	13	5.4
Completed grade school	5	2.1
Cancer Stage		
Stage 1 or 2	226	94.2
Stage 3 or 4	9	3.7
Missing	5	2.1
Type of Surgery		
Lumpectomy with node removal	184	76.7
Mastectomy with node removal	46	19.2
Simple mastectomy	10	4.2

	Study Total			
	N	*M*	*SD*	*Range*
Income ($)	168	55,164	37,117	2952–210,000
Age (years)	240	55.98	11.61	23–86

Note: No differences by study group were significant.

and antibiotic use, (b) surgical arm range-of-motion, (c) breast self-exam technique, and (d) lymphedema prevention knowledge.

Use of health services was measured with the conventional Health Service Utilization instrument by Given & Given (1993). This instrument includes items on the number of home visits, and asks questions such as, "Have you used the emergency room since your surgery?" All items require a yes or no response and are scored as 1 or 0, respectively. Due to the diverse nature of these items, internal consistency among items was not expected.

Functional status was measured by an adapted version of the instrument from the Rand Health Insurance Experiment and Medical Outcomes Research (Ware et al., 1980). The original instrument measured three dimensions of functioning: (a) physical activities, (b) balance and dexterity, and (c) upper-body self-care activities. The instrument has been tested for validity and reliability with reported alpha coefficients exceeding .90 (Jette et al., 1986; Stewart, Ware, & Barook, 1981; Ware & Sherbourne, 1992). Ten of the items used to measure functional status were taken from the physical functioning subscale of the SF-36 Health Survey (Ware, Snow, Kosinski, & Gandek, 1993). The items included were vigorous activity, moderate activity, lifting or carrying groceries, climbing several flights of stairs, climbing one flight of stairs, bending/kneeling/stooping, walking more than 1 mile, walking several blocks, walking 1 block, and bathing oneself. Respondents were asked via telephone interview to consider their functional status at two different time intervals—prior to surgery and then at the present time (4 weeks after surgery). Reliability coefficients of the adapted instrument for this study ranged from .89 to .91 on pre- and post-test measures, respectively. Scoring was done according to SF-36 instructions on a 0 to 100 scale, in which the higher number equaled better physical functioning.

Anxiety was measured by the State-Trait Anxiety Inventory, a self-report instrument (Spielberger et al., 1983). The State Anxiety scale consists of 20 statements that assess how respondents feel "right now, at this moment." The essential qualities evaluated include feelings of apprehension, tension, nervousness, and worry. The alpha coefficient for a sample of working women was .93 (Spielberger et al.). Spielberger et al. also reported evidence of concurrent, convergent, divergent, and construct validity. Both

pre- and post-test alphas for the current sample were .95 and .95, respectively.

QOL was measured with the Functional Assessment of Cancer Therapy–Breast (FACT-B) scale (Cella & Bonomi, 1994). This instrument includes six subscales that measure: (a) physical well-being, (b) social/family well-being, (c) relationship with doctor, (d) emotional well-being, (e) functional well-being, and (f) additional concerns. Items are rated on a 5-point scale, in which 0 indicates *not at all*, and 4 is *very much*. Respondents are asked to consider the previous 7 days when completing the measure. Test-retest reliability correlations ranged from .82 to .92 in a sample of 70 outpatients with various cancer diagnoses (Cella & Bonomi). The pre- and post-test alphas of the whole instrument for the current sample were .89 and .91, respectively.

Procedures

Participants were recruited from 15 surgical practices in four Midwestern communities. The nurse recruiters reviewed the surgical log and identified women scheduled for breast cancer surgery who met the study criteria. The nurse then contacted the women prior to their surgery, informed them about the study, requested their participation, and asked them to sign the consent form. (Data on women who declined participation are not available.) Once recruited, and after baseline data were collected, women were randomly assigned to the intervention or non-intervention groups. Signed consent forms were stored in a locked file at the central research office. All procedures were approved by the participating institutional review boards.

Data were collected on all participants via a combination of self-administered (written) questionnaires and telephone interviews, at two times over the course of the study (at recruitment and 4 weeks post-surgery). The rationale for this schedule was to obtain baseline data to compare with post-surgery data on the immediate efficacy of the intervention. An incentive payment of $10 was mailed to each non-intervention participant after the telephone interview was completed to demonstrate the value of her time in responding to the questionnaires and interviews. In addition, a chart audit was conducted 4 months post-surgery to determine the staging of the tumor and to gather information on any post-surgical complications.

Intervention participants (Group A) received the targeted nursing care protocol in their homes during the first 14 post-operative days, whereas Group B participants received surgeon-ordered agency home nursing care and Group C participants received no post-surgical home nursing care. The nature of the agency home nursing care was that of a generalist. Nursing care was provided by standard visiting nurse services in the various communities. The nurses did not have specialized training in post-operative breast surgery care. For example, they would visit a Group B patient as a general nurse provider of care; their previous patient may have been a diabetic, and their following patient an orthopedic case. These nurses would attend to the skilled nursing care needs of the patient that warranted insurance reimbursement for physical nursing care.

In contrast, the intervention protocol consisted of a minimum of two home visits and two phone calls by a registered nurse during the weeks immediately following surgery. In addition, each patient had 24-hour access to her nurse by pager, in the event that she had a question between nurse contacts. The nurse/patient interactions were designed to facilitate self-care and empowerment, with an effort to minimize dependence upon the nurse. The first phone call assessed any emergent concerns and was also used to schedule the first home visit. The first in-home visit occurred within 24 hours of the woman returning home after surgery. This visit focused on self-care for the drain and surgical site care, and emotional and QOL concerns. The second phone call was used to schedule the second in-home visit and to evaluate any patient concerns. The second in-home visit reinforced the holistic teaching from the first visit and also taught breast self-examination, upper body range of motion, and lymphedema protection strategies. Thus, all patients were taught not only how to care for themselves physically, but how best to be in-tune with their emotional health, in an attempt to have the fullest recovery possible. In some cases, family members were available, and the study nurse included them in the intervention to the extent they were interested and able to participate (see Wyatt & Beckrow, 2000, for a detailed description of the protocol).

Each intervention nurse received a 6-hour training program based on the standardized post-surgical protocol, so that care would be consistently delivered. In addition, each nurse was paired with a mentor nurse from the research team for the first home visit. The study nurses only cared for patients in the study and were not employed by a home care agency. They each had a copy of the protocol that they kept with them as a reference. Although nurses were available 24 hours-a-day via pagers, patients seldom contacted them during the study. This may have been because the anticipated four encounters with the nurse reduced their uncertainty about ongoing care during the immediate 14 post-operative days. All nurses had either bachelor's or master's degrees in nursing.

Data Analysis

Between-group differences on categorical variables were assessed using chi-square analyses for contingency tables; group differences for continuous variables were assessed using one-way analysis of variance (ANOVA) or multivariate analysis of variance (MANOVA). Changes over time were assessed via paired-sample t-tests. Because there were no significant baseline differences across sites, all data were analyzed together rather than by community. Similarly, the different surgeries were combined for analysis as the majority of women had a lumpectomy with lymph node dissection. In addition, there were no significant differences in outcome variables when analyzed by type of surgery.

RESULTS

Between-Group Differences

As stated previously, there were no significant presurgical differences among the three groups on any of the demographic or baseline variables. Following the intervention period, at 4-weeks post-surgery, there were no significant differences among the groups on functional status, anxiety, or total QOL, with length of hospital stay and number of nurse visits held constant as covariates. The 4-month chart audit found no significant differences among groups on further surgeries or post-operative complications.

Significant between-group differences were found related to self-care education received. Among intervention participants (Group A), a significantly greater proportion (91.3%) reported receiving education on range-of-motion exercises when compared to Groups B (75.0%) and C (61.8%) participants (χ^2 [2, $N = 223$] = 20.21, $p \le .001$). Further, among those who reported receiving education on range-of-motion, intervention participants (Group A) received a significantly greater number of teaching sessions when compared to Group B and C participants (F [2, 176] = 3.51, $p \le .05$).

Among the intervention participants (Group A), a significantly greater proportion (91.8%) reported receiving education on lymphedema prevention, than Groups B (67.8%) or C (49.1%; (χ^2 [2, N = 210] = 34.76, $p \le .001$). In addition, among those who reported receiving education, across the three groups, intervention participants (Group A) received the greatest number of teaching sessions (F [2, 155] = 4.63, $p \le .05$).

The majority of the total sample (90.0%) was discharged within the anticipated 48 hours or less after surgery. However, a significantly higher percentage (14.3%) of participants in Groups B and C combined exceeded the 48-hour stay after surgery when compared to the intervention participants (Group A; 5.8%; F [2, 240] = 6.11, $p \le .05$). When assessing all women who stayed 48 hours or less, the intervention group (Group A) stayed a significantly shorter number of hours (F [2, 234] = 6.11, $p \le .05$) than the nonintervention participants.

There were no significant differences in reported utilization of health services. However, the study

nurses made an average of 2.50 (SD = .90, with a range of 1–6) home visits per intervention participant, which was significantly fewer than the Group B participants who reported receiving an average of 6.41 (SD = 6.63, with a range of 1–40) home visits from agency nurses (F [1, 183] = 40.85, $p \le .001$).

Changes over Time

Several significant changes over time were noted. All three groups reported increased limitation in physical functioning from pre-surgery to 4 weeks post-surgery (t^A [103] = 12.67, $p \le .001$; t^B [62] = 8.34, $p \le .001$; and t^C [53] = 8.02, $p \le .001$). There was also a significant decrease in anxiety among all three groups from baseline to 4 weeks after surgery (t^A [120] = 7.02, $p \le .001$; t^B [63] = 4.43, $p \le .001$; and t^C [54] = 3.90, $p \le .001$); see Table 2).

Regarding QOL, all three groups reported significant improvements from pre-surgery to 4 weeks after surgery in emotional well-being (t^A [120] = 8.45, $p \le .001$; t^B [63] = 6.49, $p \le .001$; and t^C [54] = 5.01, $p \le .001$). The intervention and Group B participants (agency nurse) experienced improvements in two other areas, additional concerns (t^A [119] = 3.48,

TABLE A6-2

Change in Functional Status and State Anxiety by Group

SF-36 Physical Functioning Subscale (10 items). Higher scores indicate better physical functioning.

Group	Before Surgery			After Surgery		
	M	*SD*	*Range*	*M*	*SD*	*Range*
Intervention (n = 104)*	89.62	14.30	45–100	67.93	21.15	10–100
Group B[a] (n = 63)*	89.98	16.49	20–100	69.94	21.51	20–100
Group C[b] (n = 54)*	90.80	20.77	10–100	70.84	24.21	0–100
Study total (n = 221)*	90.01	16.63	10–100	69.21	21.97	0–100

State Anxiety Scale (20 items). Higher scores indicate greater anxiety.

Time	Intervention (n = 121)			Group B[a] (n = 64)			Group C[b] (n = 55)		
	M	*SD*	*Range*	*M*	*SD*	*Range*	*M*	*SD*	*Range*
Before surgery	42.34	13.71	20–78	41.12	13.39	19–75	46.13	14.20	20–80
After surgery	34.69*	12.14	20–77	35.53*	12.68	20–63	39.22*	12.64	20–80

[a]Received nursing care provided by an agency nurse.
[b]Received no nursing care.
*$p < .001$ (within group comparison).

TABLE A6-3

Quality of Life Over Time (the Higher the Mean, the Greater the Quality of Life)

	Intervention (n = 121)					
	Before Surgery			**After Surgery**		
Subscales	**M**	**SD**	**Range**	**M**	**SD**	**Range**
Physical well-being**	20.80	3.71	1–24	19.74	3.47	7–24
Social/family well-being*	19.90	4.63	8–24	20.85	3.74	6–24
Relationship with doctors	7.22	1.44	0–8	7.15	1.32	1–8
Emotional well-being***	16.22	4.86	3–24	19.32	3.92	3–24
Functional well-being	21.17	5.52	0–28	20.72	4.96	6–28
Additional concerns***	18.54	3.83	8–26	19.78	4.03	10–28
	Group B[a] (n = 64)					
Physical well-being***	21.22	2.39	14–24	19.27	4.69	5–24
Social/family well-being	20.42	4.37	7–24	21.12	3.37	10–24
Relationship with doctors	7.25	1.19	4–8	7.14	1.17	4–8
Emotional well-being***	16.20	5.06	4–24	19.36	4.14	6–24
Functional well-being	21.80	4.96	10–28	20.14	5.15	5–28
Additional concerns*	18.77	3.94	10–26	19.91	4.31	8–28
	Group C[b] (n = 55)					
Physical well-being	20.31	4.27	0–24	19.24	4.32	4–24
Social/family well-being	20.18	4.33	8–24	20.85	3.79	10–24
Relationship with doctors	7.40	1.23	2–8	7.27	1.52	1–8
Emotional well-being***	15.25	4.62	5–23	17.96	4.25	5–25
Functional well-being	20.58	6.64	1–28	19.51	5.68	1–28
Additional concerns	18.64	4.24	9–26	19.36	4.81	8–28

[a]Received nursing care provided by an agency nurse.
[b]Received no nursing care.
*p < 05 (within group comparison).
**p < .01 (within group comparison).
***p < .001(within group comparison).

$p \leq .001$; t^B [63] = 2.41, $p \leq .05$), and a significant decrease in physical well-being (t^A [119] = 3.00, $p \leq .01$; t^B [62] = 3.48, $p \leq .001$) from pre- to post-surgery that Group C participants did not report. The intervention group also reported a significant improvement from pre- to post-surgery in a third area, social/family well-being (t^A ([119] = 2.45, $p \leq .05$; see Table 3).

Chart Audit

As stated previously, there were no significant differences among the groups on further surgeries or post-operative complications. Of the total sample, 14.2% of women required one or more further surgeries for treatment of their breast cancer. Post-surgical complications that required a return visit to the surgeon were experienced by 30.4% of the sample. The most common post surgical complication, reported by 24.6% of the women, was a fluid-filled mass known as a seroma.

DISCUSSION

Although there were no significant differences among the groups on outcome variables 4 weeks post-surgery, the results of this study suggest several benefits to a targeted, in-home nursing intervention following breast cancer surgery. Women in the intervention (Group A) were significantly more likely to receive instruction on range-of-motion exercises and lymphedema prevention than those in the Groups B or C. These results serve as a manipulation check to support the unique focus of the study's intervention as compared to standard home nursing care. Enhanced instruction in these (and other) areas should improve women's self-care knowledge and ultimately, recovery after surgery.

It seems that a nursing intervention may also positively enhance QOL. Although all three groups reported improvement in emotional well-being, the intervention (Group A) and Group B participants also improved in physical well-being and additional QOL concerns. Only the study intervention group (Group A) reported a significant improvement after surgery in a third area, referred to as social/family well-being. This may be because the intervention nurses specifically focused on the various dimensions of the QOL conceptual framework (Wyatt & Friedman, 1996) used in this study, which includes social and family issues. Perhaps involving the family members in the self-care activities and discussion also had a positive impact on this area of well-being.

These findings also suggest that our specific nursing intervention protocol may be more time- and cost-effective than standard fee-for-service home nursing care. Women who received the targeted in-home nursing intervention received less than half the number of nursing visits of those receiving standard nursing care, yet achieved comparable or better physical, emotional, and educational outcomes. This finding may be partially explained by the fact that the intervention protocol encouraged independence and self-care competency for those participants.

Regardless of receiving home nursing care or no home care, all women reported limited functional status at 4 weeks after surgery. These functional limitations suggest the need for post-surgical intervention to improve functioning and physical recovery.

Future researchers must address these physical functioning and mobility needs that continue beyond 4 weeks after surgery and their impact on psychosocial issues (e.g., QOL and anxiety). With some adjustments, the intervention protocol could be expanded to support women for a longer period of time after surgery. Physical functioning could be central to the extended protocol, with special emphasis on upper body range-of-motion. This lengthened protocol could then be assessed for its impact on long-term QOL, in addition to the post-surgical sub-acute QOL, as evaluated by this study.

Finally, several limitations in research methodology must be acknowledged. All of the outcome data,

with the exception of the chart review data, were obtained from self-reported measures that may be influenced by demand characteristics (e.g., responding to please the investigator) or social desirability pressures. This may especially be an issue for the telephone interview measures. In addition, validity and reliability data are lacking for the interview measures that were developed for this study. Finally, longer-term follow-up, beyond 4 weeks post-surgery, would likely be important to better understand the efficacy of the intervention and identify the longer-term effects of short-stay surgery.

As previous researchers have shown, short-stay surgery for women with breast cancer seems to be a feasible option (Bonnema et al., 1998; Bundred et al., 1998; Burke et al., 1997; Seltzer, 1995). The drawback is that the physical and psychological needs of these women are not necessarily being met in the home, as needs vary widely from person to person (Canavan, 1997; Wang et al., 1999; Wyatt & Friedman, 1998). Through a nursing-based intervention as described in this study, women can be assured of receiving appropriate educational information that Burke et al. proposed as an essential component of feasible short-stay surgery. In addition, women can receive the support in the home that Bundred et al. found to be a crucial element of successful recovery for breast cancer patients.

Our nursing protocol represents a very different philosophy than typical agency nursing care. It empowers women to provide self-care for physical and psychological needs, rather than encouraging dependency upon the nurse, who is reimbursed per patient visit in standard nursing care. This protocol is implemented in a cost-effective manner by providing a minimum of two visits, two phone calls, and 24-hour access to a nurse through the use of a pager in the event that complications develop. It teaches women how to care for their dressing and drain, how to recognize possible signs of infection, how to manage symptoms, and how to be active participants in their own care. The intervention also addresses anxiety and QOL issues; teaches coping skills; instructs on the importance of and appropriate techniques for range-of-motion exercises, and lymphedema awareness; and provides community resources that women can access once care is complete. This approach is in contrast to traditional agency nursing care, in which, because of reimbursement issues, physical care is the focus, without the emphasis on holistic QOL teaching and management.

In summary, the results of this research may have the potential to be translated into policy for discharge planning in terms of length of hospital stay, standard of care for sub-acute post-surgical needs, and the optimal amount and type of nursing care necessary to achieve favorable outcomes and meet the needs of women following surgical treatment for breast cancer. This research lends an evidence-base for the trends currently seen in post-surgical discharge, as well as evaluating a nursing protocol with successful, cost-effective outcomes.

References

Bonnema, J., van Wersch, A. M., van Geel, A. N., Pruyn, J. F., Schmitz, P. I., & Paul, M. A. (1998). Medical and psychosocial effects of early discharge after surgery for breast cancer: A randomized trial. *British Medical Journal, 316,* 1267–1271.

Bundred, N., Maguire, P., Reynolds, J., Grimshaw, J., Morris, J., & Thomson, L. (1998). Randomized controlled trial effects of early discharge after surgery for breast cancer. *British Medical Journal, 317,* 1275–1279.

Burke, C. C., Zabka, C. L., McCarver, K. J., & Singletary, S. E. (1997). Patient satisfaction with 23-hour "short-stay" observation following breast cancer surgery. *Oncology Nursing Forum, 24,* 645–651.

Canavan, K. (1997). Nurses fight "drive-through mastectomy" trend. *The American Nurse, 29*(1), 3, 8.

Cella, D. F. & Bonomi, A. E. (1994). *Manual Functional Assessment of Cancer Therapy (FACT) scales and the Functional Assessment of HIV Infection (FAHI) scale. Version 3.* Chicago: Rush Cancer Institute.

Given, B. A. & Given, C. W. (1993). Conventional health service use. Unpublished instrument.

Gross, R. E. (1998). Current issues in the surgical treatment of early stage breast cancer. *Clinical Journal of Oncology Nursing, 2*(2), 55–63.

Hughes, L. C., Hodgson, N. A., Muller, P., Robinson, L. A., & McCorkle, R. (2000). Information needs of elderly post surgical cancer patients during the transition from hospital to home. *Journal of Nursing Scholarship, 32,* 25–30.

Jette, A. M., Davies, A. R., Cleary, P. D., Calkins, D. R., Rubenstein, L. V., & Fink, A. (1986). The Functional Status Questionnaire: Reliability and validity when used in primary care. *Journal of General Internal Medicine, 1,* 143–149.

Kambouris, A. (1995). Psychological and economic advantages of accelerated discharge after surgical

treatment for breast cancer. *The American Surgeon, 62,* 123–127.

Krug, P. (1997). Breast cancer legislation active in several states. *AORN Journal, 66,* 330–333.

Oncology Nursing Society. (1998). Advantages and disadvantages of outpatient surgery. *Oncology Nursing Society's 1998 Annual Congress Symposia Highlights, 31.*

Pederson, S. H., Douville, L. M., & Eberlein, T. J. (1994). Accelerated surgical stay programs. *Annals of Surgery, 219,* 374–381.

Seltzer, M. A. (1995). Partial mastectomy and limited axillary dissection performed as a same day surgical procedure in the treatment of breast cancer. *International Surgery, 80,* 79–81.

Spielberger, C. D., Gorsuch, R. L., Lushene, R., Vagg, P. R., & Jacobs, G. A. (1983). *Manual for the State-Trait Anxiety Inventory.* Palo Alto, CA: Consulting Psychologists Press.

Stewart, A. L., Ware, J. E., & Barook, R. H. (1981). Advances in the measurement of functional status: Construction of aggregate indexes. *Medical Care, 19,* 473–488.

Wang, X., Cosby, L. G., Harris, M. G., & Liu, T. (1999). Major concerns and needs of breast cancer patients. *Cancer Nursing, 22,* 157–163.

Ware, J., Brook, R., Davies-Avery, A., Williams, K., Stewart, A., Rogers, R., et al. (1980). *Concept utilization and measurement of health for adults in the Health Insurance Study: Vol 1. Model of health and methodology (Publication No. R-1987/1-HEW).* Santa Monica, CA: RAND Corporation.

Ware, J. E. & Sherbourne, C. D. (1992). A 36-item short form health survey (SF-36). *Medical Care, 30,* 473–483.

Ware, J. E., Snow, K. K., Kosinski, M., & Gandek, B. (1993). *SF36 Health Survey: Manual and interpretation guide.* Boston: The Health Institute, New England Medical Center.

Warren, J. L., Riley, G. F., Potosky, A. L., Klabunde, C. N., Richter, E., & Ballard-Barbash, R. (1998). Trends and outcomes of outpatient mastectomy in elderly women. *Journal of the National Cancer Institute, 90,* 833–840.

Wyatt, G. K. & Beckrow, K. C. (2000). A nursing protocol for sub-acute recovery following breast cancer surgery. *Proceedings of the 10th Biennial Conference of European Nurse Researchers, Reykjavik, Iceland 10,* 42–45.

Wyatt, G. K. & Friedman, L. L. (1996). Development and testing of a quality of life model for long-term female cancer survivors. *Quality of Life Research, 5,* 387–394.

Wyatt, G. K. & Friedman, L. L. (1998). Physical and psychological outcomes of midlife and older women following surgery and adjuvant therapy for breast cancer. *Oncology Nursing Forum, 25,* 761–768.

Feeling Safe: The Psychosocial Needs of ICU Patients

Judith E. Hupcey

Purpose: To describe the psychosocial needs of critically ill patients, including descriptions of patients' experiences when these needs are not met, and behaviors of families, friends, and ICU staff that help or impede meeting these needs.

Design: A qualitative research design was used. Participants were 45 adult critically ill patients in the medical or surgical ICU for minimum of 3 days in a large, rural American tertiary care center.

Methods: Data collection and analysis were conducted using methods of grounded theory, including theoretical sampling and the constant comparative process. Unstructured tape-recorded interviews were conducted with patients once they were stable in the ICU or immediately following their transfer to a general unit. Data were collected and analyzed simultaneously. This process continued until saturation was reached and a model of the psychosocial needs of ICU patients was developed.

Findings: The overwhelming need of ICU patients was to feel safe. The perception of feeling safe was influenced by family and friends, ICU staff, religious beliefs, and feelings of knowing, regaining control, hoping, and trusting.

Conclusions: ICU patients in this study said that feeling safe was their overarching need. Patients described feelings of distress when they did not feel safe and stated how family, staff, and religion could both positively and negatively affect this feeling. Nurses can intervene in numerous areas to foster the feeling of safety in critically ill patients.

Keywords: feeling safe, hope, trust, knowing, control, ICU patients, critically ill patients.

The experience of being critically ill has been the focus of many investigations. However, much of the research has been limited in scope, with only limited numbers or specified areas of intensive care unit (ICU) patients' psychosocial needs identified. In addition, these investigations are rarely extended beyond identification of the needs to determine how these needs are met. The purpose of this qualitative study was to investigate the psychosocial needs of critically ill patients, including these questions: (a) what are patients' experiences when their needs are not met; and (b) what do families and ICU staff do that either helps to meet or does not meet patients' needs.

Journal of Nursing Scholarship, 2000, Volume 32, Number 4, pages 361–367

BACKGROUND

Memories of the ICU Experience

ICU patients have varied memories of their ICU experiences. Some people have extensive memories, but others recall little of their ICU stay. Many of these memories include being cared for by nurses. Russell (1999) investigated the memories of ICU patients 6 months after discharge from the ICU. Patients' memories of being closely watched by both the staff and through technology added to their sense of safety. Memories of patients who were therapeutically paralyzed also included nurses who provided both emotional support and encouragement (Johnson et al., 1999). Patients in this study also remembered their families providing encouragement.

Nursing care in the ICU also was remembered as a positive experience of patients in other studies. Burfitt, Greiner, Miers, Kinney, and Branyon (1993) investigated ICU patients' perceptions of caring by nurses. They found that nurses' vigilant behaviors were of great importance. These behaviors included attentiveness, practice skills, and the extra "going out of their way." Numerous caring metaphors used by critically ill patients were identified by Jenny and Logan (1996). The significance of the care provided by nurses was evident not only in the discussion by patients about the actual care given by nurses, but also in the retelling of their distress which required nursing care. When they had unmet needs or distress, nurses provided care and often helped meet those needs.

The ICU experience for patients is not as negative as one might perceive. Compton (1991) and Elpern, Patterson, Gloskey, and Bone (1992) found that patients felt safe in the ICU. Patients did not feel frightened about their illness and many felt reassured by the skill of the nursing staff. Turner, Briggs, Springhorn, and Potgieter (1990) found that 94 of the 100 patients they interviewed perceived the ICU to be friendly and relaxed, and only 28 patients stated a fear of dying while in the unit. Many of their sample reported having confidence in the ICU staff. Positive feelings about the ICU were influenced by supportive behaviors of the nursing staff (Geary, Tringali, & George, 1997). The critically ill adults in their study had positive feelings when they felt supported and negative feelings when they did not. The supportive behaviors identified by these patients included the normal care and attention provided by nurses. These studies indicate the importance of actions of nurses in shaping positive memories of a potentially negative experience.

Nursing Interventions for ICU Patients

Nursing interventions that help patients "get through" the ICU experience also have been investigated. Interventions have been aimed at reducing anxiety (Kim, Garvin, & Moser, 1999; Updike, 1990), decreasing pain sensations, increasing sleep (Richards, 1998), and promoting positive physiological changes, such as improving heart rate and blood pressure (Updike, 1990). Interventions included music therapy (Updike, 1990), relaxation techniques, such as backrubs (Richards, 1998), and pre-ICU education for those scheduled for ICU admission following surgery (Kim et al., 1999). These interventions were beneficial, yet other psychosocial interventions also may result in positive patient outcomes. For example, hope has been found to be therapeutic to ICU patients (Cutcliffe, 1996), and may even affect survival (Morse & Dobernick, 1995). Behaviors of families and nurses appear to have a significant effect on patients' abilities to maintain hope during a critical illness (Wilkinson, 1996).

The purpose of this study was to answer the following questions: What are the psychosocial needs of ICU patients? What happens to patients when these needs are not met? How can families and nurses intervene to meet these needs?

METHODS

Design

The methods of grounded theory as described by Glaser and Strauss (1967) were used for this study. Procedures included theoretical sampling and the constant comparative process.

Sample

Following institutional review board approval, the sample was chosen using the principles of theoretical sampling as described by Glaser (1978), so that the sample was chosen based on the needs of the study. The initial sample included patients from the medical ICU who were admitted with a variety of medical conditions. As the study progressed, patients from the surgical ICU were included to broaden the scope of diagnoses. As the model was developed, additional patients were included to expand and verify the model. For example, social support from family was identified as a strong need by the patients, so patients who were identified by ICU nurses as appearing to have little or no support were asked to participate.

The total sample was 45 patients in the medical and surgical ICUs of a large, rural tertiary care medical center in the Eastern part of the United States. The sample included 20 men and 25 women. Ages ranged from 25 to 80 years, with a mean of 59. The patients had a minimum stay in the ICU of 3 days, and some were in the unit for over 1 month. The sample included patients with a wide variety of medical and surgical diagnoses.

Data Collection

Data were collected through tape-recorded, open-ended, unstructured interviews. The interview took place once the person was stable while still in the ICU or immediately following transfer to a general unit. The interviews began with the general statement: "Tell me about your hospitalization." The informants were permitted to tell their whole story before further questions were asked. When they were finished, probing questions were asked to clarify and expound on information. For example, a probing question might have been, "What helped you the most during your ICU stay?" or "What was the most upsetting part of your ICU stay?" In addition, once informants told their whole story, they were asked to help validate the emerging model. An example of such a question would be, "Other patients have said . . . ; have you had this same experience?"

The interviews lasted from 15 minutes to 1 hour. Length of time was dependent upon the condition of the patient or how long patients needed to tell their whole stories.

Interviews were transcribed verbatim with all personally identifying information removed. Following transcription, each interview was checked for accuracy by the interviewer.

Data Analysis

Analysis was achieved through the constant comparative process in which data are collected and analyzed simultaneously (Glaser & Strauss, 1967). Data were coded line-by-line, and themes were identified. As these themes were identified, they were tested against incoming data. As the themes were expounded, categories were distinguished and described. Relationships among categories were explicated and a core variable was identified and described (Chenitz & Swanson, 1986; Corbin, 1986; Glaser, 1978). Data collection continued until no new categories emerged, thus, saturation was reached.

Validity and Reliability of the Data

Threats to objectivity or confirmability, validity, and reliability of qualitative studies can occur during the design of the study, data collection, and data analysis. According to Miles and Huberman (1994) objectivity is related to freedom from researcher bias. Reliability or dependability is related to the study being reasonably consistent over time and among researchers. Validity is associated with the "truth value" (p. 278) and transferability of the findings. These issues were addressed in the study design. This investigator followed the principles of grounded theory as described by Glaser and Strauss (1967) and Glaser (1978). Sampling included a diverse group of ICU patients with a variety of diagnoses. Negative informants, that is, those patients who might have had different experiences were sought for inclusion. Interviews were critiqued for areas of bias and the transcriptions were checked for accuracy. Two researchers in addition to the primary researcher reviewed the data and participated in data analysis. During this process, the emerging model was confirmed with subsequent informants. This process yielded results that were theoretically linked to being an ICU patient and, thus, may have some transferability to other ICU contexts.

RESULTS

A model of the psychosocial needs of ICU patients was developed around the core variable of feeling safe (see Figure 1). The four categories in the model affect patients' experiences of feeling safe. The categories are knowing, regaining control, hoping, and trusting. The core variable and categories also are influenced by family and friends, ICU staff (nurses and physicians), and religion. These influencing factors provide stimuli by which the needs of ICU patients are met. In addition, family and staff interactions, which may be positive or negative, influence patients' feelings of safety and how well the patients' needs are being met.

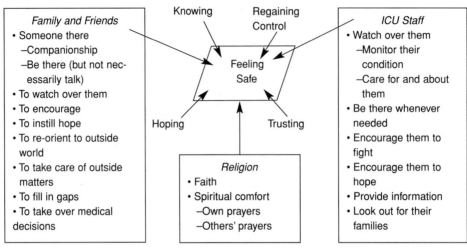

FIGURE A7-1 • Model of the psychosocial needs of ICU patients.

The model will be discussed in detail from the perspective of patients who had their needs met, thus for example, trusted the staff. The model also will be explained from the perspective of those people who did not have their needs met, did not trust, or were not in control. Both perspectives are needed to provide a full understanding of the model. In addition, the effects of family, staff, and religion will be discussed.

Needs of ICU Patients

Core Variable: Feeling Safe. The overarching need of all ICU patients in this study was to feel safe. The four categories of identified needs—knowing, regaining control, hoping, and trusting—all affected feeling safe. For example, if patients felt a loss of control during periods of confusion, they felt unsafe. Or if they lost trust in the staff, they felt unsafe. If these needs were met, patients talked about feeling safe.

Knowing. Knowing what was happening to them provided reassurance and appeared to help ICU patients "get through a terrible experience." Although patients talked about varying needs for information, those who said that they did not know or understand the whole story began to refuse treatments, fight with the staff, feel frightened, and at the extreme felt that the staff were out to get them. Patients spent enormous amounts of energy trying to pull the pieces of the ICU experience together. At times, families were the

source of this information, but some families also withheld information from patients. Those patients reported listening to the nurses and physicians during rounds and trying to piece together the information. Other patients were continually being told what was happening, but because of their medical conditions or medications they were unable to remember. One patient explained how knowing what was happening turned a frightening experience into a bearable one:

> When they tried to wean me off the breathing machine, I spent one evening very hypertensive. I was afraid to fall asleep, not knowing just what to expect. One of the nurses came in and said "[name of patient]" that machine is built so if you do not breathe, it's gonna breathe for you. It will not let you go without breathing." I didn't know that, and nobody had told me that. This information made the experience a lot easier.

Regaining Control. Regaining control of one's life was an important part of the ICU experience. Initially most patients felt a total loss of control. This loss of control related to many aspects of being a patient in the ICU. Some patients complained about their lack of control of visitors or being confined to a bed. Others had more intense feelings of a total loss of independence because they could not care for or make decisions for themselves. Patients differentiated loss of control and being out of control. Being out of control was an extremely frightening experience, while loss of control caused more frustration and a sense of insecurity. Patients expressed a turning point at which they believed that they were able to begin to regain some control. Long-term patients, such as people awaiting heart transplants, rearranged their rooms, controlled visiting times, had special meals, and negotiated with the staff about when they would have treatments. For other patients, regaining control consisted of smaller steps, such as ambulating and taking back some of the responsibilities they had delegated to family members. Patients expressed the frustration caused by loss of control. One said, "I see that it was a real emotional tragedy for me because when you come in here, the biggest problem is you lose control of your life. It's a real serious problem for me." Another said,

> I don't have any freedom. I'm confined to bed and the kids can only come in for 10 minutes at a time every hour so it's hard on them because 10 minutes is hardly worth the effort of coming in. So it's uncomfortable for them and it's very uncomfortable for me.

Hoping. Maintaining hope was imperative for ICU patients, because being hopeless meant giving up. As one patient said, "If you keep hoping, you have a chance." This sentiment was expressed by many patients who believed that they needed to maintain hope to survive. Many patients also gave examples of other patients who gave up hope and then had less than optimal outcomes. As one patient awaiting a heart transplant said:

> There were times I thought, "Is there any hope? Am I gonna make it to get the transplant?" But most of the time I was positive that I was gonna get a second chance at life. You gotta have a good frame, because if you don't have a good frame of mind it's not gonna work.

The feeling of hope came not only from within, but was greatly influenced by family, friends, religion, and the ICU staff. Continual encouragement helped patients maintain hope and fight for survival. Families tried different ways to help patients maintain hope. They talked of the outside world, brought pictures of children and grandchildren, and tried to remind patients they had something to live for. For example:

> I know there were days like there was no hope. I felt depressed and down. . . . I'm very hopeful now. I had the support of my family and the support of my best friends. Without them and their encouragement, I wouldn't have gotten through it.

Trusting. Trusting nurses and other ICU staff was essential for patients to feel safe. As patients discussed their experiences, the concept of trust was rarely mentioned unless patients distrusted. But implicit trust of the staff was evident in the descriptions given about their caregivers. Patients' discussions about nurses watching over them, meeting or attempting to meet their needs, and their full acceptance, without question, of the care given, attested to the trust placed in nurses.

> I don't know that I remember exactly what they did that helped me. But I was able to accept the fact, and have enough trust in them [nurses], that whatever they were doing was going to help me. You trust them enough to know that, whatever . . . they are doing, it's not monkeyshines. They helped you the last time and you got better. And you got better the time before that. So why not let them do what they want to do?

Patients who expressed distrust gave a different story. Instead of believing that they were being watched by nurses, they watched the nurses. They became vigilant about their care and expressed concern about the competency of the staff, a feeling never mentioned by those who trusted. These patients did not feel safe being cared for by the staff. They believed the staff were not looking out for their best interests and as a result always remained on guard. For example, "The nurses were bad. I don't know, I just had very little confidence in them and I'd be so scared to go there again." Another patient said, "I want to get out of here because I feel like I don't trust them. I don't know what they might do. . . . When I see her [one of the nurses] coming and it's like I just tense up because I'm not in no shape to, I can't defend myself."

Family and Friends, Staff, and Religious Beliefs

Feeling safe also was greatly influenced by family and friends, the staff, and for many, religion. As one patient explained: "What really gets you through this is your family, your beliefs, and the people who are here taking care of you."

Family and Friends. Family and friends were a great source of support for patients. Just their presence or "being there" made patients feel safe. Patients explained that the feeling of being watched over by family members was extremely important. Many described having family present, but not even talking, as giving them a sense of comfort. Others, whose families were not present, still felt secure by the knowledge that they were only a phone call away. One patient said,

> When you wake up when you're in intensive care, you're dozing on and off because they give you so much medication, and then when you open your eyes and see somebody you know, it feels good, reassuring or if you feel a warm hand–you know it's your son or someone—well, that really helps, it really does.

Family and friends also were important sources of encouragement. They instilled hope in patients, re-oriented them to the outside world, and encouraged them to fight. They also took care of outside matters that patients could not think about because they were so concerned with their present situation. Families also were the ties between patients and staff, and many times filled in the gaps for patients. At times, family members made decisions for patients who were either too sick or too overwhelmed to make decisions for themselves.

At times those people who were supposed to help patients feel safe were a cause of distress. Some patients complained about family members not being present when needed. Others said that their family and friends withdrew when they really needed to talk. Hiding information was another cause for concern, because it left the patient wondering, "Is something really bad wrong with me?" Patients also were distressed when their family members came in upset or crying. When this behavior occurred, one patient said, "I knew I must have looked bad."

ICU Staff. Nurses and other health care providers also were instrumental in helping patients feel safe. The feeling that staff were watching over them and caring for and about them was important to patients' sense of safety. Nurses provided support, encouraged patients to live, and to hope. The statement, "I'd call the nurse and she was there," was a common one among these patients. The following examples illus-

trate the importance of nurses in making patients feel safe: "Up here (the ICU) I feel safe. All I have to do is look funny and they know there's something wrong with me." "No matter morning, noon, or night, when I called the nurse, she was there. Just to comfort me and try to relax me so I could breathe calmly, not breathe and get in a panic, you know, and make it worse." "The nurse was a shoulder to cry on, somebody to lean on I guess. Especially at night."

In some instances the staff also caused distress for patients. Some nurses were described as not caring, being rough, not answering the call bell, not listening, not being honest, "They said it wouldn't hurt, when they knew it would," and having an "attitude." As one patient said, "She would always do things that would make me uncomfortable." When staff were rushed or overly stressed, patients felt it.

> It bothers me when they are stressed and they are asking me questions, like shooting questions and I'm trying to think and, when they are stressed and they transmit that to me. Yeah, that's one thing that I'm bothered by a lot.

Religion. Religious beliefs were not only a source of comfort but were also described as "what has gotten me through" the ICU experience. Some patients explained that the feeling they were being watched over by a higher authority provided a feeling of safety. Praying when feeling scared and knowing that others were praying for them was comforting.

DISCUSSION

Patients in this study related that feeling safe was an overwhelming need for them while they were in the ICU. Affecting the experience of feeling safe were the need to know, regain control, hope, and trust. When these needs were not met, patients did not feel safe and their experiences ranged from being upset or frustrated to being distressed, fighting, or paranoid. Family and friends, ICU staff, and religion influenced feeling safe and the meeting of these needs. Although many of the themes identified in this study have been found in earlier research, the importance of all four themes—knowing, regaining control, hoping, and trusting—and their influence on feeling safe has not been previously identified.

The concept of feeling safe in this study was similarly found in other studies of ICU patients. Feeling safe was related to the actions of nurses to foster these feelings (Compton, 1991; Elpern et al., 1992; Russell, 1999). Other researchers did not specifically identify the experience of feeling safe, but found the presence of nurses and families to be comforting for patients (Burfitt et al., 1993).

The other concepts in this study that contributed to feeling safe for the patients previously had not been investigated extensively. The concept of knowing, or more specifically, not knowing, has been examined in a few studies with the feelings of distress that were associated with that experience (Hall-Lord, Larsson, & Bostrom, 1994; Hupcey & Zimmerman, 2000; Parker, Schubert, Shelhamer, & Parillo, 1984). Hupcey and Zimmerman (2000) found that knowing for ICU patients was two components: knowing during the ICU event and knowing after the ICU stay. During the event results of not knowing included being upset, paranoid, agitated, and at times, refusing treatments. Not knowing and having confusing perceptions also led to distress in elderly ICU patients (Hall-Lord, Larsson, & Bostrom, 1994). Feeling a loss of reality and thus not knowing resulted in feelings of paranoia in a therapeutically paralyzed ICU patient (Parker, Schubert, Shelhamer, & Parrillo, 1984). The feelings of distress, confusion, and paranoia also were seen in the ICU patients in this study, during the time when they did not know what was happening to them. Communicating with ICU patients has been found to be important in enhancing the sense of knowing or understanding what is happening during an ICU admission. Russell (1999) found that adequate communication was both therapeutic and reassuring and resulted in decreased distress among ICU patients. Communication with intubated patients also has been found to be extremely important (Hafsteindóttir, 1996). Patients wanted interaction, information, and explanations even when they had impaired ability to communicate.

Patients in this study also expressed the need to regain control as part of feeling safe. The process of regaining control was seen in incremental steps throughout the ICU stay. In prior research, this concept received little attention, except related to situations of complete loss of control, such as when a patient was either confused or dependent (Hall-Lord, Larsson, & Bostrom, 1994; Laitinen, 1996). Laitenen (1996) described patients' experiences with confusion in the ICU. An important facet of confusion was

patients' memories of loss of control while confused and the embarrassment the memory of loss of control invoked. Nurses' presence during that state of confusion helped the patient feel safe. The feeling of dependency or having no control also was found to cause distress in elderly patients during an ICU stay (Hall-Lord et al., 1994) and loss of control was a major psychological stressor in patients who had cardiac surgery (Soehren, 1995). Assisting the patient to regain some control was examined by Lazure and Baun (1994) in their study of patient-controlled devices (lights for allowing visitors to enter) to indicate when the patient wanted visitors. Patients who used this device had an increased sense of control and decreased blood pressure compared to the control groups.

Little empirical work has been done related to the concept of trust with ICU patients or with hospitalized patients in general, except when included in literature about nurse-patient relationships. Hupcey, Penrod, and Morse (in press) examined the process of building and maintaining trust during acute hospitalization and found that most patients go through hospital stays with an unbroken level of trust in the staff. However, people who did not trust had experiences similar to those reported by patients in this study, that is, becoming vigilant about the care given.

Hope is another concept that has received little attention except in relation to oncology patients. Although hope was imperative for the patients in this study, few researchers have identified the benefits of supporting hope (Cirlin, 1998; Clark & Heidenreich, 1995; Cutcliffe, 1996; Johnson, Dahlen, & Roberts, 1997; Morse & Dobernick, 1995). Morse and Penrod (1999) found that hope includes a goal for the future and a path to meet that goal. Although patients in this study did not explicitly talk about the future in relation to hope, they expressed the need to hope to get through the experience, thus move toward the future.

Finally, the interrelationships between families and ICU staff were found to be an important aspect of feeling safe. Little research has been done that has indicated how these relationships affect ICU patients. Hupcey (1998, 1999) studied the interaction between nurses and families of ICU patients and strategies used by both ICU nurses and families to develop relationships. Hupcey (1999) found that although nurses' and the families' ultimate goals were to improve the patients' outcome, at times both were looking out for their own interests as well as the patients'. When ICU nurses and the families of ICU patients developed trusting relationships, families were given more of the nurse's time and were allowed to spend more time in the patient's room. In turn, families tended to become less vigilant, allowing the nurses to care for their critically ill relatives without constantly watching and questioning. A trusting relationship between families and ICU staff could enhance feelings of safety among ICU patients. As reported by patients in this study, family presence was a source of comfort, support, encouragement, and hope. Families also were found to be the link between patients and ICU staff, so the presence of families was important for these patients.

IMPLICATIONS FOR PRACTICE AND RESEARCH

Feeling safe was an overpowering need of ICU patients. Many factors influenced perceptions of feeling safe in these patients, including family and friends, staff, religion, and knowing, regaining control, hoping, and trusting. In many areas nurses can intervene to strengthen the various factors that affect feeling safe. For example, nurses can work closely with family members, building trusting relationships, so families can be incorporated as part of the team to provide support for patients. Hope also can be encouraged in families because, as Miller (1991) pointed out, hope is "contagious" and can be transmitted from the family to the patient. Another area that influenced ICU patients' perceptions of feeling safe was religion. Nurses can recommend hospital chaplains as resources for both patients and families.

The other factors that influence feeling safe—knowing, regaining control, hoping, and trusting—have not all been described so that interventions to enhance these factors can be identified or the levels of each distinguished. Once the level of trust, for example, is identified and intervention strategies described, then interventions targeted to strengthen trust can be implemented and tested using the qualitative outcome analysis (QOA) technique (Morse, Penrod, & Hupcey, 2000). With QOA, intervention strategies can be evaluated and new interventions identified and tested as clinical outcomes are assessed. For ICU patients, each of the factors that influence feeling safe—knowing, regaining control, hoping, and trusting—should be individually described

so nurses can intervene in each area to enhance feeling safe in these patients.

Hope is one aspect of feeling safe that has been adequately described and a list of specific interventions explicated. Using the hope assessment guide developed by Penrod and Morse (1997), nurses could first assess the levels of hope of ICU patients and then provide appropriate interventions to support hope in whatever form it is manifested. Through the process of QOA (Morse et al., 2000), nurses would first assess the levels of hope, identify and implement strategies to enhance hope, evaluate the outcomes of the intervention, and modify the intervention, if needed, based on the outcome.

Trust is a facet of feeling safe that is still underdeveloped; however, the trajectories of trust have been identified in hospitalized adult patients and are now being examined in other health care contexts (Hupcey et al., in press). Once this research is complete and potential intervention strategies identified for each level of trust, an assessment guide can be developed and QOA can be used to evaluate the efficacy of the interventions. Interventions to enhance trust might include showing a genuine interest in patients and showing oneself to be technically competent (Clark & Heidenreich, 1995; Hupcey et al., in press).

Control is an area that has not been adequately described, but a possible intervention identified from this study was talking to patients about their feelings related to the loss of control and independence and determining areas in which patients could be given control (such as environmental control of lights, heat, television, and curtain position). Another area found to foster feelings of control was allowing patients to make decisions related to visitors (Lazure, 1997). Knowing is an aspect of feeling safe that has been investigated by Hupcey and Zimmerman (2000). Suggested nursing interventions from this work include continuously re-orienting an intubated patient and frequently explaining details about the ICU stay to all ICU patients.

Future research should examine these underdeveloped aspects of feeling safe. As these factors are delineated, and a full range of strategies is identified and tested, the overarching need of ICU patients, that of feeling safe, can be addressed. Within this process, the influence of perceptions of feeling safe on both physiological and psychological outcomes can be evaluated.

References

Burfitt, S. N., Greiner, D. S., Miers, L. J., Kinney, M. R., & Branyon, M. E. (1993). Professional nurse caring as perceived by critically ill patients: A phenomenological study. *American Journal of Critical Care, 2,* 489–499.

Chenitz, W. C. & Swanson, J. M. (1986). Qualitative research using grounded theory. In W. C. Chenitz & J. M. Swanson (Eds.), *From practice to grounded theory* (3–15). Menlo Park, CA: Addison-Wesley.

Cirlin, H. L. (1998). Hope gives the patient the will to live. *AACN News* 15(7), 4, 14.

Clark, C. & Heidenrich, T. (1995). Spiritual care for the critically ill. *American Journal of Critical Care, 4,* 77–81.

Compton, P. (1991). Critical illness and intensive care: What it means to the client. *Critical Care Nurse, 11,* 50–56.

Corbin, J. (1986). Coding, writing memos, and diagramming. In W. C. Chenitz & J. M. Swanson (Eds.), *From practice to grounded theory* (102–120). Menlo Park, CA: Addison-Wesley.

Cutcliffe, J. (1996). Critically ill patients' perspectives of hope. *British Journal of Nursing, 5,* 674, 687–690.

Elpern, E. H., Patterson, P. A., Gloskey, D., & Bone, R. C. (1992). Patients' preference for intensive care. *Critical Care Medicine, 20,* 43–47.

Geary, P. A., Tringali, R., & George, E. (1997). Social support in critically ill adults: A replication. *Critical Care Nurse Quarterly, 20*(2), 34–41.

Glaser, B. G. (1978). *Theoretical sensitivity.* Mill Valley, CA: The Sociological Press.

Glaser, B. G. & Strauss, A. L. (1967). *The discovery of grounded theory.* Chicago: Aldine Publishing.

Hafsteindóttir, T. B. (1996). Patient's experiences of communication during the respirator treatment period. *Intensive and Critical Care Nursing, 12,* 261–271.

Hall-Lord, M. L., Larsson, G., & Bostrom, I. (1994). Elderly patients' experiences of pain and distress in intensive care: A grounded theory study. *Intensive and Critical Care Nursing, 10,* 133–141.

Hupcey, J. E. (1998). Establishing the nurse-family relationship—in the intensive care unit. *Western Journal of Nursing Research, 20,* 180–194.

Hupcey, J. E. (1999). Looking out for the patient and ourselves. The process of family integration into the ICU. *Journal of Clinical Nursing, 8,* 253–262.

Hupcey, J. E., Penrod, J., & Morse, J. M. (in press). *Meeting expectations: Establishing and maintaining trust during acute care hospitalizations.*

Hupcey, J. E., & Zimmermen, H. E. (2000). The need to know: Experiences of Critically ill patients. *American Journal of Critical Care, 9,* 192–198.

Jenny, J. & Logan, J. (1996). Caring and comfort metaphors used by patients in critical care. *Image: Journal of Nursing Scholarship, 28,* 349–352.

Johnson, K. L., Cheung, R. B., Johnson, S. B., Roberts, M., Niblett, J., & Manson, D. (1999). Therapeutic paralysis of critically ill trauma patients: Perceptions of patients and their family members. *American Journal of Critical Care, 8,* 490–498.

Johnson, L. H., Dahlen, R., & Roberts, S. L. (1997). Supporting hope in congestive heart failure patients. *Dimensions of Critical Care Nursing, 16,* 65–78.

Kim, H., Garvin, B. J., & Moser, D. K. (1999). Stress during mechanical ventilation: Benefit of having concrete objective information before cardiac surgery. *American Journal of Critical Care, 8,* 118–126.

Laitenen, H. (1996). Patients' experience of confusion in the intensive care unit following cardiac surgery. *Intensive and Critical Care Nursing, 12,* 79–83.

Lazure, L. L. A. (1997). Strategies to increase patient control of visiting. *Dimensions of critical Care Nursing, 16,* 11–19.

Lazure, L. L. A. & Baun, M. M. (1994). Increasing patient control of family visiting in the coronary care unit. *American Journal of Critical Care, 4,* 157–164.

Miles, M. B. & Huberman, A. M. (1994). *Qualitative data analysis* (2nd ed.). Thousand Oaks, CA: Sage.

Miller, J. F. (1991). Developing and maintaining hope in families of the critically ill. *AACN Clinical Issues in Critical Care Nursing, 2,* 307–315.

Morse, J. M. & Dobernick, B. (1995). Delineating the concept of hope. *Image: Journal of Nursing Scholarship, 27,* 277–285.

Morse, J. M. & Penrod, J. (1999). Linking concepts of enduring, uncertainty, suffering, and hope. *Image: Journal of Nursing Scholarship, 31,* 145–150.

Morse, J. M., Penrod, J., & Hupcey, J. E. (2000). Qualitative outcome analysis: Evaluating nursing interventions for complex clinical phenomena. *Journal of Nursing Scholarship, 32,* 125–130.

Parker, M. M., Schubert, W., Shelhamer, J. H., & Parillo, J. E. (1984). Perceptions of a critically ill patient experiencing therapeutic paralysis in an ICU. *Critical Care Medicine, 12,* 69–71.

Penrod, J. & Morse, J. M. (1997). Strategies for assessing and fostering hope: The Hope Assessment Guide. *Oncology Nursing Forum, 24,* 1055–1063.

Richards, K. C. (1998). Effect of a back massage and relaxation intervention on sleep in critically ill patients. *American Journal of Critical Care, 7,* 288–299.

Russell, S. (1999). An exploratory study of patient's perceptions, memories and experiences of an intensive care unit. *Journal of Advanced Nursing, 29,* 783–791.

Soehren, P. (1995). Stressors perceived by cardiac surgery patients in the intensive care unit. *American Journal of Critical Care, 4,* 71–76.

Turner, J. S., Briggs, S. J., Springhorn, H. E., & Potgieter, P. D. (1990). Patients' recollection of intensive care unit experience. *Critical Care Medicine, 18,* 966–968.

Updike, P. (1990). Music therapy results for ICU patients. *Dimensions of Critical Care Nursing, 9,* 39–45.

Wilkinson, K. (1996). The concept of hope in life-threatening illness. *Professional Nurse, 11,* 659–661.

Qualitative Evaluation of a School-Based Support Group for Adolescents with an Addicted Parent

Bonnie Gance-Cleveland

Background: *Adolescents with an addicted parent are at risk for physical, emotional, and social problems. They are particularly at risk for developing substance abuse. School-based support groups have been suggested as a beneficial treatment and prevention strategy.*

Objective: *To examine the features, critical attributes, processes, and benefits of school-based support groups for adolescents with an addicted parent.*

Methods: *A qualitative evaluation using the ethnographic method was conducted at two Midwestern suburban high schools.*

Results: *The study resulted in a comprehensive description of school-based support groups and an outline presenting benefits of participation for adolescents with an addicted parent. The benefits of group participation included increased knowledge, enhanced coping, increased resilience, improved relationships, and improved school performance.*

Discussion: *Findings from this study suggest that school-based support groups are beneficial to adolescents with addicted parents. Experiential knowledge is the foundation of these self-help groups. School-based support group participation enhanced self-knowledge and led to self-care and self-healing. The school-based support groups expanded the adolescents' awareness, resulting in their ability to make critical choices that facilitated changes in the dysfunctional pattern. Support group participation empowered youth to make these changes.*

Key Words: *group therapy, substance abuse, support groups.*

Significant numbers of children live with substance-abusing parents. The National Association for Children of Alcoholics has estimated there are 26.8 million children of alcoholics (COAs) in the United States, and that 11 million of these children are younger than 18 years (National Association for Children of Alcoholics [NACoA], 1998). Furthermore, 18% of adult Americans, almost one in five, lived with an alcoholic while growing up (1998). The 2001 National Household Survey on Drug Abuse reported that more than 6 million children had lived during the past year with at least one parent who abused or was dependent on drugs or alcohol (Substance Abuse and Mental Health Services Administration [SAMHSA], 2003). Among the children 5 years old and younger,

10% had a parent with substance abuse or dependence in the past year (2003).

Certain physical problems such as asthma, hypertension, abdominal pain, headaches, gastrointestinal disorders, and allergies occur more frequently among children with addicted parents (Adger, 2004). These youth have a higher incidence of emotional disorders including chemical dependence, eating disorders, low self-esteem, depression, phobias, anxiety, and suicidal behavior (Emshoff & Price, 1999; Hill, Shen, Lowers, & Locke, 2000; NACoA, 1998). Findings show that COAs exhibit more antisocial behaviors such as delinquency, rebellion, running away, social isolation, interpersonal problems, and school difficulties (Christensen & Bilenberg, 2000; Jacob & Windle, 2000; NACoA, 1998), and that they are at two-to-four times the risk of other children for developing adolescent psychiatric disorders (Lynskey, Fergussen, & Horwood, 1994). Physical and sexual abuse occurs more often among children with addicted parents. These children experience poorer family functioning and have more traumatic experiences than children in control groups (Johnson, Stiffman, Hadley-Ives, & Elze, 2001).

Finally, children with addicted parents also are at high risk for early drug and alcohol use (Hussong & Chassin, 1997). Findings show that COAs have a higher prevalence of alcohol dependence. They are four to six times more likely to develop a drinking problem than control groups (Kumpfer, 1999; Wolin & Wolin, 1995).

The average classroom has four to six children with a chemically dependent parent (NACoA, 2004). These children attend school less often, are more often late for school, and have a higher incidence of learning disabilities (NACoA, 1998; Sher, 1997). Often, these issues, coupled with the decreased availability of parents to help with homework, impair a child's ability to succeed in school. These children are in need of interventions to decrease the impact of parental addiction on their lives. Yet despite the high incidence of problems, only small percentages of children with addicted parents receive any supportive services. In a survey of substance abuse providers, 69% indicated they did not provide services to the children of their clients (Stoil, 1999).

Much of the literature on children with addicted parents suggests that school-based support groups (SBSGs) are an appropriate intervention for this vulnerable population. However, limited information is available on SBSGs and the value of this intervention. Black (2004) suggested that dealing with parental addiction as a group issue conveys a universality of experience and reduces feelings of isolation. Children are encouraged to share the dreaded family secret in a supportive and trusting atmosphere. This helps to relieve their burden and allows them to feel less alone. The goals of COA support groups are to educate, clarify, validate, problem solve, connect to support systems, assess, and protect. It was theorized that the self-help groups are based on experiential knowledge (Borkman, 1999). These groups draw on the life experiences of their members to foster nurturing support and transformation by a sharing of their experiences. The groups create more positive and less stigmatizing perspectives for their participants.

The key components of a SBSG for adolescent girls with substance-abusing parents were described as positive role modeling, sharing of problems and feelings, mutual respect and valuing of differences, health promotion, problem solving, conflict resolution, social and academic skills, accessing of community agencies, celebration, advocacy, and personal safety (Tuttle et al., 2000). Group benefits for the girls included helping them avoid risky behaviors and providing a sense of belonging. Among the additional benefits were home visits and case management (Campbell-Heider, Tuttle, Bidwell-Cerone, Richeson, & Collins, 2003). The participants completed more school, were more likely to be working or seeking employment, and had less depression and fewer pregnancies. They reported more frequent use of alcohol, but no differences in the amount consumed or in the associated problems, as compared with control subjects (Tuttle, Campbell-Heider, Bidwell-Cerone, Richeson, & Collins, 2001). The weaknesses of these studies were their retrospective design, small sample sizes, limited female participation, and lack of randomization.

Research on the effectiveness of community interventions in promoting healthy behaviors and decreasing HIV risk indicated that effective programs need to be based on theories of behavior change, to be focused on participants with similar attributes, to involve participants in planning, and to be developmentally appropriate (Stanton, Kim, Galbraith, & Parrot, 1996).

An evaluation of a school-based alcohol education curriculum for COAs reported that general education was preferred over the curriculum designed for

COAs. Significant differences were discovered when COAs found that their family's problem was shared by others. However, COAs should deal with their problems in a different fashion and reduce alcohol consumption (U.S. Department of Health and Human Services [USDHHS], 1990). A study to evaluate SBSGs designed to reduce absenteeism among elementary and middle school students reported that 60% of the participants had a substance-abusing parent. Data collected over a 3-year period showed that SBSG improved attendance (USDHHS, 1990).

A qualitative evaluation of SBSGs for COAs was conducted to identify the critical features, group processes, and relevant outcomes from the participants' and cofacilitators' perspectives. The conceptual framework that guided the study was naturalistic and interpretive. With a naturalistic approach, the investigator strives to understand the complex world as a whole and attempts to examine phenomena in natural settings without manipulation (Denzin & Lincoln, 2000). The goal is to develop an understanding from the participants' and cofacilitators' perspectives. Therefore, this study aimed to evaluate from participants' and cofacilitators' perspectives the critical features, group processes, and benefits of SBSG for adolescents with an addicted parent.

METHODS

This qualitative evaluation using ethnographic methods (Denzin & Lincoln, 2000) was conducted in a large, multicultural, Midwestern suburban school district that included students from middle- and lower-class socioeconomic backgrounds. The site was selected because it had many years of experience with SBSGs for adolescents who have addicted parents. Participant observations were conducted weekly at two high schools in the school district over one semester. Interviews were conducted with program administrators, school administrators, group cofacilitators, and participants. Theoretical sampling was used to identify participants of different ages, ethnic background, and lengths of time in the group. A focus group was conducted, and written evaluations were collected from all the participants at the final session (Table 1).

The study was approved by the institutional review board (IRB). Consent from administrators and cofacilitators along with student assent was obtained at the beginning of each interview. Parental consent was waived per IRB instruction because of the potential risk to the student, because students can consent to services, and because the study was evaluating a program in place in the school district.

Initial interviews with the program administrator and substance abuse consultant followed by examination of documents and records provided a context for the participant observations. Records and documents reviewed included the program manual, a set of minutes from a school counselor's meeting, and group evaluations from one counselor. The Federal Education Right to Privacy Act prevented the researcher from examining school documents on student performance. A total of 20 participant observations of 4 hours duration took place at two high schools with SBSGs. The observations included 5 weeks of screening students regarding their interest in group participation as well as preparation for the group, then 15 weeks of 45-minute support group sessions followed by debriefing and follow-up activities. The researcher assumed the role of cofacilitator for both groups, and was introduced to the participants as a nurse who was there to learn more about the groups.

The program administrator and a school vice principal were interviewed at the beginning of the project. The substance abuse consultant, a Master's-prepared social worker, was interviewed after each observation to clarify the observations. Interviews with the substance abuse consultant also took place at midsemester and at the conclusion of the study. A first interview examined the critical attributes and processes of the groups, a second interview focused on benefits and weaknesses of the groups, and a final interview clarified and validated the findings. Three school counselors who cofacilitate groups and three student participants were interviewed at the beginning, at the middle point, and at the conclusion of the study. Theoretical sampling was used to identify cofacilitators who were enthusiastic supporters of groups and those who had reservations. The SBSG participants were selected according to diversity in age and past experience with groups. Data saturation was reached when no new information was obtained.

A focus group evaluation was conducted at the conclusion of the support group at one high school, and all the members of the group were invited to participate. Written evaluations were obtained at the final group session at both sites. The participants'

TABLE A8-1

Demographics of Study Participants

Participant observations (N = 21)

	Male n	Male %	Female n	Female %	Total N	Total %	Latino n	Latino %	White n	White %
School 1	2	18	9	82	11	52	1	9	10	91
School 2	5	50	5	50	10	48	5	50	5	50
Total	7	33	14	66	21	100	6	29	15	71

Interviews

	Male n	Male %	Female n	Female %	Total N	Total %	Latino n	Latino %	White n	White %
Focus group School 2	n = 2 (40%)		3	60	5		2	40	3	60
Program administrator			1	100	1					100
Substance abuse consultant					1		1	100	1	100
Cofacilitators										
School 1			2	66	2				2	66
School 2			1	33	1				1	33
Students										
School 1			3	100	3		1	33	2	66
Total	n = 2 (15%)		11	85	13		4	30	9	70

Written evaluations

	Male n	Male %	Female n	Female %	Total N	Total %	Latino n	Latino %	White n	White %
School 1			3	100	3		1	33	2	66
School 2	2	40	3	60	5		2	40	3	60
Total	2	25	6	75	8		3	37	5	62

anonymity was protected by the use of code numbers on data. The data from observations, interviews, and focus groups were generated from field notes and audiotapes, then transcribed verbatim. The data were entered into the Ethnograph V4.0 to facilitate data management (Seidel, Kjolseth, & Clark, 1991).

A modified constant comparative method of analysis was used (Denzin & Lincoln, 2000; Krueger, 1995; Lincoln & Guba, 1985). The data were examined for the significant features, functions, benefits, and strengths and weaknesses of SBSGs from the perspective of the cofacilitators and participants.

Analysis of the data began with intraparticipant microanalysis, coding line by line, individual interviews, and document or record, focus group or observation. Unitizing of the data showed the contextual features and benefits that came from interviews with the administrator and the substance abuse consultant. Units of data then were categorized and examined for patterns and relation by a look at the activities, interactions, and content of the program. Integrating categories led to an explanation of the SBSG experience that included the processes, the critical attributes, and the benefits. Initially, the critical attributes and processes were blended into the same category, but comparison of new data from the interviews suggested that they were two separate but related categories. The phases of the group processes were identified during participant observation, and further clarified by interviews with the coparticipants. Benefits were identified by a look at changes in participants, expressions of change, personal growth, and increased awareness. The benefits were discovered through the focus groups and interviews with the cofacilitators and the participants, then confirmed with the written evaluations.

The literature was revisited to ensure the accuracy of the reconstruction of the experience. Final interviews with a counselor and a participant confirmed the findings and ensured the validity of the interpretation and the model for evaluation of SBSGs serving adolescents with an addicted parent.

RESULTS

Qualitative evaluation provided a description of SBSGs including the processes, phases, critical attributes, and benefits. The SBSGs each consisted of 8 to 12 students with the common problem of parental substance abuse who came together for mutual support in a process-oriented, time-limited psychoeducational group. Groups were cofacilitated by a substance abuse specialist (Master's-prepared social worker), school counselor, or school nurse. The groups met 45 minutes once a week. Attendance, varying from two to eight members, was low initially, but improved after trust was established. Groups met for 15 weeks and focused on coping skills, self-evaluation and goal setting, positive self-esteem, relationship skills, and communication skills. The participants explored how parental substance abuse affected

their lives. The purpose of the groups was described in the program manual:

> The group experience aims to break down the unspoken family rules of don't talk, don't trust, and don't feel by educating adolescents about chemical dependency; providing a consistent and predictable group environment; and by teaching coping and survival skills.

A group process with distinct phases was used to achieve this goal. The group process began with a pregroup phase of creating a group, educating the faculty and staff, obtaining referrals, and screening potential participants. In-services were provided to increase awareness of chemical dependency and its impact on the participant. Referrals came from counselors, teachers, administrators, campus supervisors, school nurses, and special education teachers. Students were contacted to determine their interest in the group. The early phase involved establishing trust, clarifying the purpose, and formulating the rules, norms, and expectations. Participants signed a contract regarding confidentiality, making up missed school work, consistent attendance, respect for other participants, and willingness to listen and share. Activities were used to facilitate introductions with good success. Both males and females shared openly as the trust was established.

During the working phase, the participants shared secrets, gained information, supported one another, critically analyzed self, identified goals, made choices, and learned to manage. As the students began to share their experiences, they identified commonalities and started to support each other. A common first step was acknowledgment of a parent's addiction. One student explained:

> When I was younger, both of my parents had problems with drugs and alcohol, so my paternal grandmother had custody of me. My dad got custody of me when my mother was in a rehab center. I always loved and idolized my mother, and I was shocked when I moved in with her and was confronted with the reality that she was an alcoholic. I felt responsible for her drinking because I had just moved in with my mother. I was faced with shattered dreams. Being in the group helps because there are other students who have the same problems.

Sharing secrets allowed the participants to support one another as they began the working phase of the group. During the working phase, the participants formulated three goals and a date for achieving the goals. They outlined the obstacles and formulated a plan for achieving the goals. The termination phase included evaluating one's progress, identifying unresolved issues, and establishing outside support. The final group session involved evaluating the group, saying goodbye, and celebrating each others' progress.

The critical attributes included recognizing commonalities, creating a caring community, establishing reciprocal relationships, recognizing patterns, and empowering students. A counselor described these attributes:

> When they join the group, the students discover there are others with the problem of parental addiction. They learn they are not the only ones dealing with this problem, and there are commonalities in the experience.

A student stated:

> The most helpful thing about group is the people, getting advice from other students, always having somebody who's gone through what you are going through.

The participants recognized that others had similar experiences and thus were able to support and challenge one another regarding damaging behavior. The group experience decreased feelings of loneliness and isolation. A focus group participant explained:

> I learned I wasn't alone. I'm not the only one; it helps to know kids of all ages are going through this, too. It feels like there are people out there like you ... and we made good friends. They are the people to trust; everyone was pretty easy to talk to because they understand my problems and can relate. You didn't feel labeled. You don't feel as weird.

The participants were particularly influenced by others who had experienced similar family problems. Finding others with common experiences allowed bonding and acceptance, which led to the second attribute: a caring community. The components of a caring community are peer support together with feeling understood, feeling cared for and wanted, and feeling sheltered and comfortable in a safe place with people you can trust. A student explained:

> People are understanding; you're able to talk freely; you get to know the people you are talking to and trust them. You feel wanted and welcome; it is sheltered, a safe place to talk. The group provides support, comfort, and advice. It helps you deal with stress.

This caring atmosphere promoted ability to move toward recognizing patterns. After participants recognized their commonalities and established trusting relationships, they began to explore their own dysfunctional patterns. As a participant described:

> I know the group is not going to solve all problems, but at least I can be aware of them. I looked at myself doing the same thing as my alcoholic parent. I was following in their footsteps.

After identifying their patterns, the participants began to make different choices and became empowered. The substance abuse specialist explained:

> I try to have every group do a panel presentation ... that is empowering to them so that they do not stay victimized. One situation that I remember was a student who had witnessed one parent murdering another parent. This student had not shared it in the group although she had alluded to some kind of secret, but she wasn't ready to tell the secret. I took her along with the other members of her group to do a panel for another school, and this student disclosed that information on the panel. I was blown away, but I think what really happened to her was that she felt a real sense of empowerment in terms of her growth, and now she was being asked to be an expert in talking about these kinds of issues. I think that security allowed her to be able to share this information, and she was able to talk about it. My philosophy is that kids become survivors. I think that getting students to do presentations is a way for them to reflect, "Yes, I had all these problems, all these issues, but I have been able to deal with them."

Allowing participants to share what they have learned empowers to recognize growth. The following benefits were identified: positive changes in behavior, increased knowledge concerning the impact of addiction, improved relationships, increased coping strategies, increased resilience, and enhanced school performance.

A participant summarized her perspective of the potential benefits:

> Group is a place for help and solutions, support, comfort, advice, and encouragement to speak up. Group provides ideas to handle stress and frustration, a strong backbone of support to overcome your problems. You talk about problems with friends, and look for a positive way to deal with things. I have tried to turn my life completely around and make progress in school. I am more focused. I have more confidence, and my concentration has improved. I'm not going to take the blame for my Mom's problems. I'm not going to be like my parents. I'm going to find a positive way to deal with things.

Increased knowledge of the impact that addiction has on the family included increased understanding of the family dynamics of addiction and the role the participant played in the addicted family.

During a support group session, the participants revealed problems in their families, describing how their parents lost jobs, homes, and families because of addiction. One participant talked about his alcoholic father and how he lost his family's trust. In addition, the participant's father lost a relationship with his sons because his older brothers did not come around anymore. One student remarked:

> My mother lost everything! Her children were taken away, she was placed in a mental hospital and she lost her home. She lost everything!

This understanding of family dynamics enhanced the ability of some students to take care of themselves and do what they needed to do to protect themselves. For example, one student said:

> My attitude has changed since I've been coming to group. I was like my Mom's Mom. I know I need to take care of myself first, and now I need to take care of my daughter. Now some minor things I let go like this past year, my Mom was in jail and I bailed her out and she left the next day and got in a fight with her boyfriend and called me to come get her again. I just tell her, "Try to figure it out."

This self-awareness changed the student's pattern of interacting with her addicted mother.

The increased understanding of addiction and its impact on various family members improved the participants' relationships. One participant said on the evaluation form:

> The major area that I've improved in is family. I have a much better relationship with my father.

Improved relationships with family members occurred as well as improved relationships with peers. Knowing that others had similar family situations enhanced the participants' connectedness and helped them to find more supportive peers.

The participants also supported one another when they were upset about a parent's drinking. When a participant began to cry while talking about her alcoholic father, the group responded by creating a telephone tree. They shared phone numbers and offered to be available to support her. Another participant suggested going to an Alateen meeting together as a group. They were given information about a local group that met on the weekends.

Increased coping strategies involved recognizing and verbalizing feelings, talking about problems, and asking for what one wanted and needed. Each participant recognized the need to take care of oneself and to decrease the caretaking of others. As the participants shared with other participants, they developed increased ability to identify options and enhanced their problem-solving abilities, resulting in decreased tension. A participant explained:

> Group helps me deal with my stress. I have always been very stressed, and I've dealt with the stress in the past by keeping it in. I developed an ulcer in junior high. I think that being able to talk about feelings and being in the group with the other students who have similar experiences has helped me with my ulcer.

Another participant talked about the power of the group in helping his pattern recognition and ability to make different choices:

> I know the group is not going to solve all problems, but at least I can be aware of them. I looked at myself doing the same thing as my alcoholic parent. I was following in their footsteps with drinking and drugging.

Participants also counseled others on effective coping strategies they had used in the past. A participant suggested to other group members:

I break large assignments into smaller pieces and do a little each night. You have to talk to your teachers about handing assignments in late if you don't have them finished. I just have to keep working until I get it all done or I won't graduate. I have to graduate.

The participants had the opportunity to recognize and share their coping strategies with others inside and outside their group. This process empowered them to recognize and make changes in behavior and enhance their coping. A participant explained:

Over spring break I went to Wyoming with my family. On Friday night my cousins were going out drinking, and I said that my parents were expecting me back so I couldn't go with them. They were drinking and driving, and they were stopped by the police for drinking under age and drinking and driving. I was really glad I didn't go with them. Also, I've talked to some of my close friends, and we've decided to start our own club for support this summer.

These participants established more supportive relationships to reinforce these healthier behaviors.

With these new coping strategies, the participants developed increased resilience. The substance abuse consultant explained it as increased self-awareness, increased self-esteem, increased assertiveness, decreased vulnerability, and decreased victimization. One student reported:

You feel more confident; your outlook on life changes. More doors open; you realize you have more options. The door to drugs and alcohol closes, [but the group] opens other doors. The drug door is slammed shut and locked, and the drinking and driving door is shut. Youth power door is open by talking to the junior high students. Weight lifting is another door open—I want to help my body not hurt it.

This increased resilience may or may not lead to a measurable change in school performance.

From the perspective of the school administration and the school community, a critical outcome was enhanced school performance. One student noted:

At the beginning of group my grades were slipping, but talking to others about how to deal with slipping grades helped me out. I adjusted to a new school . . . [other students] showed me to pay attention to what you're doing. It might have an effect on

my life later, like not being able to graduate because I'm ditching classes now. It helped me graduate.

Although there were no definitive data to support the enhanced school performance, many youth reported that benefit. Conversely, the following weaknesses were identified. Lack of support from faculty and staff was a weakness. There were questions about whether it was the school's role to offer SBSGs. Some felt that this was the family's responsibility, and that school resources should be spent differently. A lack of data showing improved school performance increased faculty resistance to the groups. An assistant principal said:

The problem with faculty support of groups is a lack of communication with staff about what is accomplished. Faculty and staff are not aware of any concrete outcomes like improved attendance, or improved grades, which would improve the credibility of the groups.

The program administrator noted:

The resistance to support groups may be due to territorial issues or the faculty and staff struggling with their own issues related to family substance abuse that makes them uncomfortable with the topic.

The resistance of the faculty may have been attributable to a lack of school performance outcomes, territorial issues, or both.

Some difficulties with support groups were identified by cofacilitators. Occasionally, group members did not follow the rules, norms, and expectations (confidentiality, respectful listening, making up course work). When participants did not follow the rules, others were possibly endangered (e.g., if students were using the group for drug connections or skipping school). In these cases, the group was discontinued. One group facilitator reported discontinuing a group because members reinforced negative behaviors (i.e., fighting among group members or disclosure of confidential information). Members were told that if they were willing to follow the rules, they could participate in a group in the future.

DISCUSSION

The study findings provide a model to use in evaluating SBSGs for adolescents with an addicted parent. Step one is identification of goals and desired outcomes derived from the program objectives. Step two is a process assessment, and step three is delineation of the perceived benefits. Step four is an outcome assessment that involves identifying appropriate tools for measuring each of the perceived benefits. Step five is assessment of the program's long-term effects, including identification of appropriate measures for documenting the long-term impact of the program on participants.

Findings from the current study validated the goals of the COA support groups described by Black (2004). Education, clarification, and validation were consistent with knowledge (e.g., solving problems with increased coping, supporting one another with support systems, identifying patterns, and making healthier choices). Similar to the theme of empowering the participants, Black (2004) stated that COA support groups empower children who have experienced powerlessness.

Critical features and processes in the current study are consistent with SBSG for adolescent girls (Campbell-Heider et al., 2003). Sharing of problems and feelings, mutual respect, and valuing of differences were consistent with secret sharing and reciprocal relationships. Likewise, Stanton et al.'s (1996) description of successful community interventions for promoting healthy behaviors included interventions based on behavior change theory, which is consistent with the self-evaluation, identification of patterns, and ability to make healthier choices found in this study.

Studies on support groups have used a variety of measures to document effects, but there has been little consistency in the results. Some of the outcomes identified in this study are consistent with the previous literature, and some are unique to this study. Increased knowledge is consistent with Borkman's (1999) experiential knowledge as a critical component of the self-help groups. Increased coping skills, interpersonal relationships, and improvement in school performance were reported in the current study for SBSGs focused on emotional distress and behavioral problems (Wassef, Mason, Collins, Van-Haalen, & Ingham, 1998). Similarly, SBSGs for depressed adolescents decreased stress and family distress (Houck, Darnell, & Lussman, 2002). The improved relationships and school performance identified in the current study were benefits of drug prevention programs. Finally, evaluation of life skills training (Botvin, Baker, Dusenbury, Botvin, & Diaz,

1995) focused on decreased substance use. The results of the current study included increased resiliency (decreased risk behaviors and substance abuse) and other broadly based benefits as outcomes.

A limitation of the study was that the researcher also was the cofacilitator of both groups, which may have influenced the participants' reports. In addition, school performance data were not examined. Improved school performance was a benefit of SBSGs reported by both participants and group cofacilitators. However, confirmation of this outcome was not possible because of Federal Education Right to Privacy Act laws.

Another limitation was that individual interviews did not include male participants, students who did not want to participate in the group experience, or those who dropped out of the group.

Findings from this study may be used to replicate groups using the model for evaluation of SBSGs involving adolescents with an addicted parent, and to educate school health professionals and policymakers regarding the value of this intervention. School-based support groups have the potential of improving outcomes for this vulnerable population.

References

Adger, H. (2004). *The role of primary care physicians.* National Association for Children of Alcoholics. Retrieved February 4, 2004, from http://www.nacoa.net/role.htm

Black, C. (2004). *COA support groups.* National Association for Children of Alcoholics. Retrieved February 4, 2004, from http://www.nacoa.net/coasupp.htm

Borkman, T. (1999). *Understanding self-help/mutual aid; Experiential learning in the commons.* Fairfax, VA: George Mason University.

Botvin, G., Baker, E., Dusenbury, I., Botvin, E., & Diaz, T. (1995). Long-term follow-up of a randomized drug abuse prevention trial in a white middle class population. *JAMA, 273,* 1106–1112.

Campell-Heider, N., Tuttle, J., Bidwell-Cerone, S., Richeson, G., & Collins, S. (2003). The buffering effects of connectedness: Teen club intervention for children of substance-abusing families. *Journal of Addictions Nursing, 14,* 175–182.

Christensen, H. & Bilenberg, N. (2000). Behavioural and emotional problems in children of alcoholic mothers and fathers. *European Child and Adolescent Psychiatry, 9,* 219–226.

Denzin, N. K. & Lincoln, Y. (2000). *Handbook of qualitative research.* Thousand Oaks, CA: Sage.

Emshoff, J. G. & Price, A. W. (1999). Prevention and intervention strategies with children of alcoholics. *Pediatrics, 103*(5 Part 2), 1112–1121.

Hill, S. H., Shen, S., Lowers, L., & Locke, J. (2000). Factors predicting the onset of adolescent drinking in families at high risk for developing alcoholism. *Biological Psychiatry, 48*(4), 265–275.

Houck, G. M., Darnell, S., & Lussman, S. (2002). A support group intervention for at-risk female high school students. *Journal of School Nursing, 18*(4), 212–218.

Hussong, A. M. & Chassin, L. (1997). Substance use initiation among adolescent children of alchoholics: Testing protective factors. *Journal of Studies on Alcohol, 58*(3), 272–279.

Jacob, T. & Windle, M. (2000). Young adult children of alcoholic, depressed, and nondistressed parents. *Journal of Studies on Alcohol, 61*(6), 836–844.

Johnson, S., Stiffman, A., Hadley-Ives, E., & Elze, D. (2001). An analysis of stressors and comorbid mental health problems that contribute to youth paths to substance-specific services. *Journal Behavioral Health Services and Research, 28*(4), 412–426.

Krueger, R. A. (1995). The future of focus groups. *Qualitative Health Research, 5*(4), 524–530.

Kumpfer, K. L. (1999). Outcome measures of interventions in the study of children of substance-abusing parents. *Pediatrics Supplement, 103*(5 Part 2), 1128–1144.

Lincoln, Y. & Guba, E. G. (1985). *Naturalistic inquiry.* Newbury Park, CA: Sage.

Lynskey, M. T., Fergussen, D. M., & Horwood, L. J. (1994). The effect of parental alcohol problems on rates of adolescent psychiatric disorders. *Addiction, 89*(10), 1277–1286.

National Association for Children of Alcoholics. (1998). *Children of alcoholics: Important facts.* Retrieved February 4, 2004, from http://www.nacoa.net/impfacts.htm

Seidel, J., Kjolseth, R., & Clark, J. A. (1991). The ethnograph applications of qualitative analysis software: A view from the field. *Qualitative Sociology, 14,* 275–-285.

Sher, K. J. (1997). Psychological characteristics of children of alcoholics. *Alcohol Health and Research World, 21,* 3.

Stanton, B., Kim, N., Galbraith, J., & Parrot, M. C. (1996). Design issues addressed in published evaluations of adolescent HIV-risk reduction intervention. *Journal of Adolescent Health, 18,* 387–396.

Stoil, M. J. (1999). *Educational support services needed for children of addicted parents.* Chicago, IL: Society for Public Health Education. Retrieved November 6, 1999, from www.nacoa.net/SOPHE.htm

Substance Abuse and Mental Health Services Administration (SAMHSA). (2003). The National Household Survey on Drug Abuse 2001 report: *Children living with substance-abusing or substance-dependent parents.* Rockville, MD: SAMHSA, United States Department of Human Health Services. Retrieved October 23, 2003, http://www.DrugAbuseStatistics.samhsa.gov

Tuttle, J., Bidwell-Cerone, S., Campbell-Heider, N., Richeson, G., & Collins, S. (2000). Teen club: A nursing intervention for reducing risk-taking behavior and improving well-being in female African American adolescents. *Journal of Pediatric Health Care 14*(1), 103–108.

Tuttle, J., Campbell-Heider, N., Bidwell-Cerone, S., Richeson, G., & Collins, S. (2001). Nursing intervention for adolescent children of substance abusing parents: A study of five-year outcomes. *Adolescent and Family Health, 2*(1), 47.

U.S. Department of Health and Human Services. (1990). *Communities creating change.* Rockville, MD: National Institutes of Health: RP0768.

Wassef, A., Mason, G., Collins, L., VanHaalen, J., & Ingham, D. (1998). Effectiveness of one-year participation in school-based volunteer facilitated peer support groups. *Adolescence, 33*(129), 91–97.

Wolin, S. & Wolin, S. (1995). Resilience among youth growing up in substance-abusing families. *Pediatric Clinics of North America, 42,* 415–429.

Non-somatic Effects of Patient Aggression on Nurses: A Systematic Review

Ian Needham, Christopher Abderhalden,
Ruud J. G. Halfens, Joachim E. Fischer, Theo Dassen

Aim: This paper describes a systematic review of the predominant non-somatic effects of patient assault on nurses.

Background: Patient aggression towards nurses is a longstanding problem in most nursing domains. Although reports on the consequences of physical aggression are more numerous, the non-physical effects create much suffering.

Method: A systematic review of literature from 1983 to May 2003 was conducted using the Medline, CINAHL, PsychINFO, and PSYINDEX databases. Articles from international journals in English or German and reporting at least three non-somatic responses to patient aggression were included.

Findings: The electronic search produced 6616 articles. After application of the inclusion and exclusion criteria, 25 texts from eight countries and four domains of nursing remained. Twenty-eight main effects were found, and these were categorized using a system suggested by Lanza and including bio-physiological, emotional, cognitive, and social dimensions. The predominant responses were anger, fear or anxiety, post-traumatic stress disorder symptoms, guilt, self-blame, and shame. These main effects occurred across most countries and nursing domains.

Conclusion: Despite differing countries, cultures, research designs, and settings, nurses' responses to patient aggression are similar. Standardized questionnaires could help improve estimations of the real prevalence of non-somatic effects. Given the suffering caused by non-somatic effects, research should be aimed at preventing patient aggression and at developing better ways to prepare nurses to cope with this problem.

Key Words: aggression, violence, assault, nursing, victim, systematic review, post-traumatic stress disorder.

INTRODUCTION

Patient violence is a long-standing problem in nursing (Hansen 1996), especially in psychiatric nursing, in accident and emergency nursing, and in the care of the elderly. Research on physical injuries inflicted on health care staff by patients is common (Noble & Rodger 1989, Hanson & Balk 1992, Bensley et al. 1997, Lee et al. 1999). Rates for physical injury range from 2% (Noble & Rodger 1989) to 16% (Carmel & Hunter 1993). A recent study conducted in Germany revealed that 10% of health care workers (predominantly nurses) needed medical treatment after

Journal of Advanced Nursing, 2005, Volume 49, Number 3, pages 283–296

assault, and one nurse contracted life-threatening injuries (Richter & Berger 2000).

However, serious injuries occur much more rarely than minor ones with little or no physical injury (Fottrell 1980, Whittington & Wykes 1992). In a study of psychiatric patients' violence to staff, only 2% of the assaults led to major physical injuries as compared with 59% which induced no detectable injury (Noble & Rodger 1989). Non-somatic effects of aggression have been deemed by nurses themselves and by the literature as petty and not worthy of serious research (Haller & Deluthy 1988, Whittington & Wykes 1992). The primacy of physical injury is illustrated by Rippon (2000), who reports that after a sexual assault one nurse received no support; however, after being punched by a patient she was assisted.

The terminology on aggressive behavior varies considerably. Some researchers apply the term *assault* solely to the physical dimension (Owen et al. 1998), but for others verbal acts constitute assault (Chambers 1998, Vanderslott 1998, Gates et al. 1999). Sometimes sexual harassment (Vanderslott 1998) or unwanted sexual acts (Flannery et al. 1995) are used in conjunction with aggressive patient behavior. Other authors leave the definition of patient aggression to the victims (Hauck 1993). Differing operational definitions render data collection and the comparison of aggression rates difficult.

Research has demonstrated that psychological and emotional wounds may linger on and interfere with normal working and leisure lifestyles for months or years after the incident (Rippon 2000), with 49% of nurses in a study on assaults by psychiatric patients expressing the belief that it takes several months to recover emotionally from an assault (Baxter et al. 1992). One study (Richter & Berger 2000) reports that 14% of assaulted staff suffer from some severe symptoms of post-traumatic stress disorder (PTSD), and another study on short- and long-term effects of patient assault reports that some nurses suffer from moderate to severe PTSD at 1 year following the attack (Ryan & Poster 1989). On an organizational level, Richter notes that the effects of psychological sequelae for the organization cannot be estimated (Richter 1998).

Aim

The aim of this literature review was to identify and categorize the predominant non-somatic effects of patient assault on nurses.

Search Methods

We conducted an electronic search, used citations found in relevant articles, and consulted experts in the field for suggestions about texts. Texts fully or partially devoted to emotional, psychological, biopsychological, or social sequelae of patient aggression on nurses and written or published between 1983 and May 2003 in English or German were sought, as shown in Table 1.

The electronic search aimed at inclusiveness and sensitivity (Greenhalgh 2001) in order to cover a broad range of nursing populations and settings. This strategy was adopted because no indexing or Medical Subject Headings (MESH) terms exist for non-somatic consequences of patient aggression towards carers. The search included the databases MEDLINE (PUBMED online), Cumulative Index of Nursing and Allied Health Literature (CINAHL), PsychINFO, and PSYINDEX, with the search strategy tailored to the data bank in question. The search strategy for PUBMED for example, was: {[Aggression (MESH:NOEXP) or violence (MESH:NOEXP or dangerous behavior (MESH)] and [psychiatry (MESH) or health facilities (MESH) or health personnel (MESH) or nursing (MESH) or nursing, practical (MESH)]}.

Non-somatic effects were defined according to the categorization of Lanza (1992), which entails biophysiological, emotional, cognitive, and social reactions. As Lanza did not elaborate on the four categories, the following conceptualizations are employed in this review:

- Bio-physiological effects refer to non-visible somatic responses in a physiologically involuntary fashion.
- Emotions are sentiments not associated with any kind of psychological or psychiatric pathology but rather are common or 'normal' feelings.

TABLE A9-1

Inclusion Criteria

- Articles in English or German
- Articles containing at least three empirically acquired non-somatic effects
- Articles published between 1983 and May of 2003

- Cognition is defined as a non-emotive mode of perceiving, including perception of self or referring to a person's system of beliefs or convictions.
- Social interaction refers to interpersonal exchange.

Results

The electronic search revealed 6616 articles. After excluding articles in languages other than German and English and abstracts or those without authors, 3009 remained. After inspection of the titles, keywords, and abstracts, hard copies were acquired for the 114 articles deemed suitable for the review. All these were assessed according to the inclusion and exclusion criteria by at least two members of the research group. The reasons for the 91 exclusions are shown in Table 2. Two unpublished studies (Hauck 1993, Vincent et al. 2000) were drawn to our attention by experts. The 25 articles included in this review are characterized and arranged in alphabetical order [at the end of this article]. The main non-somatic effects, according to the categories suggested by Lanza, are presented according to the nursing domains (psychiatric, emergency, residential and gerontological, general and mixed nursing settings) in Table 3.

Bio-physiological Effects

Anxiety or fear is the most frequently reported bio-physiological effect. Anxiety may occur in a generalized form (Lanza 1983, Ryan & Poster 1989, Whittington & Wykes 1992) and fear may relate, for example, to the workplace (Bin Abdullah et al. 2000, Arnetz & Arnetz 2001), or patients (Fernandes et al. 2002). Fear can be differentiated as fear of the perpetrator of other patients (Lanza 1983, Whittington & Wykes 1992, Hauck 1993), fear for oneself or one's family (Fry et al. 2002), fear of permanent side effects of the assault or of becoming physically dependent on others (Lanza 1983), fear of retaliation towards the aggressor (Lanza 1983, Ryan & Poster 1989), or fear of co-workers or of the future (Hauck 1993). The reported rates of fear range from 12.4% (Richter & Berger 2000) to 49% (Arnetz & Arnetz 2001) ($n = 85$ and 8531, respectively). Guilt or self-blame or shame is also a prominent reaction to aggression reported in a majority of the studies. Some nurses feel guilty for not handling the situation in a more appropriate way (Hauck 1993).

Patient aggression may lead in a minority of cases to a fully-established PTSD or isolated symptoms of this. PTSD is a long-lasting anxiety response following a traumatic or catastrophic event, and consists of various symptoms in the following groups: persistent re-experience of the traumatic event (e.g. including images, thoughts, or perceptions, recurrent distressing dreams), persistent avoidance of trauma-associated stimuli (e.g. thoughts, feelings, or conversations, efforts to avoid activities, places, or people that arouse recollections of the trauma, inability to recall an important aspect of the trauma), and persistent symptoms of increased arousal such as difficult falling or staying asleep (American Psychiatric Association 1994). Isolated PTSD symptoms have been reported implicitly or explicitly by numerous authors (Table 3). Caldwell reports that 137 of 224 (56.1%) traumatized clinical staff in psychiatry contracted some PTSD symptoms but only 22 (9.8) suffered the full clinical PTSD (Caldwell 1992). In a study of aggression victims in a German psychiatric setting not a single person suffered from fully-established PTSD (Richter & Berger 2000), which demonstrates the need to differentiate between isolated symptoms and all three dimensions of PTSD.

TABLE A9-2	
Articles Excluded From the Review	
Reason for Exclusion	*n*
Articles containing no non-somatic effects	61
Articles containing <3 non-somatic effects	10
Articles containing no empirical data or containing insufficient description of methods	12
Articles reiterating other findings published elsewhere	8
Total	91

Cognitive Effects

Various threats to personal integrity or pride are reported, with some victims perceiving themselves as disrespected, unappreciated, violated, robbed of their rights (Gates et al. 1999), humiliated (Lanza et al. 1991, Hauck 1993), compromised (Chambers 1998), or intimidated, harassed and threatened (Fry et al. 2002). Others perceive themselves as being at the mercy of the perpetrator (Hauck 1993), whilst yet others experience disbelief that the assault occurred (Ryan & Poster 1989, Adams & Whittington 1995, Chambers 1998, May & Grubbs 2002, Hislop & Melby 2003). Denial or rationalization of the assault (Lanza 1983) or disbelief at being involved in the incident (Chambers 1998) may also occur. Some incidents can lead to a radical transformation of the conception of the world, with some victims stating that nothing will ever be the same again (Hauck 1993), that the event has a disruptive meaning (Flannery et al. 1995), or that the world has become less predictable (Hauck 1993; Gates et al. 1999) or threatening (Hauck 1993).

Emotional Effects

Emotional reactions constitute the greatest variety of symptoms, with anger being the most frequently reported. Anger may be directed towards the nurses themselves, superiors (Hauck 1993) or the institution (Hauck 1993, Chambers 1998). The range of percentages of nurses experiencing anger is greatest in emergency services, with rates from 14% ($n = 763$) (Fernandes et al. 2002) to 68.6% ($n = 35$) (Bin Abdullah et al. 2000). Two groups of authors report higher anger rates following verbal aggression than physical aggression (O'Connell et al. 2000, Fernandes et al. 2002). Feelings of guilt and self-blame are sometimes reinforced by superiors placing the blame for assaults on the victims (Hauck 1993). Guilt sometimes occurs in conjunction with shame (Åström et al. 2002) and may lead to impairment in self-confidence (Hauck 1993). The other emotional effects are shown in Table 3.

Social Effects

Assaults can affect (Gates et al. 1999, Suserud et al. 2002) or undermine (Flannery et al. 1995) the nurse-patient relationship and lead to behaviors such as less eagerness to spend time with residents, less willingness to answer residents' call lights (Gates et al. 1999), avoiding patients (Flannery et al. 1995, Levin et al. 1998), or adopting a passive role (Chambers 1998). Some nurses report becoming callous towards patients (Levin et al. 1998).

Nurses' perceptions of their job competency and security at or satisfaction with the workplace may be affected. Some of the assaulted nurses question the normality of a job in which workers are assaulted (Hauck 1993), or even consider changing jobs (Lanza 1983, Bin Abdullah et al. 2000). Some actually change ward or employer (O'Connell et al. 2000). Many assault victims feel insecure at work (Hauck 1993, Bin Abdullah et al. 2000, Vincent et al. 2000, May & Grubbs 2002), more vulnerable (Lanza 1983, Fry et al. 2002), or less in control (Lanza et al. 1991).

Patient aggression and assault can lead to real or perceived impairments in professional performance, leading nurses to doubt the quality of their work (Bin Abdullah et al. 2000), their competency (Whittington & Wykes 1992), or perceive themselves as having failed.

Other Effects

The following effects of aggression on nurses were reported fewer than three times in the 25 articles used in this review: bio-physiological (decreased energy, hyper vigilance and hyper alertness), cognitive (impaired concentration, increased cautiousness), emotion (burn-out, feeling confused, crying, feeling sorry for the perpetrator, dependency, depression, distress, embarrassment, laughter, numbness, resignations, thoughts of suicide, and vulnerability), and social (impaired expression of feelings, changed or impaired relationships to co-workers or family members, stigmatization of victims).

DISCUSSION

The aim of this review was to identify and categorize the non-somatic effects of patient violence on nurses. The review produced 28 predominant non-somatic effects, which were categorized according to the system suggested by Lanza (1992). The effects were derived from studies conducted in eight countries and four settings. If we had employed the 114 texts considered prior to the application of the exclusion criteria, the number of effects would have been greater. The variability of nurses' reactions, vocabulary in which nurses express their reactions, and lack of standardization of terms expressing reaction are

TABLE A9-3

Synopsis of the Most Prominent Non-somatic Symptoms

	Domain	Country	Bio-physiological					PTSD			Cognitive			
			Anxiety or Fear	Body Tension	Disquiet/Irritability	Headache	Sleep Disorder, Nightmares	Stress	Avoidance	Increased Arousal	Persistent Re-experience	Disbelief	Personal Integrity Threatened	Transformed Perception
Adams and Whittington (1995)	P	UK							•		•	•		
Caldwell (1992, p. 825)	P	USA							•	•	•			
Flannery et al. (1991, p. 294)	P	USA	•				•			•	•			
Flannery et al. (1995, p. 36)	P	USA							•		•			•
Fry et al. (2002, p. 711)	P	AUS	•				•						•	
Hauck (1993, p. 300)	P	CH	•	•	•			•		•	•		•	•
Lanza et al. (1991, p. 56)	P	USA						•					•	•
Lanza (1983, p. 336)	P	USA	•	•	•	•	•		•	•		•		
Murray and Snyder (1991)	P	USA												

TABLE A9-3

Synopsis of the Most Prominent Non-somatic Symptoms (*continued*)

					Emotional								Social		
Anger	Apathy, Indifference	Apprehension, Distress, Upset	Exhaustion, Fatigue, Strain	Frustration	Guilt, Self-Blame, Shame	Helplessness	Hurt, Insult, Disappointment	Powerlessness	Resentment, Annoyance	Sadness, Unhappiness	Shock, Surprise	Doubts on Job Appropriateness	Relationship to Patient Impaired	Professional Performance Impaired	Insecurity at Work
		•													
														•	
•		•							•		•				•
									•			•		•	•
•												•		•	
•	•		•		•	•				•	•			•	
				•						•					
•					•	•					•				
•		•			•							•		•	•

TABLE A9-3

Synopsis of the Most Prominent Non-somatic Symptoms (*continued*)

	Domain	Country	Bio-physiological					Stress	PTSD		Cognitive			
			Anxiety or Fear	Body Tension	Disquiet/Irritability	Headache	Sleep Disorder, Nightmares		Avoidance	Increased Arousal	Persistent Re-experience	Disbelief	Personal Integrity Threatened	Transformed Perception
Richter and Berger (2000, p. 302)	P	D	•			•			•	•	•			
Ryan and Poster (1989, p. 259)	P	USA	•	•								•		
Whittington and Wykes (1992)	P	UK	•		•		•				•			
Bin Abdulla et al. (2000, p. 444)	E	SGP				•				•				
Fernandez et al. (2002, p. 763)	E	CDN	•		•	•						•		
Hislop and Melby (2003, p. 982)	E	UK										•		
Levin et al. (1998, p. 388)	E	USA		•						•				

TABLE A9-3

Synopsis of the Most Prominent Non-somatic Symptoms (*continued*)

	Emotional												Social			
Anger	Apathy, Indifference	Apprehension, Distress, Upset	Exhaustion, Fatigue, Strain	Frustration	Guilt, Self-Blame, Shame	Helplessness	Hurt, Insult, Disappointment	Powerlessness	Resentment, Annoyance	Sadness, Unhappiness	Shock, Surprise	Doubts on Job Appropriateness	Relationship to Patient Impaired	Professional Performance Impaired	Insecurity at Work
•				•				•							
														•	
•											•			•	
•					•			•		•					
•				•	•	•		•	•					•	
•	•			•	•	•		•		•				•	

TABLE A9-3

Synopsis of the Most Prominent Non-somatic Symptoms (*continued*)

	Domain	Country	Bio-physiological					PTSD			Cognitive			
			Anxiety or Fear	Body Tension	Disquiet/Irritability	Headache	Sleep Disorder, Nightmares	Stress	Avoidance	Increased Arousal	Persistent Re-experience	Disbelief	Personal Integrity Threatened	Transformed Perception
Suserud et al. (2002, p. 776)	E	S									•			
Åström et al. (2002)	R	S	•											
Chambers (1998, p. 264)	R	UK	•					•	•			•	•	
Gates et al. (1999, p. 251)	R	USA	•							•			•	•
O'Connell et al. (2000)	G	AUS	•											
Arnetz & Arnetz (2001, p. 374)	M	S	•											
May & Grubbs (2002, p. 768)	M	USA	•									•		
Menckel & Viitsara (2002, p. 753)	M	S			•									
Vincent et al. (2000, p. 2003)	M	DK	•	•										
Studies reporting effect			15	5	5	3	4	3	6	9	9	6	5	4

P, psychiatric setting; E, accident and emergency; R, residential/gerontological setting; M, mixed settings; G, general; PTSD, post-traumatic stress disorder.
Countries: AUS, Australia; CH, Switzerland; CDN, Canada; D, Germany; DK, Denmark; S, Sweden; SGP, Singapore; UK, United Kingdom; USA, United States of America.

TABLE A9-3

Synopsis of the Most Prominent Non-somatic Symptoms (*continued*)

	Emotional												Social			
Anger	Apathy, Indifference	Apprehension, Distress, Upset	Exhaustion, Fatigue, Strain	Frustration	Guilt, Self-Blame, Shame	Helplessness	Hurt, Insult, Disappointment	Powerlessness	Resentment, Annoyance	Sadness, Unhappiness	Shock, Surprise	Doubts on Job Appropriateness	Relationship to Patient Impaired	Professional Performance Impaired	Insecurity at Work
•				•	•	•	•		•			•			•
							•			•			•		
								•							•
•				•		•	•			•					
•															
•	•		•					•							•
•															
•															
•															
17	3	4	3	6	8	6	3	5	5	6	4	4	5	6	6

three possible reasons for the great number of responses. Because of the semantic proximity of some effects (e.g. guilt, self-blame, and shame), we summarized some effects into categories in the synoptic table (Table 3). This procedure is a trade-off between semantic precision and a manageable number of effects.

The most frequently reported effects are anger, anxiety (fear), and guilt (self-blame, shame). The data in Table 3 suggest that these three primary reactions occur in all domains and in most countries. Anger and anxiety are considered relatively normal reactions and should not be confused with pathology. Guilt, self-blame, and shame may be linked to nurses' double role—maintaining one's own rights whilst offering the best quality of care—in dealing with aggressive patients. Chambers (1998) remarks on some nurses' tendency to blame themselves, to assume responsibility, and often to set themselves unrealistically high standards when attempting to deal with violent patients. Murray and Snyder (1991) report on health care workers' high expectations of themselves. Such high moral standards, whilst being laudable, may lead to the ethical dilemma of endeavoring to fulfill professional moral standards whilst concurrently wishing to safeguard and maintain the nurse's own rights.

Powerlessness is reported in the articles from all nursing domains except psychiatry. This finding may be associated with the socialization and education of psychiatric nurses. Given the high rates of aggression in psychiatric nursing this may indicate habituation to or better personal and structural resources for managing patient aggression.

Because of the focus of the review on adverse effects on assaulted nurses, no references to those on whom patient aggression and assault have little or no effect are included in this paper. Certain nurses are apparently not affected (Lanza 1983, Vincent et al. 2000) and it is conceivable that patient aggression may have a positive effect (e.g. strengthening of certain personality traits) on some. As Flannery notes, 65% of nurses saw some meaning in the assault (Flannery et al. 1991) and regarding intention to leave the job, one group of authors notes that 54% of nurses had never considered doing this because of violence.

Limitations

Several methodological limitations apply to this systematic review. There is always the danger of missing relevant literature. This is possibly the case with some articles we discovered in languages (Finnish, Swedish) beyond our scope. It is also difficult to detect unpublished literature on the subject under scrutiny. Thus, in spite of the fact that two unpublished studies are included, and notwithstanding good feedback from international experts on the comprehensiveness of our search (Greenhalgh 2001), some selection bias may have occurred.

The 28 predominant effects found here are the result of a simple enumeration process and do not reflect any association with severity of suffering of the victims. The number and quality of non-somatic reactions of anxiety and fear also seem to be affected by the research question and study design. An illustration of this difficulty is the non-somatic reactions of anxiety or fear: possible explanations for the differing rates of anxiety or fear ranging from 2.7% (trainee nursing aides) to 40.0% experienced caring staff are sampling (assaulted vs. non-assaulted, convenience vs. randomized sample), status (trainee vs. experienced), age of participants, setting (high level aggressions care settings such as psychiatry or accident and emergency), or definition of threat, aggression, violence, and attack. A similar caveat applies to anger as the most frequently reported effect: whilst anger is reported in accident and emergency and general and mixed nursing settings, it only occurs in some psychiatric settings. This finding can be explained by the fact that most authors not reporting anger in psychiatric nursing (Caldwell 1992, Whittington & Wykes 1992, Adams & Whittington 1995, Flannery et al. 1995, Richter & Berger 2000) conducted studies placing the emphasis on PTSD or related concepts. It must also be stressed that the apparent concentration of PTSD symptoms in the domain of psychiatric nursing (Table 3) may possibly be a product of researchers' interest in this syndrome rather than an expression of real rates in this nursing domain.

The studies employing qualitative research methods used in this review (Hauck 1993, Chambers 1998, Hislop & Melby 2003) produced on average 10.3 non-somatic effects as compared to 5.8 in quantitative studies, indicating that an open response format may influence the reporting of experienced effects.

Although we sought to counteract these problems by stringent application of the inclusion and exclusion criteria (Greenhalgh 2001), the results must be interpreted with caution.

CONCLUSIONS

However, in spite of these shortcomings, this review demonstrates various points. Nurses' reactions to patient aggression are complex and encompass a broad spectrum of non-somatic reactions. This finding is reflected in a comment by Chambers (1998, p. 433) that nurses involved in the management of aggressive patients are involved in a 'complex mesh of feelings and interrelated experiences, some of which appear to contradict others'. In spite of individual variability in nurses' reactions to patient aggression, some reactions seem to be consistent between countries and nursing settings.

Although evidence on the real frequencies and prevalence rates of non-somatic effects of patient aggression on nurses is inconclusive, the most pre-dominantly reported consequences are anger, fear or anxiety, PTSD symptoms, guilt, self-blame, and shame. These effects exist despite differing countries, cultures, and nursing settings. The use of standardized instruments and representative samples would be helpful to derive material suitable for comparison and meta-analysis. Given the effects of patient aggression on nurses and the subsequent suffering further research should concentrate on interventions to prevent patient aggression and to prepare nurses to cope with such effects.

What is already known about this topic

- Patient aggression is a problem for nurses in many nursing domains.
- Physical consequences are well reported in the literature and are acknowledged as causing serious injury.
- Many non-somatic effects are known but are seen as less serious, although they also cause much suffering.

What this paper adds

- The predominant non-somatic effects of patient aggression from eight countries in four domains of nursing are anger, fear or anxiety, post-traumatic stress disorder symptoms, guilt, self-blame, and shame.
- The low occurrence or lack of some non-somatic effects such as frustration or powerlessness in psychiatric settings is possibly attributable to professional socialization, or to habituation towards handling aggression in this nursing domain.
- Identification of the methodological constraints which prevent comparisons across settings and strategies for future research.

AUTHORS' CONTRIBUTIONS

All listed authors have contributed directly to this study and this paper. IN contributed to conception of study, electronic and hand search, coding, writing of manuscript; CA contributed to cross validation of coding procedures with IN, electronic search, retrieval of articles, assistance in structuring data presentation, and writing of manuscript; RJGH contributed to design and supervision of search strategy, critical review of manuscript; JEF contributed to supervision of data analysis and integration, critical review of manuscript; TD contributed to supervision of the project, critical inspection of manuscript.

References

Adams J. & Whittington R. (1995). Verbal aggression to psychiatric staff: Traumatic stressor or part of the job? *Perspectives in Psychiatric Care, 2,* 171–174.

American Psychiatric Association (1994). *Diagnostic and statistical manual of mental disorders* (4th ed.). Washington, DC: Author.

Arnetz J. E. & Arnetz B. B. (2001). Violence towards health care staff and possible effects on the quality of patient care. *Social Science and Medicine, 52,* 417–427.

Åström S., Bucht G., Eisemann M., Norberg A., & Saveman B. I. (2002). Incidence of violence towards staff caring for the elderly. *Scandinavian Journal of Caring Sciences, 16,* 66–72.

Baxter E., Hafner R. J., & Holme G. (1992). Assaults by patients: The experience and attitudes of psychiatric hospital nurses. *Australian and New Zealand Journal of Psychiatry, 26,* 567–573.

Bensley L., Nelson N., Kaufman J., Silverstein B., Kalat J., & Shields, J. W. (1997). Injuries due to assaults on psychiatric hospital employees in Washington State. *American Journal of Industrial Medicine, 1,* 92–99.

Bin Abdullah A. M., Khim L. Y. L., Wah L. C., Bee O. G., & Pushpam S. (2000). A study of violence towards nursing staff in the emergency department. *Singapore Nursing Journal, 27,* 30–37.

Caldwell M. F. (1992). Incidence of PTSD among staff victims of patient violence. *Hospital and Community Psychiatry, 43,* 838–839.

Carmel H. & Hunter M. (1993). Staff injuries from patient attack: five years' data. *The Journal of the American Academy of Psychiatry and the Law, 21,* 485–493.

Chambers N. (1998). 'We have to put up with it—don't we?' The experience of being the registered nurse on duty, managing a violent incident involving an elderly patient: A phenomenological study. *Journal of Advanced Nursing, 27,* 429–436.

Fernandes C. M., Raboud J. M., Christenson J. M., Bouthillete F., Bullock L., Ouellet L., & Moore C. F. (2002). The effect of an education program on violence in the emergency department. *Annals of Emergency Medicine, 39,* 47–55.

Flannery R., Fulton P., Tausch J., & DeLoffi A. (1991). A program to help staff cope with psychological sequelae of assaults by patients. *Hospital and Community Psychiatry, 41,* 935–938.

Flannery R., Hanson M., & Penk W. (1995). Patients' threats. Expanded definition of assault. *General Hospital Psychiatry, 17,* 451–453.

Fottrell E. (1980). A study of violent behaviour among patients in psychiatric hospitals. *British Journal of Psychiatry, 136,* 216–221.

Fry A. J., O'Riordan D., Turner M., & Mills K. L. (2002). Survey of aggressive incidents experienced by community mental health staff. *International Journal of Mental Health Nursing, 11,* 112–120.

Gates D. M., Fitzwater E., & Meyer U. (1999). Violence against caregivers in nursing homes: Expected, tolerated, and accepted. *Journal of Gerontological Nursing, 4,* 12–22.

Greenhalgh T. (2001). *How to read a paper: The basics of evidence-based medicine.* (2nd ed.). London: BMJ Books.

Haller R. & Deluthy R. (1988). Assaults on staff by psychiatric in-patients: A critical review. *British Journal of Psychiatry, 152,* 174–179.

Hansen B. (1996). Workplace violence in the hospital psychiatric setting. An occupational health perspective. *American Association of Occupational Health Nurses Journal, 4,* 575–580.

Hanson R. & Balk J. (1992). A replication study of staff injuries in a state hospital. *Hospital and Community Psychiatry, 43,* 836–837.

Hauck M. (1993). *Die Wut bleibt—Gewalt von Patienten gegenüber Pflegenden (The anger remains—Patient violence towards nurses).* Kaderschule für die Krankenpflege, Aarau.

Hislop E. & Melby V. (2003). The lived experience of violence in accident and emergency. *Accident and Emergency Nursing, 11,* 5–11.

Lanza M. L. (1983). The reactions of nursing staff to physical assault by a patient. *Hospital Community Psychiatry, 34,* 44–47.

Lanza M., Kayne H., Hicks C., & Milner J. (1991). Nursing staff characteristics related to patient assault. *Issues in Mental Health Nursing, 12,* 253–265.

Lanza M. L. (1992). Nurses as patient assault victims: An update, synthesis, and recommendations. *Archives of Psychiatric Nursing, 5,* 163–171.

Lee S. S., Gerberich S. G., Waller L. A., Anderson A., & McGovern P. (1999). Work-related assault injuries among nurses. *Epidemiology, 10,* 685–691.

Levin P. F., Hewitt J. B., & Misner S. T. (1998). Insights of nurses about assault in hospital-based emergency departments. *Image Journal of Nursing Scholarship, 30,* 249–254.

May D. D. & Grubbs L. M. (2002). The extent, nature, and precipitating factors of nurse assault among three groups of registered nurses in a regional medical center. *Journal of Emergency Nursing, 28,* 11–17.

Menckel E. & Viitasara E. (2002). Threats and violence in Swedish care and welfare—magnitude of the problem and impact on municipal personnel. *Scandinavian Journal of Caring Sciences, 16,* 376–385.

Murray G. & Snyder J. C. (1991). When staff are assaulted. A nursing consultation support service. *Journal of Psychosocial Nursing and Mental Health Services, 29,* 24–29.

Noble P. & Rodger S. (1989). Violence by psychiatric in-patients. *British Journal of Psychiatry, 155,* 384–390.

O'Connell B., Young J., Brooks J., Hutchings J., & Lofthouse J. (2000). Nurses' perceptions of the nature and frequency of aggression in general ward settings and high dependency areas. *Journal of Clinical Nursing, 9,* 602–610.

Owen C., Tarantello C., Jones M., & Tennant C. (1998). Violence and aggression in psychiatric units. *Psychiatric Services, 49,* 1452–1457.

Richter D. (1998). Gewalt und Gewaltprävention in der psychiatrischen Pflege: Eine Übersicht über die Literatur. In: *Gewalt in der psychiatrischen Pflege.* Huber, Bern.

Richter D. & Berger K. (2000). Physische und psychische Folgen bei Mitarbeitern nach einem Patientenübergriff: Eine prospektive Untersuchung in sechs psychiatrischen Kliniken. *Arbeitsmedizin, Sozialmedizin, Umweltmedizin, 35,* 357–362.

Rippon T. J. (2000). Aggression and violence in health care professions. *Journal of Advanced Nursing, 31,* 452–460.

Ryan J. A. & Poster E. C. (1989). The assaulted nurse: Short-term and long-term responses. *Archives of Psychiatric Nursing, 3,* 323–331.

Suserud B. O., Blomquist M., & Johansson I. (2002). Experiences of threats and violence in the Swedish ambulance service. *Accident and Emergency Nursing, 10,* 127–135.

Vanderslott J. (1998). A study of incidents of violence towards staff by patients in an NHS Trust hospital. *Jour-nal of Psychiatric and Mental Health Nursing, 5,* 291–298.

Vincent C., Perlt D., Sorensen S., & Winther L. (2000). *Violence Against Trainees—A questionnaire study* (p. 38). Socialt Udviklingscenter SUS, Copenhagen.

Whittington R. & Wykes T. (1992). Staff strain and social support in a psychiatric hospital following assault by a patient. *Journal of Advanced Nursing, 17,* 480–486.

Articles Used in the Systematic Review

Author and Year	Setting, Subjects, Sample	Study Type, Aim, Definition	Instrument, Analysis	Main Results Related to Non-somatic Effects
Adams and Whittington (1995)	Sixty-eight psychiatric nursing staff, UK, c	Prospective survey on verbal abuse and threats: TV	IRF, RIES, descriptive statistics, testing	Fifty episodes of verbal aggression reported by 20 nurses evoked intrusion and avoidance symptoms resulting in a score of 30.9 on the RIES, whilst an earlier study produced a RIES score of 10.3 following physical aggression.
Arnetz and Arnetz (2001)	8531 (rr 61–76%) general hospital staff, S, c	Action research on association between patient violence and care quality: T, no definition of violence	Quality of care instrument, descriptive statistics, and testing	284 hospital staff (12%) had experienced violence in the preceding year with the most common reactions being anger, sadness, disappointment, and fear. Other reactions were post-violence cautiousness, fear, less enjoyment working with patients. Workplace violence was significantly related to non-somatic symptoms.
Åström et al. (2002)	506 (rr 78%) nursing staff in residential settings, S, c	Cross-sectional survey on incidence of violence and staff's emotional reactions: no definition	Questionnaire, descriptive statistics	A considerable number of nurses report aggression consequences such as powerlessness (56%), unhappiness (51%), and anger (49%). Shame (11%) and guilt (15%) were also reported.
Bin Abdullah et al. (2000)	35 (rr 86%) emergency staff, CNG, c	Survey on prevalence and effects of patient violence, PV	Questionnaire, descriptive statistics	94% reported psychological effects following patient violence including anger and irritability (69%), feelings of insecurity (69%), depression (3%), and anxiety (9%).
Caldwell (1992)	224 (rr 45%) mental health staff, USA, c	Survey on violence, consequences and debriefing: no definition	Questionnaire, descriptive statistics	62% (*n* = 138) of staff gave accounts of critical violence incidents with 61% reporting PTSD symptoms. 10% (23) met the criteria for PTSD.

(Continued)

Articles Used in the Systematic Review (*continued*)

Author and Year	Setting, Subjects, Sample	Study Type, Aim, Definition	Instrument, Analysis	Main Results Related to Non-somatic Effects
Chambers (1998)	5 assaulted gerontological nurses, UK, c	Phenomenological study on experiences with violence: no definition	In-depth interviews, Colaizzi analysis	An exhaustive description of the experience of managing violent patients is given which includes experiences of powerlessness, resentment, resignation, and anger by the nurses.
Fernandes et al. (2002)	106 (rr 65%) emergency department staff in CND, c	Survey on perceived incidence and consequences of violence: no definition	Questionnaire, descriptive statistics	Nurses reported consideration of job change (38%), short, medium, and long-term impaired job performance (25%, 24%, and 19%, respectively), fear of patients (73%), and impaired job satisfaction (74%).
Fernandes et al. (2002)	667 (rr 84% emergency department staff, CND, c	Prospective survey on the effects of violence management: PV	Questionnaire, descriptive statistics	Surveys were conducted at baseline and at 3 and 6 months post-training with nurses constituting 56%, 55%, and 66% of the samples, respectively. The impacts of verbal and physical violence are feeling upset, blame, fear of being alone with patient, increased irritability, anger, and headache.
Flannery et al. (1991)	62 assaults on health care workers in a mental hospital, USA, c	Prospective survey on effects of an intervention for the assaulted, VP	Interviews, description of effects	During interviews conducted as part of the 'Assaulted Staff Action Program' (ASAP) the victims reported on experiencing fright, anger, apprehension, sleep disturbances, intrusive memories, recall of traumatic incidents, and hyper vigilance.
Flannery et al. (1995)	19 assaults on psychiatric staff, USA, c	Prospective survey on frequency and impact of threats on carers, T	PTSD monitoring, descriptive statistics	Some of the nurses involved in 19 cases of severe threat experienced PTSD-like symptoms ($n = 9$) and disruption in mastery and meaning ($n = 11$).
Fry et al. (2002)	Community mental health staff ($n = 92$, rr 77%) AUS, c	Survey on characteristics of aggressive incidents and staff experiences with aggression, PV	Questionnaire based on the OAS, descriptive statistics	Respondents of the cross-sectional survey reported anxiety (44%), emotional distress (35%), feelings of vulnerability, violation of psychological integrity (9%) (including intimidation, harassment, and threat), and fear. Other experiences were e.g. nightmares, thoughts about further attacks, or preoccupation with risk and safety. 'Less common' reactions were e.g. surprise annoyance, shock, laughter, or burnout.

Articles Used in the Systematic Review (*continued*)

Author and Year	Setting, Subjects, Sample	Study Type, Aim, Definition	Instrument, Analysis	Main Results Related to Non-somatic Effects
Gates et al. (1999)	60 nursing home nurses, USA, c	Focus group on perceptions of violence: PTV	Structured questions, content analysis, descriptive depiction of effects	In focus groups the victims of patient aggression report on the following feelings: hurt, anger, frustration, resentments, sadness, feelings of hurt and unpredictability, lack of respect, shock, madness fear, feeling ban, and ambivalence.
Hauck (1993)	7 assaulted psychiatric nurses, CH, c	Content analysis on the experience of assaulted nurses: no definition	Open interview, coding, categorizing procedures	Assaulted nurses reported anger, resentment, guilt/self-blame, numbness, exhaustion/fatigue, threats to personal integrity, transformed perception, impaired capacity to express feelings, stigmatization, doubts on job appropriateness, and feelings of workplace insecurity impairment in professional performance.
Hislop and Melby (2003)	Accident and emergency nurses ($n = 26$, rr 95%), UK, c	Phenomenological inquiry into the lived experience of violence: PTV	Giorgi method of analysis	The core category 'why me?' of the lived experience of A&E nurses includes frustration, powerlessness, incapacity to understand being the target of aggression, embarrassment, and anger. In the core category 'sense of isolation' respondents report feeling being left totally alone (by management) and fear (of personal injury).
Lanza et al. (1991)	21 (rr unclear) psychiatric nurses, USA, sampling unclear	Prospective survey on characteristics of assaulted nurses: no definition	VIS, NSCF, descriptive statistics	Of the seven assaulted nurses 30% felt more apprehensive, 10% more vulnerable, 10% less in control, 10% intended job change, and 10% experienced strained family relationships.
Lanza et al. (1983)	40 assault nurses in psychiatry, USA, c	Explorative survey summarizing reactions to assault	Questionnaire, descriptive statistics	After administration of a questionnaire with 108 possible response reactions numerous short-and long-term emotional, social, bio-physiological, and cognitive reactions were found (e.g. anger, helplessness, anxiety, or changes in relationships to others). Some nurses were not prone to reaction after assault.
Levin et al. (1998)	22 emergency department nurses, USA, c	Focus groups on nurses' views on assaults: P	Coding procedures, descriptive depiction of effects	Victims reported long-term chronic pain, muscle tension, loss of sleep, nightmares, flashback, anger, withdrawal from patients, callousness, burnout, impairment of personal relationships

(Continued)

Articles Used in the Systematic Review (*continued*)

Author and Year	Setting, Subjects, Sample	Study Type, Aim, Definition	Instrument, Analysis	Main Results Related to Non-somatic Effects
May and Grubbs (2002)	86 (rr 69%) general, emergency, ICU nurses, USA, c	Survey on patient assaults on nurses: PTV	HASN, descriptive statistics, ANOVA	Victims of patient violence experiences: decreased job satisfaction (65%), anger (66%), anxiety (53%), fear (36%), emotional distress (36%), disbelief (34%), powerlessness (23%), and impaired job confidence (20%).
Menckel and Viitasara (2002)	2380 (rr 85%) care workers, S, stratified sampling	Survey on prevalence and consequences of threats and violence: no definition of violence	Questionnaire, descriptive depiction of effects	Of the 2380 subjects 696 were nurses. The care givers' most common reactions to violence were: anger (41%), irritation (38%), sadness (35%), helpless or insulted (~33%), or frustration.
Murray and Snyder (1991)	19 (rr 54%) assaulted psychiatric staff, USA, c	Survey to assess stress at 6 weeks post-assault: P	Questionnaire, descriptive depiction of effects	83% of assaulted nurses reported reactions of frustration, anger, self-criticism, disbelief, and sadness.
O'Connell et al. (2000)	209 (rr 52%) general nurses, AUS, r	Survey on the perception and experience of violence: no definition	Questionnaire, descriptive statistics	95% of the sample had experienced verbal or physical aggression in the past year. Reactions to verbal violence were: anger (71%), anxiety (29%), embarrassment (31%), fear (22%), frustration (73%), guilt (9%), helplessness (36%), hurt (47%), resentment (42%), or feeling burnt out (58%). Nurses having experienced physical aggression reported lesser percentages on the above effects.
Richter and Berger (2000)	85 (rr 50%) assaulted psychiatric workers in D, c	Prospective survey on patient assault and consequences: P	Interview, PTSD questionnaire, descriptive statistics	The 85 assaulted carers (all bar two nurses) experienced shock (44%), despondency (7%), fear (12%). PTSD symptoms were also experienced: re-experience (11%), avoidance (1%), and increased irritability (4%). None of the assaulted fulfilled all three criteria constituting a complete clinical PTSD.
Ryan and Poster (1989)	61 assaulted nursing staff, USA, c	Prospective longitudinal survey on assault effects: PT	ARQ, ATPAQ, interview, inferential statistics	The following reactions to violence were found: anger (40–50%), anxiousness, feeling sorry for the perpetrator, feelings of inadequacy in preventing the aggressive incident (30–40%), increased body tension and awareness (40–50%), with social

Articles Used in the Systematic Review (*continued*)

Author and Year	Setting, Subjects, Sample	Study Type, Aim, Definition	Instrument, Analysis	Main Results Related to Non-somatic Effects
				and cognitive responses having been experienced at 'a lower rate'.
Suserud et al. (2002)	66 (rr 92%) ambulance service nurses, S, c	Survey on experiences with threats and violence: T, no clear definition of violence	Questionnaire, descriptive depiction of effects	Ambulance nurses having experienced violence perceived impairment of performance, anger, feeling confounded, shock, impairment of nurse-patient relationship, and difficulty to concentrate.
Vincent et al. (2000)	660 (rr 69%) health care trainees; DK, c	Survey on assault consequences: PTSV	Questionnaire, descriptive statistics	Trainees in social work (428), nursing (228), and nursing aides (184) participated. Of the 660 students 428 had experienced violence or threats of violence. The main experiences were: body tension, anxiety/fear (4.8%), anger (17.1%), powerlessness, indifference, exhaustion/fatigue, feelings of workplace insecurity.
Whittington and Wykes (1992)	23 assaulted nurses, one assaulted doctor, UK, c	Prospective longitudinal survey on post-assault strain and support: P	SSEV, SQ, VSQ, inferential statistics	Victims of patient violence were interviewed three times (<72 hours, 7, and 14 days). The following non-somatic responses varied individually in intensity across time: sleep disorder, nightmares, anxiety/fear, exhaustion, with fatigue and irritability being the most prominent reactions.

rr, response rate; c, convenience sample; P, physical; V, verbal; T, threat.
Countries: AUS, Australia; CH, Switzerland; CDN, Canada; D, Germany; DK, Denmark; S, Sweden; SGP, Singapore; UK, United Kingdom; USA, United States of America.
ARQ, Assault Response Questionnaire; ATPAQ, Attitudes Toward Patient Physical Assault Questionnaire; HASN, Hospital Assault Survey for Nurses; IRF, Incident Report Form; NSCF, Nursing Staff Characteristics Form; OAS, Overt Aggression Scale; PTSD-Interview, Post-Traumatic Stress Disorder Interview, German version; RIES, Revised Impact of Events Scale; SQ, Strain Questionnaire; SSEV, Spielberger's Self Evaluations Questionnaire; VIS, Victim Interview Schedule; VSQ, Victim Support Questionnaire.

Demographic Characteristics as Predictors of Nursing Students' Choice of Type of Clinical Practice

Abstract: This descriptive study examined predictors of nursing students' choice of field of clinical practice using a convenience sample of 30 baccalaureate students in a Midwestern university. Students voluntarily completed a written questionnaire and responded to a subjective question about experiences influencing their choice of field. Students favored acute settings such as intensive care and emergency rooms over less acute settings, and their age and self-rating of health were related to these choices. Three types of experiences were described as meaningful contributors to choice of field of practice.

The nursing shortage is of grave concern to the public and to the profession of nursing itself, and nursing workforce planning is a priority. Nursing workforce planning needs to address the numbers of nurses prepared and the level of nursing preparation at the international level, as well as nationally (Hegyvary, 2006; Peterson, 2005). In considering nursing workforce needs, one needs to consider not just the numbers of nurses, but also the choice of clinical practice of those nurses. While declining enrollments in schools of nursing affect the availability of nurses in all settings, settings that are less "popular" among new graduates will be even harder hit by this shortage. This includes long-term health care settings and primary care settings. The needs for nurses in these types of settings vary from country to country. For example, in South Africa, the number of nursing positions in hospitals is much smaller than those in primary health clinics. In contrast, in the United States, the aging population makes needs in long-term care facilities greater than those in primary care.

BACKGROUND

In the United States, the general public's image of nursing continues to be the dedicated individual providing bedside nursing for acute health problems. Often the only image nursing students have of the field as they begin their education comes from television shows such as *Scrubs* or *Gray's Anatomy*. These portrayals usually project an image of nurses as either oversexed or always in the midst of life-threatening crises. The impact of such portrayals of nurses is reflected in the common situation when students, who think they may be interested in primary care or public health nursing "someday," often plan to do "real nursing" in a hospital first. As long-term planning for the nursing workforce continues, it will be important to be able to predict which students are more likely to fill gaps in the different and varied fields of nursing practice. This will allow nursing programs to target student recruitment toward those students most likely to move into clinical practice settings with the greatest need. Therefore, this study examined the relationships among nursing students' demographic characteristics and their choice for practice following graduation. Specifically, the study addressed the following three questions.

1. Are age, gender, race, and marital status associated with choice of first clinical practice after graduation?
2. Do older students and those with higher levels of perceived well-being select primary care settings for clinical practice after graduation more often than do younger students and those with lower levels of well-being?
3. What student experiences bring meaning to their choices of field of nursing practice?

METHODS

Sample

This study used a convenience sample of undergraduate baccalaureate nursing students in the second semester of their junior year of their program. The students were completing a required research course. The NLN-accredited nursing program located in a large Midwestern university enrolls 120 undergraduate students each year. The university draws students from throughout the Midwest and reports a generally diverse student body, including representative numbers of Latino and black students. Programs to earn a bachelor's degree in nursing include a traditional four-year program, an RN to BSN program, and an LPN to BSN program. Students in all three of these programs take the research course that provided the sample for this study. Participation in the study was voluntary, and completion of the questionnaire was anonymous. A total of 30 out of 33 students participated.

Procedure

An independent faculty member who was not teaching the course administered the questionnaires, and the subjects placed the questionnaires in a sealed box themselves. Subjects were told that the questionnaire was part of the nursing department's efforts to plan future programs. In order to avoid any overt breach in confidentiality, all students remained in the classroom while the questionnaires were being completed, and all students placed questionnaires in the box, whether or not they had completed the questionnaire.

Measures

The entire questionnaire consisted of three sections. The first section asked about demographic characteristics, the second section asked about post-secondary education, perceived well-being, and planned choice of career, and the last section asked about subjects' preferences of automobiles. The last section was included to be used as a class exercise for the research course itself. Each section is described below.

Demographic characteristics included in this study were age, gender, and marital status. Each of these variables could reflect selected life experiences of students that might influence their choice of practice site after graduation.

The section asking about post-secondary education, well-being, and planned career choice included items asking about completion of previous technical programs, or associate or undergraduate degrees. Subjects were asked if they were currently licensed to practice as either an LPN or RN and to give the total number of years of post-secondary education they had completed. Well-being was measured on a four-point scale rating perceived health as excellent, good, fair, and poor (Kaplan & Camacho, 1983). This single self-report item has been used in a number of studies, including the Human Population Laboratory Studies in Alameda County, CA (Kaplan & Camacho, 1983). The item has demonstrated reliability and validity. It has been shown to be strongly related to a persons' baseline physical health status, and to be significantly related to different mortality rates for both men and women of all ages who perceived their health as excellent versus poor (Kaplan & Camacho, 1983).

The last questions in the second section of the questionnaire asked subjects about their anticipated choice of field of nursing immediately post graduation and long-term. Responses were selected from a list of nursing career options, eliminating the need to code individual responses. Subjects also were asked a single open-ended qualitative question, "What experiences in your life have led to your anticipated choice for field of nursing practice?" Subjects were provided with a single page of lined paper for this response.

The third section of the questionnaire regarding automobile preferences included questions about ownership of an automobile, and a rating on a 10-point scale of the condition of that automobile or how much they want an automobile if they do not own one. Subjects were asked to rank their color preferences for automobiles, and to answer a series of dichotomous questions about their use of various forms of transportation.

The questionnaire was reviewed for face validity by three undergraduate faculty of nursing. It was then pilot-tested with a sample of five graduate student nurses in their research course in order to assure clarity and relevancy. Only very minor changes in language resulted from this pilot test.

Analysis

Only the results from the first two sections of the questionnaire are reported here. Objective data from the questionnaires were analyzed using SPSS (Statistical Package for the Social Sciences) software program. Written subjective responses were directly transcribed and were analyzed using common phenomenological methods (Boyd & Munhall, 1993). Analysis included data reduction, identification of common themes, and conclusion drawing and was aided by use of QRS NUD.IST (Non-Numerical Unstructured Data Indexing Searching and Theory-building Multi-Functional) software program.

RESULTS

The sample included 30 undergraduate baccalaureate nursing students, 25 female and 5 male. Ninety percent were single ($n = 27$) and the average age of subjects was 23 ($SD = 2$).

The majority of the subjects (60%) were traditional four-year baccalaureate students; however, subjects did represent all of the different programs offered. Many subjects had completed more than three years of post-secondary education ($M = 3.5, SD = 1$). Only 20% of subjects rated their own health as "fair or poor." Students' choices of field of nursing immediately post graduation and for a long-term career are reported in Table 1. In both cases, the majority of students selected acute care settings, with an emphasis on intensive care and emergency department care as their anticipated field of nursing.

Choice of field or setting was dichotomized for acute setting versus non-acute setting for additional

TABLE B-1

Students' Choices of Field of Nursing

Field of Choice	Number (%) Selecting Field Immediately Post Graduation	Number (%) Selecting Field as Long-Term Goal
Intensive Care (adult)	18 (60%)	9 (30%)
Neonatal or Pediatric Intensive Care	3 (10%)	6 (20%)
Emergency Department	3 (10%)	9 (30%)
Obstetrics	1 (3%)	0
Medical/Surgical	0	0
Pediatrics	2 (7%)	2 (7%)
Health Department	0	0
Long-Term Care, Nursing Home	2 (7%)	0
Primary Care Clinic or Health Care Provider Office	1 (3%)	4 (13%)

analysis. There was a significant difference in age of subjects who selected the two settings ($t = 2.4, p < .05$), with younger students selecting acute fields of practice. There also was a significant difference in rating of health ($t = 2.1, p < .05$), with subjects who rated their health higher choosing acute care fields of practice more than those with lower levels of self-rated health. Lastly, there was an association between type of nursing program and choice of field of study ($\text{Chisq}_{[10, N=30]} = 23, p < .05$). There was no significant association between race or gender and choice of field of study, and no differences in number of years of post-secondary education and field of study. Logistic regression indicated that only age of subject and rating of health statistically contributed to the odds of

selecting a non-acute care field of study when age, health rating, and type of nursing program were entered. One-way analysis of variance indicated that students who were older were more likely to be in the LPN to BSN program or the RN to BSN program.

Analysis of subjective findings yielded three distinct themes that represent the meaning of life experiences related to choice of field of nursing. The themes and selected quotes from subjects are included in Table 2. The first theme was personal life experiences such as illness or death of a loved one, or their own acute illness. Subjects described experiences with nurses in the emergency room and the hospital and how these gave unique meaning to the health crisis being faced.

TABLE B-2

Definitions of Themes and Examples That Represent Meaning of Experiences in Relation to Choice of Nursing Field

Themes	Examples of Experiences
Personal Life Experience: Direct interactions with health care providers and the health care system surrounding student's own health or that of others	"Seeing how those nurses took care of my mother as she lay there unconscious with so many tubes and machines hooked to her made me decide right then and there that this was what I wanted to do."
	"It was the nurse holding my hand as the doctor in the emergency room told me about my brother that made it possible for me to keep going. I want to be like that nurse and help others in such terrible times of life."
	"After I got home from the hospital a nurse came to visit and change my dressing. She was so caring and kind and gentle. Taking nursing into people's homes is what I want to do."
Experiences with Nursing Role Models: Direct interactions with significant others who are nurses	"My aunt was a nurse. She always was so strong and sure of herself—I wanted to be just like her and work in the emergency department."
	"In our town Mrs. Timms was the person everyone went to with a question or for help. It seemed like her being a nurse just made her able to help everyone. Mrs. Timms worked in the Health Department Clinic so that seems to me to be a good place to practice nursing."
Experiences with Fictional Media: Vicarious experiences of providing nursing care in certain settings as described or depicted in books, television, and the movies	"Watching the nurses in *ER;* they always knew what was going on and were really there for the patients—that is why I want to practice in the emergency room."

The second theme was direct experiences with family or close friends who provided nursing care in the field chosen by the subject. Subjects described love and respect and a desire to follow in the footsteps of these role models that had influenced their plans for field of nursing.

The last theme was experiences with fictional media including novels, movies, and television shows. These subjects described being moved and excited by descriptions or scenes showing nurses providing care in the fields they expected to choose post graduation.

DISCUSSION

Overall, students in this study identified that their choice of nursing field was intensive care and emergency room care. Maternity care and care of children were the second most commonly identified fields, with public health, primary care, and long-term care the least frequently chosen. Objectively, the major demographic characteristic that was associated with choice of acute care field of practice was age, with younger nursing students more frequently choosing acute fields compared with older students. Students who were older were more likely to be in the RN to BSN program or the LPN to BSN program, and therefore type of baccalaureate program was also related to choice of field. Lastly, self-rating of health was related to choice of field of practice, with students who rated themselves in better health being more likely to choose acute care fields.

Subjectively, students described experiences in their personal lives, with role models and with fictional characters as meaningful in their decisions about choice of field. Age of students may very well relate to these types of experiences, since one would expect that older students would be more likely to have a range of personal life experiences with various fields of nursing. Younger students are more likely to have primarily experienced health care in the acute setting, if at all, and may well depend on role models and fictional characters more than older students. Certainly, the fictional characters available to these students would create an emphasis on acute settings. The differences in self-rating of health further support this idea, since students who are in poor health are more likely to have personal experiences with a variety of health care fields, not just acute care. The subjective transcribed data was not connected to the objective demographic data, so it was not possible to explore these possibilities more completely.

Given the changes in health care in this country and throughout the world, and the increased emphasis on primary health care and early discharge from hospitals, it is clear that not all graduates who wish to practice in intensive care and emergency rooms will be able to do so. Nursing programs that are particularly concerned about shortages in non-acute settings may be able to expand this workforce by focusing their recruitment efforts on older students and by further developing or expanding RN to BSN and LPN to BSN programs. In addition, nursing needs to make fields of nursing other than acute care more visible to the public at large in order to widen the number of meaningful experiences nursing students might have that will affect their choice of field of practice.

References

Boyd, C. O. & Munhall, P. L. (1993). Qualitative research proposals and reports. *NLN Publications, 19*(2535), 424-453.

Hegyvary, S. T. (2006). Editorial: Roots of the shortage. *Journal of Nursing Scholarship, 33*(3), 204.

Kaplan, B. A. & Camacho, T. (1983). Perceived health and mortality: A nine-year follow-up of the Human Population Laboratory cohort. *American Journal of Epidemiology, 111*, 292-304.

Peterson, C. A. (2005). In short supply: Around the work, the need for nurses grows. *American Journal of Nursing, 101*(9), 61.

Sample In-Class Data Collection Tool

This questionnaire is for use in this research class only. Completing the questionnaire is entirely voluntary. If you do choose to fill out the questionnaire, please answer each question fully and thoughtfully.

DO NOT PUT YOUR NAME ON THIS FORM

Section One

What is your AGE in years? _____

Are you   MALE   FEMALE (circle one)

What is your MARITAL STATUS? (check one) ____ Single

____ Married

____ Divorced or Widowed

____ Partnered

Section Two

How many YEARS school have you <u>completed</u> since finishing high school? _____

In general, how would you rate your OVERALL HEALTH? (circle one)

Excellent   Good   Fair   Poor

Below, you will find a list of possible fields for nursing practice. Please check which one you want as your FIRST CHOICE for practice when you graduate from this nursing program. CHECK ONLY ONE!

____ Emergency Department

____ Health Department

____ Intensive Care Unit for Adults

____ Long-Term Care, Nursing Home

____ Medical/Surgical Unit

____ Neonatal or Pediatric Intensive Care

____ Obstetrics

____ Pediatric Unit

____ Primary Care Clinic or Health Care Provider Office

Below, you will find the same list of fields of nursing. This time, please check which one you want as your FIRST CHOICE for practice as a **long-term goal**.

____ Emergency Department

____ Health Department

____ Intensive Care Unit for Adults

____ Long-Term Care, Nursing Home

____ Medical/Surgical Unit

____ Neonatal or Pediatric Intensive Care

____ Obstetrics

____ Pediatric Unit

____ Primary Care Clinic or Health Care Provider Office

On the back of this questionnaire, please describe <u>the one major experience</u> in your life that has led you to select the field of nursing that you indicated above.

Section Three

Do you currently own a car? (check one)   ___ YES   ___ NO

- IF "YES," please answer the following questions about the car you own.
- If "NO," please answer the following questions for the car you expect to own in the immediate future.

Is the car (check one)   ____ NEW   ____ USED

Please **rate** the overall condition of the car you own or expect to own in the <u>immediate</u> future by circling ONE rating from the scale below.

1   2   3   4   5   6   7   8   9   10
Terrible   OK   Excellent

Please select your preferences for the CAR OF YOUR DREAMS:

Color (write in your primary color choice) _____

Type (such as SUV, sedan, convertible) _____

Transmission type (check one)   ____Automatic   ____ Standard 5 speed

Engine cylinders (check one)   ____ 4 cylinder ____ 6 cylinder ____ 8 cylinder ____ Unknown

From a range of 0% to 100%, how often do you wear seatbelts while riding or driving in a vehicle? _____ % of the time.

Thank you for completing this questionnaire, which we will use for practice in this class only.

Case Number	Marital Status	Health Rating	Case Number	Marital Status	Health Rating
1	Single	4	16	Married	3
2	Married	3	17	Single	4
3	Divorced/widowed	3	18	Single	3
4	Married	2	19	Divorced/widowed	3
5	Married	1	20	Single	4
6	Single	3	21	Married	3
7	Single	1	22	Married	2
8	Single	4	23	Single	3
9	Single	4	24	Single	2
10	Divorced/widowed	3	25	Single	3
11	Married	2	26	Divorced/widowed	4
12	Single	3	27	Single	3
13	Single	3	28	Single	3
14	Single	2	29	Married	2
15	Married	2	30	Married	3

Historical Analysis of Siderail Use in American Hospitals

Barbara L. Brush, Elizabeth Capezuti

Purpose: *To explore the social, economic, and legal influences on siderail use in 20th century American hospitals and how use of siderails became embedded in nursing practice.*

Design: *Social historical research.*

Methods: *Numerous primary and secondary sources were collected and interpreted to illustrate the pattern of siderail use, the value attached to siderails, and attitudes about using siderails.*

Findings: *The persistent use of siderails in American hospitals indicates a gradual consensus between law and medicine rather than an empirically driven nursing intervention. Use of siderails became embedded in nursing practice as nurses assumed increasing responsibility for their actions as institutional employees.*

Conclusions: *New federal guidelines, based on reports of adverse consequences associated with siderails, are limiting siderail use in hospitals and nursing homes across the United States. Lowering siderails and using alternatives will depend on new norms among health care providers, hospital administrators, bed manufacturers, insurers, attorneys, regulators, and patients and their families.*

Throughout most of the 20th century, the use of siderails as safeguards against patients' falls from hospital beds has spurred debate. Although researchers and practitioners have argued the merits and pitfalls of siderail use, few have explored how use of siderails evolved and gradually became embedded in nursing practice. Raising bed siderails remains the most frequently used intervention to prevent bed-related falls and injuries among hospitalized patients and institutionalized older adults (Capezuti, 2000; Capezuti & Braun, 2001).

Examining the social, economic, and legal influences on siderail use in 20th century American hospitals, we explored the centrality of the hospital bed to the mission and purpose of nursing and the shifting focus of bedside care from patient comfort to patient safety. We argue that use of siderails has been based more on a gradual consensus between law and medicine than on empirical evidence for nursing practice. Nonetheless, nurses, as hospital employees, adopted siderail use as part of their standard of bedside care (Barbee, 1957).

Social historical research methods were used to collect and interpret data. Thus, the pattern of siderail use, the value attached to siderails as an example of benevolent care, and attitudes about raising siderails were examined as they evolved and shifted over time. Primary sources included medical trade catalogs, hospital procedure manuals, newsletters, photography, and other archival materials from the New York Academy of Medicine, the College of Physicians in Philadelphia, and the Center for the Study of the History of Nursing at the University of Pennsylvania. Journal articles, government documents, published histories of hospital bed design, and nursing and medical texts provided additional sources of data.

THE HOSPITAL BED AS CENTRAL TO NURSING'S MISSION

In 1893, Isabel Adams Hampton made clear, in a chapter devoted entirely to hospital beds, that nurses were the overseers of beds and their occupants. As she put it, "A nurse who works over [beds] daily ought to be a fair judge of what is required in the way of a bed for the sick" (Hampton, 1893, p. 75). Hampton charged nurses to coordinate bed type to patient condition, maintain a neat and uniform bed appearance at all times, and ensure patient comfort during the period of recuperation.

In Hampton's day, the ideal bed was 6 feet 6 inches long, 37 inches wide, and 24–26 inches from the floor (Hampton, 1893). Although similar in length and width to standard twin beds in homes, hospital beds were approximately 6–8 inches higher to facilitate patient care and prevent unnecessary strain on nurses. Because beds were a fixed "nursing" height, stools were often used to accommodate patients as they transferred from bed.

Bed height, more than any other bed dimension, has consistently influenced bedside nursing care in American hospitals and long-term care facilities. Bed height and the outcomes of bed-related falls in hospitals have been the basic issues underlying numerous legislative and practice initiatives in the 20th century. Despite changes meant to remedy injurious outcomes from bed-related falls, however, patients falling from high beds are deemed at risk for increased morbidity and mortality (O'Keeffe, Jack, & Lye, 1996). Bed siderails, initially used as a temporary means to prevent confused, sedated, or elderly patients from falling from bed, are now permanent

fixtures on most institutional beds (Braun & Capezuti, 2000; Capezuti & Braun, 2001). Their increased use in the latter half of the 20th century reflects a shifting emphasis from patient comfort to patient safety as hospitals, evolving from charitable institutions to modern medical centers, became increasingly subject to litigation (Stevens, 1989).

"Rendering the Obstinate Docile"

Bed siderails were rarely available on adult hospital beds until the 1930s. More common were cribs or children's beds equipped with full or partial crib sides, which, similar to siderails, were meant to protect infants and young children from falling from or leaving beds unattended. The primary intervention for agitated, confused, or other adults considered at risk of falling from bed was nurses' provision of "careful and continuous watchfulness" (Merck Manual, 1934, p. 36).

Haigh and Hayman's (1936) study of 116 "out of bed" incidents at the University Hospital of Cleveland, however, provided early evidence of siderail use to control adult patient behavior and prevent deleterious outcomes. The authors reported that in 31% of bed-related falls at the study institution, patients climbed over siderails, and an additional 7% removed a physical restraint and then proceeded over the rails before falling. Although siderails, as well as rails in combination with restraints, were ineffective in preventing falls or deterring patients from leaving beds unassisted, the nurse and physician authors concluded that siderails were a reasonable precautionary measure against falls from bed as well as necessary adjuncts in "rendering the obstinate docile" (Haigh & Hayman, 1936, p. 45).

When first used, siderails, also known as sideboards or side restraints, were not permanently fastened to hospital beds. Instead, they were accessories that nurses physically attached to beds when they deemed necessary or when prescribed by a physician (Tracy, 1942). Securing these devices was a time-consuming and cumbersome procedure that often required at least two people (Manley, 1944).

In the 1940s, siderail use on adult hospital beds gradually became the subject of legal action against personal injury and death. In 1941, for example, the parents of 21-year-old Edgar Pennington sued Morningside Hospital after their son fell from bed and sustained a fatal head injury (Morningside Hospital

v. Pennington et al., 1941). When Mr. Pennington was initially hospitalized, his bed siderails were raised because of his irrational behavior. A few days later and presumably calmer, his siderails were removed and his left leg was chained to the bed instead. The plaintiffs argue that the nurses' failure to maintain siderails on their son's bed caused him to sustain his fatal fall. Whether his leg was still chained to the bed when he was found "with his bloody head on the concrete floor" was unsubstantiated. Ultimately, the case was dismissed.

A year earlier, the surviving husband of Jennie Brown Potter sued the Dr. W. H. Groves Latter-Day Saints Hospital for his wife's fall-related death, claiming that the hospital's failure to attach sideboards to her bed constituted negligence. As in Morningside Hospital v. Pennington et al. (1941), the court ruled for the defendant, citing lack of evidence that standard of due care required the hospital to place sideboards on patients' beds (Potter et al. v. Dr. W. H. Groves, 1940).

The Nurse's Role in Hospital Safety

By the 1950s, siderail use became more visibly linked to institutional liability. Numerous factors contributed to this transition. First, many states adopted laws overturning charitable hospitals' immunity from the negligence of their employees, necessitating hospitals' purchase of expensive insurance policies (Hayt, Hayt, & Groeschel, 1952). Second, a severe post-war nursing shortage limited nurses' ability to provide previous levels of watchfulness over patients in their charge (Lynaugh & Brush, 1996). Finally, bed manufacturers expanded their focus in advertising to include patient safety along with patient comfort and rest. Consequently, institutional beds equipped with permanent full-length siderails became more readily available (Hospitals, 1954). Nurses raised siderails on patients' beds to reassure the public and hospital administrators that even if nurses were in short supply, at least patients were secure in their beds (Aberg, 1957; Barbee, 1957).

Ludham (1957) reinforced this notion in one of the first reported studies of hospital insurance claims involving bed incidents. In his study of 7,815 "out-of-bed" incidents in California hospitals, Ludham found that, although 63% (4,893) of reported incidents occurred when siderails were raised, claims paid by insurance companies increased ten-fold when falls

occurred in the absence of raised siderails. The imbalance in jury awards was largely attributed to the perception that raising siderails was a demonstrable effort, however unproved, to protect patients from falls and serious injury. With no supporting evidence, Ludham nonetheless echoed previous claims (Aston, 1955; Price, 1956) that out-of-bed incidents with raised siderails caused less severe injury because patients had something to grasp when falling. He recommended that hospitals establish standing orders or policies requiring siderail use with certain types of patients (e.g., sedated, confused, "older") as a national standard of hospital practice. Locally, the Council on Insurance of the California Hospital Association urged its hospitals to permanently attach siderails to every bed "as rapidly as possible" (Ludham, 1957, p. 47).

Professional journal articles and nursing texts also regularly encouraged nurses to use siderails as part of their therapeutic actions (Aberg, 1957; Harmer & Henderson, 1952; Price, 1954), especially because of the claim that "bedfalls, together with hot-water bottle burns account for more lawsuits involving nurses than all other risks combined" (Hayt, Hayt, Groeschel, & McMullan, 1958, p. 206). Although the standard hospital bed height was "not always comfortable to the patient (but) convenient for the nurse and the doctor" (Harmer & Henderson, 1952, p. 126), siderails, defined as restraints or restrictive devices, were advocated in the prevention of falls and injury from these high beds (Hayt, Hayt, & Groeschel, 1952; McCullough & Moffit, 1949; Price, 1954).

Meanwhile, bed manufacturers continued to sell to "safety-minded hospital administrators" (Hospitals, 1954, p. 197). The Hard Manufacturing Company's "Slida-Side" offered permanent siderails on every hospital bed, and the Inland Bed Company guaranteed portable siderails to "provide safety for your patients, protection for your hospital" (Hospitals, 1954, p. 194). Both the Hall Invalid Bed and the Simmons Vari-Hite bed could be manually lowered from the standard height of 27 inches to the "normal home bed height" of 18 inches (Hospitals, 1950). They were considered safer for two reasons: they eliminated the need for "slipping, tilting footstools," and they allowed patients to get up from a familiar bed height without calling for the nurse (Hospitals, 1950, pp. 87, 102). Thus, and most important, the Simmons Company reported, the Vari-Hite bed reduced "the likelihood of falling and serious injury" (Hospitals, 1950, p. 87).

The Hill-Rom Company also advertised its Hilow Beds as the pinnacle of modernization and fall prevention because the crank-operated bed could be lowered to 18 inches, making patients less likely to misjudge the distance to the floor, lose their balance, and fall (Hospitals, 1955). To make their point that lower beds eliminated the need for full siderails to prevent bed-related falls and injuries, advertisements depicted the Vari-Hite and Hall Invalid beds without siderails and the Hilow Bed with a half rail meant to assist patients to transfer independently.

Despite the availability of lower and variable height beds that eliminated the need for siderails, that were comfortable for patients, and increased nursing efficiency, fixed "nursing height" beds with permanent full-length siderails were used more regularly than were these new inventions (Smalley, 1956). The "common sense" notion that siderails were safety devices led to hospital-wide policies that standardized their use. Because nurses and hospital administrators failed to question siderail efficacy in preventing bedside falls, they also failed to use alternatives. Gradually, hospital-based nurses in the 1950s raised siderails to substitute for their physical presence at the bedside and to protect hospitals' legal interests.

The Standard of Good Nursing Practice

An escalating nurse shortage in the 1960s and 1970s, coupled with changes in hospital architecture from multipatient wards to semiprivate and private patient rooms, prompted the continued use of siderails, as well as other physical restraints, as substitutes for nursing observation. By the 1980s, falls, especially from beds, were identified as a major hospital liability issue (Rubenstein, Miller, Postel, & Evans, 1983). In 1980 the National Association of Insurance Commissioners reported that falls represented 10% of all paid claims between 1975 and 1978; absence of siderails was identified as a principal justification. As a result, "routine use of bedrails" became "the standard of good nursing practice" (Rubenstein et al., 1983, p. 273).

As siderail use became common nursing practice, particularly to prevent falls among older patients, its scientific rationale was brought into question. Rubenstein and colleagues (1983) at Harvard Medical School labeled the continued use of siderails, in the absence of supporting data, an example of "defensive medicine" (p. 273). In other words, raising siderails was practice based on consensus rather than on scientific evidence. Based largely on legal action against hospitals and their personnel, siderail use became a means to promote patients' "right" to safety during hospitalization and nurses' "responsibility" to keep patients safe (Anonymous, 1984; Horty, 1973).

Shifting decisions about patient safety to nurses shifted liability from physicians to institutions. As a result, institutions took greater precautions to ensure that patients, especially the elderly, did not fall. Raising siderails for individuals deemed vulnerable to injury or death, in addition to using physical restraints for immobilization, reinforced the opinion that siderails and restraints were benevolent interventions (Cohen & Kruschwitz, 1997; Strumpf & Tomes, 1993). Although nurse attorney Jane Greenlaw found medication to be a major cause of negligence related to siderail use, she also noted the importance of a patient's mental state in determining liability. She noted, "Where it can be shown that a patient was senile, irrational, confused, or otherwise impaired, this can affect the hospital's duty to safeguard the patient" (Greenlaw, 1982, p. 125), and "Nursing responsibility to evaluate each person's safety and to act accordingly, regardless of whether the attending physician has done so" (Greenlaw, 1982, p. 127).

The nurse's duty to render independent judgment about siderail use was evident in the 1977 fall and injury case of John Wooten. Eighty-three-year-old Wooten suffered a severe head injury after falling at the Memphis, Tennessee Veterans Administration Hospital. During the evening, Wooten had risen from his bed unattended and walked a short distance before falling. Before the fall, Wooten's physician deemed him "stable" and gave an order for "bedrest with bedside commode and up in chair three times per day" (Anonymous, 1984, p. 4). Despite the physician's medical opinion, the U.S. District Court of Tennessee ruled that hospital personnel were negligent in caring for Wooten because his condition "mandated the use of siderails" (Anonymous, 1984, p. 4). The Court held that raised siderails was a reminder for patients to call nurses when they needed assistance to transfer from bed. Moreover, because Wooten was "older", he was at greater risk for confusion and disorientation. The Court awarded $80,000 in damages.

In 1981, 80-year-old Esther Polonsky was injured during her stay at Union Hospital in Lynn, Massachusetts, upon attempting to use the bathroom during the night. Several hours before the incident, the nurse had administered 15 milligrams of Dalmane to Polonsky to aid sleep. The Appeals Court of Massachusetts found that because the nurse failed to raise her bed siderails, a confused and disoriented Polonsky fell and fractured her right hip. She recovered $20,000 in damages (Regan, 1981).

While Polonsky's fall was directly linked to her medication, the case of Catherine Kadyszeski, like that of Wooten, illustrated the ageism often associated with siderail use (Tammelleo, 1995). Kadyszeski was 67 years old in 1985 when she fractured her left hip in a bathroom-related fall at New York's Ellis Hospital. Although heavily sedated with Demerol, Vistaril, and Phenobarbital, Kadyszeski did not win her claim on the basis of oversedation. Rather, the hospital was found negligent for failing to comply with its own rule that siderails be raised for all patients over age 65.

The continued use of siderails and restraints in the 1980s and 1990s sharply contrasted with new ideas about the importance of mobility during recuperation from acute illness or surgery (Allen, Glasziou, & Del Mar, 1999). The trend toward decreasing bedrest and increasing ambulation in hospitalized patients did not translate to the care of frail elders (Creditor, 1993; Sager et al., 1996). While younger patients' beds were equipped with half instead of full-length siderails to facilitate transfers, older patients continued to be immobilized in bed, in large part because nurses equated full siderail use with greater patient protection (Rubenstein et al., 1983). Even as negative consequences of immobilizing hospital elders, such as deconditioning, pressure ulcers, and pneumonia, were reported in the literature (Creditor, 1993; Hoenig & Rubenstein, 1991; Inouye et al., 1993; Sager et al., 1996), the use of siderails in this population did not abate.

IMPLICATIONS FOR CURRENT PRACTICE

Reports of siderail-related entrapment injuries and deaths over the past decade (Food and Drug Administration, 1995; Parker & Miles, 1997; Todd, Ruhl, & Gross, 1997) continue to challenge perceptions of siderails as safety devices. Many legal claims are not being won against hospitals for siderail misuse (Braun & Capezuti, 2000; Capezuti & Braun, 2001). The Health Care Finance Administration (HCFA) has issued surveyor guidelines redefining siderails as restraints when they impede the patient's desired movement or activity, such as getting out of bed (U.S. Department of Health & Human Services, 2000). The fundamental goal of these guidelines is to deter health care providers from routinely using siderails. Instead, they encourage a thorough assessment of patients' individualized needs and consideration of alternative interventions to siderail use (Capezuti et al., 1999; Capezuti, Talerico, Strumpf, & Evans, 1998). More broadly, the HCFA guidelines will likely influence siderail use by hospitals accredited through the Joint Commission on Accreditation of Healthcare Organizations (JCAHO, 1996). Because JCAHO must, at a minimum, meet applicable federal law and regulation, new standards, consistent with HCFA regulations, likely will be promulgated in the near future (Capezuti & Braun, 2001).

The acceptance and use of alternatives to siderails, however, will depend on a new consensus among health care providers, hospital administrators, bed manufacturers, insurers, attorneys, regulators, and patients and their families. To reach consensus, all parties need to understand how and why siderails became common practice in the first place and why, despite evidence to the contrary, they remain firmly entrenched as acceptable bedside care. Rethinking siderail use, especially with the elderly, will require new incentives for their discontinuation. The new guidelines by HCFA (U.S. Department of Health & Human Services, 2000) are a beginning step in this direction.

Bed manufacturers have also reintroduced adjustable low-height beds, similar to the models first proposed in the 1950s. These "new" beds, as well as siderails with narrower rail gaps, will be on the market over the next few years. Financing the purchase of this equipment and retrofitting outdated bed systems will likely raise new concerns about siderail-related liability (Braun & Capezuti, 2000; Capezuti & Braun, 2001). Nurse researchers are in key positions to evaluate how legislative and manufacturing trends affect clinical outcomes.

Given the gradual evolution of siderail use in American hospitals, nurses can anticipate that attitudes and practices about use of siderails will not change quickly or easily. Changing views and practices of siderail use will require reinterpretation of nursing care standards and benevolent care. Given the evidence of these shifting ideas and practices now (Braun & Capezuti, 2000; Capezuti & Braun, 2001; Capezuti, 2000; Donius & Rader, 1994), new perceptions and habits will develop. Those changes should be based on empirical outcomes rather than on untested consensus.

References

Aberg, H. L. (1957). The nurse's role in hospital safety. *Nursing Outlook, 5,* 160–162.

Allen, C., Glasziou, P., & Del Mar, C. (1999). Bed rest: A potentially harmful treatment needing more careful evaluation. *Lancet, 354,* 1229–1233.

Anonymous. (1984, February). Hospital policy re: "siderails" nurses' responsibility [Journal article]. *Regan Report on Nursing Law, 24,* 4.

Aston, C. S., Jr. (1955). Grasping bars means added safety. *Hospitals, 29,* 102–104.

Barbee, G. C. (1957). More about bedrails and the nurse. *American Journal of Nursing, 57,* 1441–1442.

Braun, J. A. & Capezuti, E. (2000). The legal and medical aspects of physical restraints and bed siderails and their relationship to falls and fall-related injuries in nursing homes. *DePaul Journal of Healthcare Law, 3,* 1–72.

Capezuti, E. (2000). Preventing falls and injuries while reducing siderail use. *Annals of Long-Term Care, 8*(6), 57–63.

Capezuti, E., Bourbonniere, M., Strumpf, N., & Maislin, G. (2000). Siderail use in a large urban medical center (Abstract). *The Gerontologist, 40*(Special Issue, 1), 117.

Capezuti, E. & Braun, J. A. (2001). Medicolegal aspects of hospital siderail use. *Ethics, Law, and Aging Review, 7,* 25–57.

Capezuti, E., Talerico, K. A., Cochran, I., Becker, H., Strumpf, N., & Evans, L. (1999). Individualized interventions to prevent bed-related falls and reduce siderail use. *Journal of Gerontological Nursing, 25,* 26–34.

Capezuti, E., Talerico, K. A., Strumpf, N., & Evans, L. (1998). Individualized assessment and intervention in bilateral siderail use. *Geriatric Nursing, 19*(6), 322–330.

Cohen, E. S., & Kruschwitz, A. L. (1997). Restraint reduction: Lessons from the asylum. *Journal of Ethics, Law, and Aging, 3,* 25–43.

Creditor, M. C. (1993). Hazards of hospitalization of the elderly. *Annals of Internal Medicine, 118,* 219–223.

Donius, M. & Rader, J. (1994). Use of siderails: Rethinking a standard of practice. *Journal of Gerontological Nursing, 20,* 23–27.

Food and Drug Administration. (1995, August 23). *FDA Safety Alert: Entrapment hazards with hospital bed side rails.* Rockville, MD: U.S. Dept. of Health and Human Services, Public Health Service, Center for Devices and Radiological Health.

Greenlaw, J. (1982, June). Failure to use siderails: When is it negligence? *Law, Medicine & Health Care, 10*(3), 125–128.

Haigh, C. & Hayman, J. M., Jr. (1936). Why they fell out of bed. *The Modern Hospital, 47,* 45–46.

Hampton, I. A. (1893). *Nursing: Its principles and practice.* Philadelphia: W. B. Saunders.

Harmer, M. & Henderson, V. (1952). *Textbook of the principles and practice of nursing.* New York: Macmillan.

Hayt, E., Hayt, L. R., & Groeschel, A. H. (1952). *Law of hospital and nurse.* New York: Hospital Textbook Co.

Hayt, E., Hayt, L. R., Groeschel, A. H., & McMullan, D. (1958). *Law of hospital and nurse.* New York: Hospital Textbook Co.

Hoenig, H. M. & Rubenstein, L.Z. (1991). Hospital-associated deconditioning and dysfunction. *Journal of the American Geriatrics Society, 39,* 220–222.

Horty, J. F. (1973). Hospital has duty to maintain premises, but employees have duty to be cautious. *Modern Hospital, 120,* 50.

Hospitals. (1950). Hall Invalid Bed; Simmons Vari-Hite [Advertisements]. *Hospitals, 24,* 86–87, 102.

Hospitals. (1954). Inland Bed Company; Hard Slida-Side [Advertisements]. *Hospitals, 28,* 19, 197.

Hospitals. (1955). Hill-Rom Hilow Beds [Advertisement]. *Hospitals, 29,* 161.

Inouye, S. K., Wagner, D. R., Acampora, D., Horwitz, R. I., Cooney, L. M., Hurst, L. D., et al. (1993). A predictive index for functional decline in hospitalized elderly medical patients. *Journal of General Internal Medicine, 8,* 645–652.

Joint Commission on Accreditation of Healthcare Organizations (JCAHO). (1996). *Comprehensive accreditation manual for hospitals (restraint and seclusion standards plus scoring: Standards TX7.1–TX7.1.3.3, 191–193j).* Oakbrook Terrace, IL: Author.

Ludham, J. E. (1957). Bedrails: Up or down? *Hospitals, 31,* 46–47.

Lynaugh, J. E. & Brush, B. L. (1996). *American nursing: From hospitals to health systems.* Cambridge, MA: Blackwell.

Manley, M. E. & The Committee on Nursing Standards, Division of Nursing, Department of Hospitals. (1944). Chapter VI: Preparation and care of beds. In *Standard nursing procedures of the department of hospitals, city of New York* (pp. 109–125). New York: Macmillan.

Merck & Company. (1934). *The Merck manual of therapeutics and materia medica* (6th ed.). Rahway, NJ: Author.

McCullough, W. & Moffit, M. (1949). *Illustrated handbook of simple nursing.* New York: McGraw-Hill.

Morningside Hospital & Training School for Nurses v. Pennington et al., 189 Okla. 170, 114P.2d 943 (1941).

National Association of Insurance Commissioners. (1980). *Medical claims: Medical malpractice closed claims, July 1, 1975 through June 30, 1978* (Vol. 2). Brookfield, WI: Author.

O'Keeffe, S., Jack, C. I., & Lye, M. (1996). Use of restraints and bedrails in a British hospital. *Journal of the American Geriatrics Society, 44,* 1086–1088.

Parker, K. & Miles, S. H. (1997). Deaths caused by bedrails. *Journal of the American Geriatrics Society, 45,* 797–802.

Potter et al. *v. Dr. W. H. Groves Latter-Day Saints Hospital,* 99 Utah 71, 103 P.2d 280 (1940).

Price, A. L. (1954). *The art, science and spirit of nursing.* Philadelphia: W. B. Saunders.

Price, A. L. (1956). Short side guards are safer. *Hospital Management, 82,* 86–89.

Regan, W. A. (1981). Legal case briefs for nurses. *Regan Report on Nursing Law, 21,* 3.

Rubenstein, H. S., Miller, F. H., Postel, S., & Evans, H. B. (1983). Standards of medical care based on consensus rather than evidence: The case of routine bedrail use for the elderly. *Law, Medicine & Health Care, 11,* 271–276.

Sager, M. A., Franke, T., Inouye, S. K., Landefeld, C. S., Morgan, T. M., Rudbert, M. A., et al. (1996). Functional outcomes of acute medical illness and hospitalization in older persons. *Archives of Internal Medicine, 156,* 645–652.

Smalley, H. E. (1956). Variable height bed: A study in patient comfort and efficiency in care. *Hospital Management, 82,* 42–43.

Stevens, R. (1989). *In sickness and in wealth: American hospitals in the twentieth century.* New York: Basic Books.

Strumpf, N. E. & Tomes, N. (1993). Restraining the troublesome patient: A historical perspective on a contemporary debate. *Nursing History Review, 1,* 3–24.

Tammelleo, A. D. (1995). Siderails left down—patient falls from bed: "Ordinary negligence" or "malpractice"? *Regan Report on Nursing Law, 36,* 3.

Todd, J. F., Ruhl, C. E., & Gross, T. P. (1997). Injury and death associated with hospital bed side-rails: Reports to the U.S. Food and Drug Administration from 1985–1995. *American Journal of Public Health, 87,* 1675–1677.

Tracy, M. A. (1942). *Nursing: An art and a science.* St. Louis, MO: CV Mosby.

U.S. Department of Health & Human Services. (2000, June). *Health Care Financing Administration, guidance to surveyors. Hospital conditions of participation for patients' rights* (Rev. 17). Retrieved from http://www.hcfa.gov/quality/4b.htm

Abstract: a summary or condensed version of the research report. Chapter 1, p. 15.

Aggregated data: data that are reported for an entire group rather than for individuals in the group. Chapter 11, p. 262.

Analysis of variance (ANOVA): a statistical test for differences in the means in three or more groups. Chapter 5, p. 102.

Anonymous: a participant in research is anonymous when no one, including the researcher, can link the study data from a particular individual to that individual. Chapter 7, p. 150.

Assent: to agree or concur; in the case of research, assent reflects a lower level of understanding about the meaning of participation in a study than consent. Assent is often sought in studies that involve older children or individuals who have a level of impairment that limits their ability but does not preclude their understanding of some aspects of the study. Chapter 7, p. 157.

Assumptions: ideas that are taken for granted or viewed as truth without conscious or explicit testing. Chapter 11, p. 254.

Audit trail: written and/or computer notes used in qualitative research that describe the researcher's decisions regarding both the data analysis process and collection process. Chapter 8, p. 171.

Beta (β) value: a statistic derived from regression analysis that tells us the relative contribution or connection of each factor to the dependent variable. Chapter 5, p. 104.

Bias: some unintended factor that confuses or changes the results of the study in a manner that can lead to incorrect conclusions; bias distorts or confounds the findings in a study, making it difficult to impossible to interpret the results. Chapter 6, p. 123.

Bivariate analysis: statistical analysis involving only two variables. Chapter 4, p. 69.

Categorization scheme: an orderly combination of carefully defined groups where there is no overlap among the categories. Chapter 4, p. 70.

Central tendency: a measure or statistic that indicates the center of a distribution or the center of the spread of the values for the variable. Chapter 4, p. 80.

Clinical trial: a study that tests the effectiveness of a clinical treatment; some researchers would say that a clinical trial must be a true experiment. Chapter 9, p. 222.

Cluster sampling: a process of sampling in stages, starting with a larger element that relates to the population and moving downward into smaller and smaller elements that identify the population. Chapter 6, p. 127.

Codebook: a record of the categorization, labeling, and manipulation of data for the variables in a quantitative study. Chapter 11, p. 260.

Coding: reducing a large amount of data to numbers or conceptual groups (*see* data reduction) in qualitative research; giving individual datum numerical values in quantitative research. Chapter 4, p. 71.

Coercion: the involvement of some element that controls or forces someone to do something. In the case of research, coercion occurs if a patient is forced to participate in a study to receive a particular test or service, or to receive or not to receive the best quality of care. Chapter 7, p. 152.

Comparison group: a group of subjects that differs on a major independent variable from the study group, allowing comparison of the subjects in the two groups in terms of a dependent variable. Chapter 9, p. 212.

Conceptual framework: an underlying structure for building and testing knowledge that is made up of concepts and the relationships among the concepts. Chapter 10, p. 231.

Conceptualization: a process of creating a verbal picture of an abstract idea. Chapter 3, p. 53.

Conclusions: the end of a research report that identifies the final decisions or determinations regarding the research problem. Chapter 2, p. 23.

Confidentiality: assurance that neither the identities of participants in the research will be revealed to anyone else, nor will the information that participants provide individually be publicly divulged. Chapter 7, p. 150.

Confidence intervals: the range of values for a variable, which would be found in 95 out of 100 samples; confidence intervals set the boundaries for a variable or test statistic. Chapter 5, p. 93.

Confirmation: the verification of results from other studies. Chapter 3, p. 51.

Confirmability: the ability to consistently repeat decision-making about the data collection and analysis in qualitative research. Chapter 8, p. 170.

Construct validity: the extent to which a scale or instrument measures what it is supposed to measure; the broadest type of validity that can encompass both content- and criterion-related validity. Chapter 8, p. 184.

Content analysis: the process of understanding, interpreting, and conceptualizing the meanings imbedded in qualitative data. Chapter 4, p. 70.

Content validity: validity that establishes that the items or questions on a scale are comprehensive and appropriately reflect the concept they are supposed to measure. Chapter 8, p. 183.

Control group: a randomly assigned group of subjects that is not exposed to the independent variable of interest to be able to compare that group to a group that is exposed to the independent variable; inclusion of a control group is a hallmark of an experimental design. Chapter 9, p. 212.

Convenience sample: a sample that includes members of the population who can be readily found and recruited. Chapter 6, p. 121.

Correlation: the statistical test used to examine how much two variables covary; a measure of the relationship between two variables. Chapter 5, p. 98.

Correlational studies: studies that describe interrelationships among variables as accurately as possible. Chapter 9, p. 213.

Covary: when changes in one variable lead to consistent changes in another variable; if two variables covary, then they are connected to each other in some way. Chapter 5, p. 98.

Credibility: the confidence that the researcher and user of the research can have in the truth of the findings of the study. Chapter 8, p. 172.

Criteria for participation: factors that determine how individuals are selected for a study; they describe the common characteristics that define the target population for a study. Chapter 6, p. 118.

Criterion-related validity: the extent to which the results of one measure match those of another measure that is also supposed to reflect the variable under study. Chapter 8, p. 184.

Cross sectional: a research design that includes the collection of all data at one point in time. Chapter 9, p. 210.

Data: the information collected in a study that is specifically related to the research problem. Chapter 2, p. 25.

Data analysis: a process that pulls information together or examines connections between pieces of information to make a clearer picture of all the information collected. Chapter 2, p. 25.

Data reduction: organizing large amounts of data, usually in the form of words, so that it is broken down (or reduced) and labeled (or coded) to identify to which category it belongs. Chapter 4, p. 71.

Data saturation: the point at which all new information collected is redundant of information already collected. Chapter 4, p. 72.

Deductive knowledge: a process of taking a general theory and seeking specific observations or facts to support that theory. Chapter 10, p. 229.

Demographics: descriptive information about the characteristics of the people studied. Chapter 4, p. 83.

Dependent variable: the outcome variable of interest; it is the variable that depends on other variables in the study. Chapter 4, p. 74.

Descriptive design: research design that functions to portray as accurately as possible some phenomenon of interest. Chapter 9, p. 204.

Descriptive results: a summary of results from a study without comparing the results with other information. Chapter 2, p. 26.

Directional hypothesis: a research hypothesis that predicts both a connection between two or more variables and the nature of that connection. Chapter 10, p. 241.

Discussion: the section of a research report that summarizes, compares, and speculates about the results of the study. Chapter 3, p. 50.

Distribution: the spread among the values for a variable. Chapter 4, p. 78.

Dissemination: the spreading or sharing of knowledge; communication of new knowledge from research so that it is adopted in practice. Chapter 11, p. 261.

Electronic databases: categorized lists of articles from a wide range of journals, organized by topic, author, and journal source available on CDs or online. Chapter 1, p. 14.

Error: the difference between what is true and the results from the data collection. Chapter 8, p. 165.

Ethnography: qualitative research methods used to participate or immerse oneself in a culture in order to describe it. Chapter 9, p. 206.

Evidence-based nursing (EBN): the process that nurses use to make clinical decisions and to answer clinical questions about delivery of care to patients. Chapter 1, p. 4.

Experimental designs: quantitative research designs that include manipulation of an independent variable, a control group, and random assignment to groups. Chapter 9, p. 195 & 214.

Experimenter effects: a threat to external validity that occurs when some characteristic of the researchers or data collectors themselves influences the results of the study. Chapter 9, p. 203.

External validity: the extent to which the results of a study can be applied to other groups or situations; how accurate the study is in providing knowledge that can be applied outside of or external to the study itself. Chapter 9, p. 198.

Factor analysis: a statistical procedure to help identify underlying structures or factors in a measure; it identifies discrete groups of statements that are more closely connected to each other than to all the other statements. Chapter 5, p. 105.

Field notes: documentation of the participant's tone, expressions, and associated actions, and what is going on in the setting at the same time; they are a record of the researcher's observations about the overall setting and experience of the data collection process while in that setting or field itself; field notes are used to enrich and build a set of data that is thick and dense. Chapter 8, p. 168.

Five human rights in research: rights that have been identified by the American Nurses Association guidelines for nurses working with patient information that may require interpretation; they include the right to self-determination, the right to privacy and dignity, the right to anonymity and confidentiality, the right to fair treatment, and the right to protection from discomfort and harm (ANA, 1985). Chapter 7, p. 148.

Frequency distribution: a presentation of data that indicates the spread of how often values for a variable occurred. Chapter 4, p. 78.

Generalizability: the ability to say that the findings from a particular sample can be applied to a more general population; *see* Generalization. Chapter 6, p. 131.

Generalization: the ability to say that the findings from a particular study can be interpreted to apply to a more general population. Chapter 3, p. 54.

Grounded theory: a qualitative research method that is used to study interactions to understand and recognize linkages between ideas and concepts, or to put in different words, to develop theory; the term *grounded* refers to the idea that the theory that is developed is based on or grounded in participants' reality. Chapter 9, p. 207.

Group interviews: the collection of data by interviewing more than one participant at a time. Chapter 8, p. 168.

Hawthorne effect: a threat to external validity that occurs when subjects in a study change simply because they are being studied, no matter what intervention is applied; reactivity and the Hawthorne effect are the same concept. Chapter 9, p. 202.

Historical research method: a qualitative research method used to answer questions about linkages in the past to understand the present or plan the future. Chapter 9, p. 208.

History: a threat to internal validity that occurs because of some factor outside those examined in a study, affecting the study outcome or dependent variable. Chapter 9, p. 200.

Hypothesis: a prediction regarding the relationships or effects of selected factors on other factors under study. Chapter 2, p. 34.

Independent variables: those factors in a study that are used to explain or predict the outcome of interest; independent variables also are sometimes called *predictor variables* because they are used to predict the dependent variable. Chapter 4, p. 74.

Inductive knowledge: a process of taking specific facts or observations together to create general theory. Chapter 10, p. 229.

Inference: the reasoning that goes into the process of drawing a conclusion based on evidence. Chapter 4, p. 67.

Informed consent: the legal principle that an individual or his or her authorized representative is given all the relevant information needed to make a decision about participation in a research study and is given a reasonable amount of time to consider that decision. Chapter 7, p. 148.

Instrument: a term used in research to refer to a device that specifies and objectifies the process of collecting data. Chapter 8, p. 175.

Instrumentation: a threat to internal validity that refers to the changing of the measures used in a study from one time point to another. Chapter 9, p. 200.

Institutional review board (IRB): a group of members selected for the explicit purpose of reviewing any proposed research study to be implemented within an institution or by employees of an institution to ensure that the research project includes procedures to protect the rights of its subjects; the IRB is also charged to decide whether or not the research is basically sound in order to ensure potential participants' rights to protection from discomfort or harm. Chapter 7, p. 148.

Internal consistency reliability: the extent to which responses to a scale are similar and related. Chapter 8, p. 181.

Internal validity: the extent to which we can be sure of the accuracy or correctness of the findings of a study; how accurate the results are within the study itself or internally. Chapter 9, p. 198.

Internet: the network that connects computers throughout the world. Chapter 1, p. 12.

Inter-rater reliability: consistency in measurement that is present when two or more independent data collectors agree in the results of their data collection process. Chapter 8, p. 180.

Items: the questions or statements included on a scale used to measure a variable of interest. Chapter 8, p. 176.

Key words: terms that describe the topic or nature of the information sought when searching a database or the Internet. Chapter 1, p. 14.

Knowledge: information that furthers our understanding of a phenomenon or question. Chapter 1, p. 11.

Likert-type scale: a response scale that asks for a rating of an item on a continuum that is anchored at either end by opposite responses. Chapter 8, p. 177.

Limitations: the aspects of how the study was conducted that create uncertainty concerning the conclusion that can be derived from the study as well as the decisions that can be based on it. Chapter 2, p. 24.

Literature review: a synthesis of existing published writings that describes what is known or has been studied regarding the particular research question or purpose. Chapter 2, p. 33; Chapter 10, p. 234.

Longitudinal research design: a research design that includes the collection of data over time. Chapter 9, p. 210.

Matched sample: the intentful selection of pairs of subjects that share certain important characteristics to prevent those characteristics from confusing what is being explained or understood within the study. Chapter 6, p. 124.

Maturation: a threat to internal validity that refers to changes that occur in the dependent variable simply because of the passage of time, rather than because of some independent variable. Chapter 9, p. 200.

Mean: the arithmetic average for a set of values. Chapter 4, p. 80.

Measurement effects: a threat to external validity because various procedures used to collect data in the study changed the results of that study. Chapter 9, p. 202.

Measure of central tendency: a measure that shows the common or typical values within a set of values; central tendency measures reflect the "center" of a distribution, or the center of the spread; the mean, the mode, and the median are the three most commonly used. Chapter 4, p. 80.

Measures: the specific method(s) used to assign a number or numbers to an aspect or factor being studied. Chapter 2, p. 31.

Median: a measure of central tendency that is the value in a set of numbers that falls in the exact middle of the distribution when the numbers are in order. Chapter 4, p. 80.

Member checks: a process in qualitative research where the data and the findings from their analysis are brought back to the original participants to seek their input as to the accuracy, completeness, and interpretation of the data. Chapter 8, p. 172.

Meta-analysis: a quantitative approach to knowledge by taking the numbers from different studies that addressed the same research problem and using statistics to summarize those numbers, looking for combined results that would not happen by chance alone. Chapter 2, p. 40.

Metasynthesis: a report of a study of a group of single research studies using qualitative methods. Chapter 2, p. 40.

Methods: the methods section of a research report describes the overall process of implementing the research study, including who was included in the study, how information was collected, and what interventions, if any, were tested. Chapter 2, p. 28.

Mixed methods: some combination of research methods that differ in relation to the function of the design, the use of time in the design, or the control included in the design. Chapter 9, p. 219.

Mode: the value for a variable that occurs most frequently. Chapter 4, p. 80.

Model: the symbolic framework for a theory or a part of a theory. Chapter 9, p. 213.

Mortality: a threat to internal validity that refers to the loss of subjects from a study due to a consistent factor that is related to the dependent variable. Chapter 9, p. 201.

Multifactorial: a study that has a number of independent variables that are manipulated. Chapter 9, p. 215.

Multivariate: more than two variables; multivariate studies examine three or more factors and the relationships among the different factors. Chapter 2, p. 27.

Nondirectional hypothesis: a research hypothesis that predicts a connection between two or more variables but does not predict the nature of that connection. Chapter 10, p. 241.

Nonparametric: a group of inferential statistical procedures that are used with numbers that do not have the bell-shaped distribution or that are categorical or ordinal variables. Chapter 5, p. 94.

Nonprobability sampling: a sampling approach that does not necessarily assure that everyone in the population has an equal chance of being included in the study. Chapter 6, p. 123.

Normal curve: a type of distribution for a variable that is shaped like a bell and is symmetrical. Chapter 4, p. 79.

Novelty effects: a threat to external validity that occurs when the knowledge that what is being done is new and under study somehow affects the outcome, either favorably or unfavorably. Chapter 9, p. 203.

Null hypothesis: a statistical hypothesis that predicts that there will be no relationship or difference in selected variables in a study. Chapter 5, p. 106.

Operational definition: a variable that is defined in specific, concrete terms of measurement. Chapter 8, p. 163.

Parametric: a group of inferential statistical procedures that can be applied to variables that are (1) normally distributed and (2) interval or ratio numbers such as age or intelligence score. Chapter 5, p. 94.

Participant observation: a qualitative method where the researcher intentionally imbeds himself or herself into the environment from which data will be collected and becomes a participant. Chapter 8, p. 168.

Peer review: the critique of scholarly work by two or more individuals who have at least equivalent knowledge regarding the topic of the work as the author of that work. Chapter 10, p. 237.

Phenomenology: a qualitative method used to increase understanding of experiences as perceived by those living the experience; assumes that lived experience can be interpreted or understood by distilling the essence of that experience. Chapter 9, p. 205.

Pilot study: a small research study that is implemented for the purpose of developing and demonstrating the effectiveness of selected measures and methods. Chapter 11, p. 267.

Population: the entire group of individuals about whom we are interested in gaining knowledge. Chapter 6, p. 116.

Power analysis: a statistical procedure that allows the researcher to compute the size of a sample needed to detect a real relationship or difference, if it exists. Chapter 6, p. 131.

Practice: actions that are planned and implemented exclusively for the enhancement of health and the improvement of the well-being of an individual. Chapter 7, p. 147.

Predictor variables: those factors in a study that are expected to affect the dependent variable in a specified manner; predictor variables are also called *independent variables*. Chapter 4, p. 74.

Pre-test/post-test: a research design that includes an observation both before and after the intervention. Chapter 9, p. 215.

Primary sources: use of sources of information as they were originally written or communicated. Chapter 10, p. 236.

Printed indexes: written lists of professional articles that are organized and categorized by topic and author, covering the time period from 1956 forward. Chapter 1, p. 12.

Probability: the percent of the time that the results found would have happened by chance alone. Chapter 5, p. 92.

Probability sampling: strategies to assure that every member of a population has an equal opportunity to be in the study. Chapter 6, p. 125.

Problem: section of a research report that describes the gap in knowledge that will be addressed by the research study, or a statement of the general gap in knowledge that will be addressed in a study. Chapter 2, p. 33.

Procedures: specific actions taken by researchers to gather information about the problem or phenomenon being studied. Chapter 2, p. 31.

Prospective designs: a research design that collects data about events or variables moving forward in time. Chapter 9, p. 210.

Purposive sample: inclusion in a study of participants who are intentionally selected because they have certain characteristics that are related to the purpose of the research. Chapter 6, p. 121.

p value: a numerical statement of the percentage of the time the results reported would have happened by chance alone. For example, a p value of .05 means that in only 5 out of 100 times would one expect to get the results by chance alone. Chapter 2, p. 27.

Qualitative methods: approaches to research that focus on understanding the complexity of humans within the context of their lives and tend to focus on building a whole or complete picture of a phenomenon of interest; qualitative methods involve the collection of information as it is expressed naturally by people within the normal context of their lives. Chapter 2, p. 28.

Quality improvement: a process of evaluation of health care services to see if they meet specified standards or outcomes of care. Chapter 12, p. 281.

Quality improvement study: a study that evaluates whether or not certain expected clinical care was completed. Chapter 2, p. 43.

Quantitative methods: approaches to research that focus on understanding and breaking down the different parts of a picture to see how they do or do not connect; quantitative methods involve the collection of information that is very specific and limited to the particular pieces of information being studied. Chapter 2, p. 29.

Quasi-experimental designs: a research design that includes manipulation of an independent variable but will lack either a control group or random assignment. Chapter 9, p. 215.

Questionnaire: a written measure that is used to collect specific data, usually offering closed or forced choices for answers to the questions. Chapter 8, p. 176.

Quota sampling: selection of individuals from the population who have one or more characteristics that are important to the purpose of the study; these characteristics are used to establish limits or quotas on the number of subjects who will be included in the study. Chapter 6, p. 124.

Random assignment: the process ensuring that subjects in a study all have an equal chance of being in any particular group within the study. The sample itself may be one of convenience or purposive, so there may be some bias influencing the results. But, since that bias is evenly distributed among the different groups to be studied, it will not unduly affect the outcomes of the study. Chapter 6, p. 129.

Random selection: the process of creating a random sample; selection of a subset of the population where all the members of the population are identified, listed, and assigned a number and then some device, such as a random number table or a computer program, is used to select who actually will be in the study. Chapter 6, p. 125.

Reactivity effects: threats in external validity that refer to subjects' responses to being studied. Chapter 9, p. 202.

Regression: a statistical procedure that measures how much one or more independent variables explain the variation in a dependent variable. Chapter 5, p. 103.

Reliability: the consistency with which a measure can be counted on to give the same result if the aspect being measured has not changed. Chapter 8, p. 180.

Repeated measures: designs that repeat the same measurements at several points in time. Chapter 9, p. 211.

Replication: a study that is an exact duplication of an earlier study; the major purpose of a replication study is confirmation. Chapter 3, p. 52.

Research design: the overall plan for acquiring new knowledge or confirming existing knowledge; the plan for systematic collection of information in a manner that assures the answer(s) found will be as meaningful and accurate as possible. Chapter 9, p. 195.

Research hypothesis: a prediction of the relationships or differences that will be found for selected variables in a study. Chapter 5, p. 106; Chapter 10, p. 239.

Research objectives: clear statements of factors that will be measured in order to gain knowledge regarding a research problem; similar to the research purpose, specific aims, or research question. Chapter 10, p. 234.

Research problem: a gap in existing knowledge that warrants filling and can be addressed through systematic study. Chapter 10, p. 227.

Research purpose: a clear statement of factors that are going to be studied in order to shed knowledge on the research problem. Chapter 10, p. 232.

Research questions: statements in the form of questions that identify the specific factors that will be measured in a study and the types of relationships that will be examined to gain knowledge regarding a research problem; similar to the research objectives, purposes, and specific aims. Chapter 10, p. 239.

Research utilization: the use of research in practice. Chapter 12, p. 276.

Response rate: the proportion of individuals who actually participate in a study divided by the number who agreed to be in a study but did not end up participating in it. Chapter 6, p. 137.

Results: a summary of the actual findings or information collected in a research study. Chapter 2, p. 25.

Retrospective designs: quantitative designs that collect data about events or factors going back in time. Chapter 9, p. 210.

Rigor: a strict process of data collection and analysis as well as a term that reflects the overall quality of that process in qualitative research; rigor is reflected in the consistency of data analysis and interpretation, the trustworthiness of the data collected, the transferability of the themes, and the credibility of the data. Chapter 8, p. 170.

Risk:benefit ratio: a comparison of how much risk is present for human subjects compared to how much benefit there is to the study. Chapter 7, p. 150.

Sample: a subset of the total group of interest in a research study; the individuals in the sample are actually studied to learn about the total group. Chapter 2, p. 30; Chapter 6, p. 116.

Sampling frame: the pool of all potential subjects for a study; that is, the pool of all individuals who meet the criteria for the study and, therefore, could be included in the sample. Chapter 6, p. 124.

Sampling unit: the element of the population that will be selected for study; the unit depends on the population of interest and could be individuals, families, communities, or outpatient prenatal care programs. Chapter 6, p. 129.

Saturation: a point in qualitative research where all new information collected is redundant of information already collected; *see* Data saturation. Chapter 4, p. 72; Chapter 6, p. 122.

Scale: a set of written questions or statements that in combination are intended to measure a specified variable. Chapter 8, p. 176.

Secondary sources: someone else's description or interpretation of a primary source. Chapter 10, p. 236.

Selection bias: when subjects have unique characteristics that in some manner relate to the dependent variable, raising a question as to whether the findings from the study were due to the independent variable or to the unique characteristics of the sample. Chapter 9, p. 201.

Selectivity: the tendency of certain segments of a population agreeing to be in studies. Chapter 6, p. 137.

Semistructured questions: questions asked in order to collect data that specifically targets objective factors of interest. Chapter 8, p. 175.

Simple random sampling: a sample in which every member of the population has an equal probability of being included; considered the best type of sample because the only factors that should bias the sample will be present by chance alone, making it highly likely that the sample will be similar to the population of interest. An approach for acquiring the population of interest in which the researcher uses a device such as a random number table or computer program to randomly select subjects for a study. Chapter 6, p. 125.

Significance: a statistical term indicating a low likelihood that any differences or relationships found in a study happened by chance alone. Chapter 2, p. 27.

Skew: a distribution where the middle of the distribution is not in the exact center; the middle or peak of the distribution is to the left or right of center. Chapter 4, p. 81.

Snowball sampling: a strategy for recruiting individuals in a study that starts with one participant or member of the population and then uses that member's contacts to identify other potential participants. Chapter 6, p. 121.

Specific aim: clear statements of the factors to be measured and the relationships to be examined in a study to gain new knowledge about a research problem; similar to research purpose, objectives, or questions. Chapter 10, p. 234.

Speculation: a process of reflecting on the results of a study and putting forward some explanation for them. Chapter 3, p. 53.

Standard deviation: a statistic that is the square root of the variance; it is computed as the average differences in values for a variable from the mean value; a big standard deviation means that there was a wide range of values for the variable; a small standard deviation means that there was a narrow range of values for the variable. Chapter 4, p. 77.

Stratified random sampling: an approach to selecting individuals from the population by dividing the population into two or more groups based on characteristics that are considered important to the purpose of the study and then randomly selecting members within each group. Chapter 6, p. 125.

Structured questions: questions that establish what data is wanted ahead of the collection and do not allow the respondent flexibility in how to answer. Chapter 8, p. 175.

Study design: the overall plan or organization of a study. Chapter 3, p. 57.

Systematic review: the product of a process that includes asking clinical questions, doing a structured and organized search for theory-based information and research related to the question, reviewing and synthesizing the results from that search, and reaching conclusions about the implications for practice. Chapter 2, p. 40.

Systematic sampling: an approach to selection of individuals for a study where the members of the population are identified and listed and then members are selected at a fixed interval (such as every fifth or tenth individual) from the list. Chapter 6, p. 127.

Testing: a threat to internal validity where there is a change in a dependent variable simply because it is being measured or due to the measure itself. Chapter 9, p. 200.

Test-retest reliability: consistency in the results from a test when individuals fill out a questionnaire or scale at two or more time points that are close enough together that we would not expect the "real" answers to have changed. Chapter 8, p. 181.

Themes: results in qualitative research that are ideas or concepts that are implicit in the data and are recurrent throughout the data; abstractions that reflect phrases, words, or ideas that appear repeatedly as a researcher analyzes what people have said about a particular experience, feeling, or situation. A theme summarizes and synthesizes discrete ideas or phrases to create a picture out of the words that were collected in the research study. Chapter 2, p. 26; Chapter 4, p. 72.

Theory: an abstract explanation describing how different factors or phenomena relate. Chapter 2, p. 33; Chapter 10, p. 228.

Theoretical definition: a conceptual description of a variable. Chapter 8, p. 163.

Theoretical framework: an underlying structure that describes how abstract aspects of a research problem interrelate based on developed theories. Chapter 10, p. 231.

Transferability: the extent to which the findings of a qualitative study are confirmed or seem applicable for a different group or in a different setting from where the data were collected. Chapter 8, p. 171.

Triangulation: a process of using more than one source of data to include different views, or literally to look at the phenomenon from different angles. Chapter 8, p. 172.

Trustworthiness: the honesty of the data collected from or about the participants. Chapter 8, p. 170.

***t* test:** a statistic that tests for differences in means on a variable between two groups. Chapter 5, p. 96.

Univariate analysis: statistical analysis about only one variable. Chapter 4, p. 69.

Unstructured interviews: questions asked in an informal open fashion without a previously established set of categories or assumed answers, used to gain understanding about a phenomenon or variable of interest. Chapter 8, p. 167.

Validity: how accurately a measure actually yields information about the true or real variable being studied. Chapter 8, p. 182.

Variable: some aspect of interest that differs among different people or situations; something that varies: it is not the same for everyone in every situation. Chapter 4, p. 68.

Variance: the diversity in data for a single variable; a statistic that is the squared deviations of values from the mean value and reflects the distribution of values for the variable. Chapter 4, p. 76.

Visual analog: a response scale that consists of a straight line of a specific length that has extremes of responses at either end but does not have any other responses noted at points along the line. Subjects are asked to mark the line to indicate where they fall between the two extreme points. Chapter 8, p. 177.

Withdrawal: a right of human subjects to stop participating in a study at any time without penalty until the study is completed. Chapter 7, p. 152.

INDEX